Treatment of Panic Disorder

A Consensus Development Conference

Treatment of Panic Disorder
A Consensus Development Conference

Edited by

Barry E. Wolfe, Ph.D.
Chief
Psychosocial Treatment Research Program
Clinical Treatment Research Branch
Division of Clinical and Treatment Research
National Institute of Mental Health
National Institutes of Health
Rockville, Maryland

Jack D. Maser, Ph.D.
Chief
Anxiety and Somatoform Disorders Program
Division of Clinical and Treatment Research
National Institute of Mental Health
National Institutes of Health
Rockville, Maryland

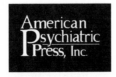

American Psychiatric Press, Inc.

Washington, DC
London, England

Note: The authors have worked to ensure that all information in this book concerning drug dosages, schedules, and routes of administration is accurate as of the time of publication and consistent with standards set by the U.S. Food and Drug Administration and the general medical community. As medical research and practice advance, however, therapeutic standards may change. For this reason and because human and mechanical errors sometimes occur, we recommend that readers follow the advice of a physician who is directly involved in their care or the care of a member of their family.

Manufactured in the United States of America on acid-free paper
First Edition
97 96 95 94   4 3 2 1

American Psychiatric Press, Inc.
1400 K Street, N.W., Washington, DC   20005

The views expressed in this book are those of the authors only and are not necessarily those of the National Institutes of Health or the National Institute of Mental Health.

Library of Congress Cataloging-in-Publication Data
Treatment of panic disorder : a consensus development conference /
   [edited by] Barry E. Wolfe, Jack D. Maser.
        p.   cm.
   Includes bibliographical references and index.
   ISBN 0-88048-685-6 (alk. paper)
   1. Panic disorders--Treatment--Congresses.   I. Wolfe, Barry.
II. Maser, Jack D.
   [DNLM: 1. Panic Disorder--therapy--congresses.   WM 172 T7847
1994]
RC535.T74   1994
616.85′22306--dc20
DNLM/DLC
for Library of Congress   93-17653
                                                                           CIP

British Library Cataloguing in Publication Data
A CIP record is available from the British Library.

Contents

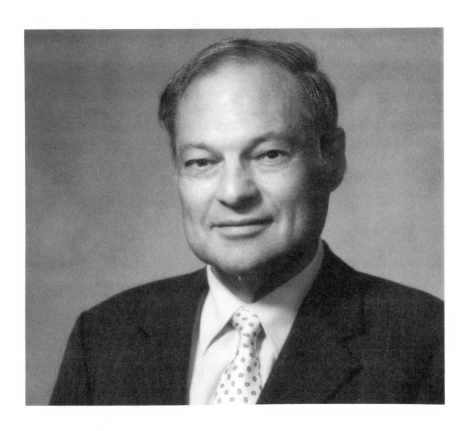

Dedication
To Gerald L. Klerman, M.D.

During the preparation of this volume, Gerald L. Klerman, M.D., died. He left behind a grieving family, numerous colleagues and friends, and a vacuum in psychiatric research that will be difficult to fill. Among those friends and colleagues are the contributors to and editors of this book.

That he was a student of psychopharmacology and psychosocial treatment was amply demonstrated throughout his unusually productive and brilliant career. We have chosen four examples of this dual interest to demonstrate our point.

From 1988 to 1990 Dr. Klerman was president of the Association for Clinical Psychosocial Research, and from 1976 to 1977 he was president of the American College of Neuropsychopharmacology. In 1977, for his research on the interaction of drugs and psychotherapy in the treatment of depression, he was awarded the American Psychiatric Association Foundation Fund Prize for Research in Psychiatry. Under a similar justification, he was given the highly prestigious Ana Monika Award in 1986. Our last example comes from the list of editorial boards on which he was asked to serve. Two of these are *Social Psychiatry* and *Psychopharmacologia*.

Proponents of both psychosocial and psychopharmacological treatments looked to Gerry for wisdom and good judgment in deciding difficult issues, for vision in sensing where the resources of a field might best be directed, and for a sense of historical context so that past mistakes would not be repeated.

He had the breadth and scope of knowledge to understand the strengths and limitations of each treatment modality, and he used his intelligence to define each position more clearly than did the advocates.

From 1977 to 1980, during the Carter Administration, he served as Administrator of the Alcohol, Drug Abuse, and Mental Health Administration, and in that capacity he was our boss. We remember him with fondness as well as for the dramatic improvements that he made in the functioning of our branch of government.

We were sorry to see him step down from the administrator's job; now we mourn his passing. By dedicating this book to him, we hope to celebrate his life.

J.D.M. and B.E.W.

Contributors

Michaela Amering, M.D.
Department of Psychiatry, University of Vienna, Vienna, Austria

James C. Ballenger, M.D.
Professor and Chairman, Department of Psychiatry
and Behavioral Sciences; Director, Institute of Psychiatry,
Medical University of South Carolina, Charleston, South Carolina

David H. Barlow, Ph.D.
Distinguished Professor of Psychology, Department of Psychology,
State University of New York at Albany, Albany, New York

Dianne L. Chambless, Ph.D.
Professor, Department of Psychiatry, The American University,
Washington, DC

David M. Clark, D.Phil.
Wellcome Principal Research Fellow, Department of Psychiatry,
University of Oxford, Warneford Hospital, Oxford, England

Abby J. Fyer, M.D.
Associate Professor of Clinical Psychiatry, Columbia University; Co-Director,
Anxiety Disorders Clinic, New York State Psychiatric Institute

Martha M. Gillis, M.A.
Research Assistant, Department of Psychology, The American University,
Washington, DC

Jack M. Gorman, M.D.
Professor of Clinical Psychiatry, College of Physicians and Surgeons
at Columbia University; Chief, Department of Clinical Psychobiology,
New York State Psychiatric Institute, New York, New York

George R. Heninger, M.D.
Professor and Associate Chairman for Research and Director,
Abraham Ribicoff Research Facilities, Connecticut Mental Health Center,
Department of Psychiatry, Yale University, New Haven, Connecticut

Wayne Katon, M.D.
Professor of Psychiatry; Chief, Division of Consultation Liaison Psychiatry;
Director, Health Services and Epidemiology, Department of Psychiatry,
University of Washington Medical School, Seattle, Washington

Heinz Katschnig, M.FD.
Professor of Psychiatry and Head, Department of Psychiatry,
University of Vienna, Vienna, Austria

Gerald L. Klerman, M.D.[1]
Professor of Psychiatry; Associate Chairman for Research, Cornell University
Medical College, Payne Whitney Clinic, New York, New York

Andrew Leon, Ph.D.
Assistant Professor of Psychiatry, Cornell University Medical College,
Payne Whitney Clinic, New York, New York

Michael R. Liebowitz, M.D.
Professor of Clinical Psychiatry, Columbia University; Co-Director,
Anxiety Disorders Clinic, New York State Psychiatric Institute

Richard A. Lucas, M.A.
Research Assistant, Laboratory for the Study of Anxiety Disorders,
Department of Psychology, The University of Texas at Austin, Austin, Texas

Jack D. Maser, Ph.D.
Chief, Anxiety and Somatoform Disorders Program,
Division of Clinical and Treatment Research,
National Institute of Mental Health, National Institutes of Health,
Rockville, Maryland

Larry K. Michelson, Ph.D.
Professor of Psychology, Department of Psychology,
The Pennsylvania State University, University Park, Pennsylvania

S. Rachman, Ph.D.
Professor, Psychology Department, University of British Columbia, Vancouver,
British Columbia, Canada

Karl Rickels, M.D.
Stuart and Emily Mudd Professor of Human Behavior, Professor of Psychiatry,
Department of Psychiatry, University of Pennsylvania, Philadelphia,
Pennsylvania

Edward Schweizer, M.D.
Associate Professor of Psychiatry, Department of Psychiatry,
University of Pennsylvania, Philadelphia, Pennsylvania

---

[1] Deceased.

M. Katherine Shear, M.D.
Associate Professor of Psychiatry, University of Pittsburgh, Pittsburgh, Pennsylvania

Lisa Spielman, Ph.D.
Research Assistant, Cornell University Medical College, Payne Whitney Clinic, New York, New York

Michael J. Telch, Ph.D.
Associate Professor, Director, Laboratory for the Study of Anxiety Disorders, Department of Psychology, The University of Texas at Austin, Austin, Texas

Myrna M. Weissman, Ph.D.
Professor of Epidemiology in Psychiatry and Chief, Division of Clinical and Genetic Epidemiology, College of Physicians and Surgeons of Columbia University, New York State Psychiatric Institute, New York, New York

Barry E. Wolfe, Ph.D.
Chief, Psychosocial Treatment Research Program, Clinical Treatment Research Branch, Division of Clinical and Treatment Research, National Institute of Mental Health, National Institutes of Health, Rockville, Maryland

Section I

Introduction

Chapter 1

Origins and Overview of the Consensus Development Conference on the Treatment of Panic Disorder

Barry E. Wolfe, Ph.D., and
Jack D. Maser, Ph.D.

With or without agoraphobia, panic disorder is a debilitating mental illness that may afflict as many as 3 million people in the United States in the course of their lifetime (based on an adult population of 184,000,000). Its treatment, however, has stimulated one of the most heated controversies in psychiatry and clinical psychology. Until recently, attempts to achieve agreement on what treatments are efficacious have been fraught with difficulty. Part of the problem has been fealty to disciplinary perspective, whether biological or psychosocial; another part of the problem has been the absence of a sufficient data base. In the last two decades, we have seen changes in both problems: there has been an increased willingness of proponents of one treatment approach to explore the possible benefits of other treatment approaches, and there has been a significant growth of the data base. These changes make consensus among divergent positions possible.

This volume contains the presentations given at the National Institutes of Health/National Institute of Mental Health (NIH/NIMH) Consensus Development Conference on the Treatment of Panic Disorder, held September 25–27, 1991. In many respects, this corpus of evidence summarizes the state-of-the-science on the diagnosis, classification, etiology, and treatment of panic disorder.

The views expressed in this chapter are those of the authors only, and do not necessarily reflect those of the National Institute of Mental Health.

Our goal is to provide the reader with the same information provided to the Consensus Development Panel. The reader can then determine for himself or herself whether the panel's statement, presented in its entirety in the last chapter, represents a reasonable consensus on the treatment of panic disorder patients. An invaluable bibliography that was provided to the panel is included at the end of this book.

The cardinal symptoms of panic disorder are unexpected panic attacks and the anticipatory fear of recurring panic attacks. About one-third of panic disorder patients develop agoraphobia, which essentially involves a fear of venturing too far from a self-defined safety zone. The designation of panic disorder as a mental disorder in the *Diagnostic and Statistical Manual of Mental Disorders,* Third Edition (DSM-III; American Psychiatric Association 1980) is little more than a decade old, but the exponential growth of research interest in this disorder has been astonishing. The bibliography at the end of this book includes over 1,400 citations that were produced on the disorder between January 1985 and July 1991.

Rationale for a Consensus Development Conference

Throughout the 1970s and 1980s, parallel research literatures appeared on the treatment of panic disorder and agoraphobia, complete with nonconverging and competing conceptions of etiology, treatment approach, and mechanisms of change. The emerging biomedical view was that panic was the core element of panic disorder, which was presumed to have a biological etiology, and that agoraphobia occurred secondary to the anticipatory fear of future panic attacks. Behavior therapists focused primarily on the phobic avoidance behavior associated with agoraphobia, which was viewed as an equal element of a tripartite conception of the disorder: panic attacks, anticipatory anxiety, and phobic avoidance.

Prior to 1983, proponents of the two positions barely spoke the same language or spoke to each other, and they rarely read research reports produced by the opposite camp. However, they all had one common need: assessment. All clinical researchers need to measure disorders, their target symptoms, and dysfunctional behaviors as well as treatment-related behavioral changes. Such a focus on assessment is necessary—first to characterize the sample being studied so that replication is possible, and second to determine whether some independent variable (e.g., treatment) has produced a change in the behavior that was originally measured. This common need was the impetus for the growing rapprochement between the psychological and biomedical camps.

By the time DSM-III-R (American Psychiatric Association 1987) was published, panic attacks were generally considered to be central to panic disorder and agoraphobic avoidance behavior was considered to be a secondary manifestation. Nonetheless, three related anxiety disorders were included in DSM-III-R: panic disorder without agoraphobia, panic disorder with agoraphobia, and agoraphobia without a history of panic attacks.

During the 1980s, the rapprochement between the cognitive-behavior and biomedical perspectives allowed the discussion to progress from problems of mutual interest to collaboration on research projects. NIMH, which had been instrumental in bringing about this nascent collaborative spirit, deemed that the time might be appropriate to hold a consensus development conference. In November 1989, a planning meeting, attended by experts in psychological and pharmacological treatments for panic, was convened for the purpose of determining whether the time was, in fact, propitious for a consensus development conference. The participants agreed on the need for and timeliness of such a conference, and the planning of the particulars began immediately.

Format of the Consensus Development Conference

The NIH/NIMH Consensus Development Conference on the Treatment of Panic Disorder was another effort by NIMH to continue dialogue between the cognitive-behaviorists and the psychopharmacologists. The format of the consensus development conference was seen as an excellent means of letting each camp put its best data forward, thereby indicating that both had something legitimate to say. One concern was that too many unresolved controversies existed for any consensus to be reached, but this concern proved unfounded. More obvious objectives were to 1) evaluate the claims of treatment efficacy, 2) sharpen the scientific questions being asked, and 3) elucidate issues for future research.

With the collaboration of NIMH staff, the conference was organized by the NIH's Office of Medical Applications of Research (OMAR), an office that was created in response to a congressional mandate for scientists to evaluate new medical technologies. Eighteen speakers representing primarily the cognitive-behavior and biomedical perspectives presented data-based papers on the diagnosis, classification, epidemiology, etiology, and treatment of panic disorder with and without agoraphobia. These presentations occupied about one and a half days and included time for discussion and questions from the panel, other presenters, and the audience.

The consensus panel was comprised of experts in psychology, psychiatry, cardiology, internal medicine, and methodology, as well as members of the general public. Although panel members often had expertise in specific mental disorders (e.g., borderline personality disorder, major depression), none was a recognized expert in panic disorder. The panelists' job was to listen to, evaluate, and weigh the evidence. Then they were to formulate a consensus statement (see Chapter 18) that addressed the following five questions:

1. What are the epidemiology, natural history, and course of panic disorder with and without agoraphobia? How is this disorder diagnosed?
2. What are the current treatments? What are the short-term and long-term effects of acute and extended treatment of this disorder?
3. What are the short-term and long-term adverse effects of these treatments? How should they be managed?
4. What are considerations for treatment planning?
5. What are the significant questions for future research?

Organization of This Book

An Overview of Panic Disorder

In Chapters 2 through 4, the diagnosis, natural history, epidemiology, genetics, and primary care of panic disorder are addressed. That panic disorder is a distinct mental disorder is generally accepted; however, controversy continues to flare over the criteria by which panic disorder with and without agoraphobia is diagnosed. In Chapter 2, Liebowitz and Fyer delineate three sets of variables that remain controversial—threshold, boundary, and cognitive issues—in the definition of the disorder. Their chapter presents the difficulties associated with the current criteria for 1) distinguishing panic disorder from panic attacks that occur in normal populations; 2) defining boundaries between panic disorder and other anxiety disorders, such as specific phobias; and 3) the extent to which cognitive factors should be used in the definition of the disorder. In addition, the authors discuss some of the solutions contemplated by the American Psychiatric Association's task force on the forthcoming DSM-IV. The point is that the existing criteria are adequate for the prototypical cases of panic disorder with and without agoraphobia, but are problematic for the "marginal" cases (i.e., those at the boundary between normality and panic disorder, on the one hand, and panic disorder and other anxiety disorders, on the other).

In Chapter 3, Weissman reviews the limited amount of data available on the epidemiology and genetics of panic disorder from the Epidemiologic Catchment Area (ECA) study (Robins and Regier 1991). She reports that about one-quarter of the 18,000 subjects of the study felt they were nervous people, about 9% had isolated panic attacks, and 1.5% met the DSM-III criteria for panic disorder at some time in their life. About one-third of the subjects with panic disorder and one-half with panic attacks also met criteria for agoraphobia. Weissman points out that these rates are similar to the rates found in several countries around the world, including such places as New Zealand, Germany, Korea, and Canada. The one exception appears to be Taiwan, where there are lower rates for most psychiatric disorders, including panic disorder.

The epidemiological data also indicate that, apart from being a serious disturbance in and of itself, panic disorder has a major impact on the patient's quality of life. The disorder is associated with poor physical and emotional health, increased risk of alcohol abuse, marital and financial problems, increased medication and emergency room use, and suicide attempts. Such data verify that panic disorder is a serious mental disorder.

Weissman's review of family and twin studies shows substantial evidence for the familial nature of panic disorder. These data suggest a possible genetic etiology, but the mode of transmission is still unclear. Several genetic linkage studies are under way that may provide further clarification of this issue within the next 5 years.

Data from epidemiological studies and mental health services research indicate that a large number of patients with mental disorders are treated within the nonpsychiatric general medical care system. These patients typically use twice as much medical care as patients without mental illness. Thus, the premise that enhanced diagnosis of patients with panic disorder will lead to more appropriate and effective care for these patients appears supported by Weissman's epidemiological data.

In Chapter 4, Katon focuses on a primary care–psychiatric management module of panic disorder. This module is composed of four essential steps: 1) case identification, 2) clinical history and assessment, 3) patient treatment planning, and 4) specific treatment modalities. Noteworthy among the recommendations in Katon's module is the need to assess more than just panic symptomatology and panic attacks. It is important to assess family history, stressful life events, temperamental factors, the patient's history of developmental vulnerabilities, and the patient's health concerns and attributions about the nature of the illness. This advice is good not only for the practitioner, but also for the clinical investigator, who should routinely assess such areas.

Pharmacological Treatments

Although evidence of effective pharmacotherapy for panic was first presented by Klein and his colleagues in the 1960s, it was not until the late 1970s and early 1980s that clinicians recognized several classes of medications as effective panic block-ades, including tricyclic antidepressants, monoamine oxidase inhibitors, and high-potency benzodiazepines. Recent research has focused on 1) the relative effectiveness of the various medications, 2) how to extend the efficacy of treatment beyond the acute phase by increasing dosage or prolonging the length of treat-ment, 3) how to ameliorate side effects and withdrawal problems, and 4) an investigation of combined pharmacological and psychosocial treatments, as com-pared with isolated administration of each modality. Ballenger concludes his excellent review of the literature in Chapter 5 with the contention that "there is no best medicine for all patients." He reports some encouraging evidence that main-tenance treatment (given during months 3 to 12) enhances the benefits of al-prazolam and imipramine for panic disorder patients, and that combined psychosocial and pharmacological treatment may be superior to either given alone. But several unresolved issues remain. Ballenger's list includes 1) matching treatment to the patient, 2) determining the optimal length of treatment, 3) reducing the relapse rate, and 4) developing effective treatments for patients resistant to initial pharmacotherapy.

The long-term outcome of treated and untreated panic disorder patients has little empirical data associated with it. In Chapter 6, Katschnig and Amering review research on both issues and find that in seven follow-up studies of un-treated panic disorder patients, about one-half showed evidence of recovery or much improvement. These studies, however, were conducted before 1980 when panic disorder became part of the DSM nomenclature, and also prior to the widespread use of panic medication. In addition, any reported recovery percent-age from these studies is thrown into question by the heterogeneity of these samples.

Katschnig then reports the findings of his long-term follow-up study of patients who had participated in the Cross-National Collaborative Panic Study and were treated psychopharmacologically. The data he and Amering presented to the panel were based on 220 of 367 patients who could be re-interviewed. During the poststudy year, only 24% had experienced no panic attacks. That percentage increased to 39% between the poststudy and current year. Although Katschnig views these results with optimism, they do suggest that much more work is needed to develop treatments that produce more enduring benefits. The more pessimistic view is that between 61% and 76% of patients treated in the Cross-National Study continued to have panic attacks.

Pharmacological treatments are effective in reducing or eliminating panic attacks, but they are also attended by a number of problems, including relapse and disturbing side effects. According to Gorman in Chapter 7, new medications are being sought, primarily to reduce the side effect profile. Although the ultimate goal of such research is to find a medication that would "cure" panic disorder, most research has more limited objectives. New antipanic medications that have fewer side effects, more rapid onset of action, and the capacity to be administered over long periods of time to patients who relapse frequently after discontinuation of the medication are being sought. Gorman focuses on the serotonin reuptake inhibitors that show promise in panic blockade. He cites two uncontrolled studies documenting that fluoxetine is effective in blocking panic. Serotonin reuptake inhibitors are particularly promising because of their favorable side effect profile.

The other class of medications that has been the subject of several investigations is the high-potency benzodiazepines. The success of alprazolam ran counter to the common belief that benzodiazepines were not useful in the treatment of panic. Gorman cites research on the effectiveness of lorazepam, clonazepam, and adinazolam. In contrast, the hypertensive drugs have shown modest antipanic effects, and other antidepressants, such as trazodone and bupropion, appear to be ineffective.

The discovery of an effective treatment always seems to precede our understanding of the mechanisms underlying the treatment's efficacy. This phenomenon appears to be the case whether the treatment is psychological or biological. In Chapter 8 Heninger provides an overview of the research on neurobiological mechanisms that shows that panic attacks can be generated by the administration of pharmacological, physiological, and environmental stimuli, and can be reduced by different pharmacological agents. These data point to the involvement of multiple neurobiological mechanisms.

Various brain neurotransmitter systems have been implicated in the genesis and modulation of anxiety and panic, including the gamma-aminobutyric acid–benzodiazepine complex (GABA-BZ), the noradrenergic (NE), serotonergic (5-hydroxytryptamine [5-HT]), purinergic, and several peptide systems. Because of the intricately interactive nature of all of these systems, Heninger posits an integrated model involving GABA-BZ system modulation of the NE and 5-HT systems, including neuropeptide transmitter input to the hippocampus and amygdala. Such a model would account for the multiple pathways involved in the pathogenesis of anxiety and panic disorder, as well as for the panic-inducing effects of certain pharmacological stimuli and panic-reducing effects of pharmacological treatment. Heninger proposes—and we heartily concur with—the investigation of neurobiological variables in psychosocial treatment studies. Heninger's other suggestion for future research is equally germane: "Since the pharmacological treatments are thought to mostly block symptom expression at a secondary level, future research should increasingly investigate the more fundamental molecular biological abnormalities involved."

Psychological Treatments

As mentioned earlier, parallel literatures had been developed in the 1970s and 1980s on the pharmacological and psychological treatments of panic disorder and agoraphobia. Whereas pharmacotherapies focused on the panic attacks, psychological treatments focused on the agoraphobic avoidance behavior. A variety of exposure methods were developed, tested, and found efficacious in the treatment of phobic avoidance behavior. But as panic attacks emerged as a central feature of the disorder (now called *panic disorder with agoraphobia*), it became clear to clinical investigators that more attention needed to be paid to the reduction or elimination of panic. Exposure-based methods were producing clinically significant improvement in 60%–75% of treated patients, but 80% of these patients had residual symptoms and about 35% were obtaining little benefit from these treatments.

Barlow's presentation in Chapter 9 focuses on the work of his clinic and that of other centers that, in recent years, have developed closely related antipanic, cognitive-behavior treatment packages. During the 1980s, Barlow and his associates developed a treatment package that included breathing retraining, interoceptive exposure, and cognitive restructuring that was particularly aimed at the catastrophic misinterpretations of frightening bodily sensations. Barlow's clinic as well as others around the world are reporting similar success rates with cognitive-behavior therapy, rates that approach 90% of patient samples achieving freedom from panic attacks by the end of treatment. More recently, Barlow reported the first systematic 2-year follow-up study of patients treated in his clinic; he found that 81% of patients treated by his panic control treatment remained panic-free at the 24-month assessment. Barlow qualifies these excellent results with evidence that panic attack reduction in isolation is a rather narrow target in many cases of panic disorder with agoraphobia, and that more comprehensive approaches may be required to increase the numbers of patients whose functioning returns to within the normal range.

In Chapter 10, Clark covers somewhat similar ground to Barlow's, but with a greater emphasis on the cognitive component of the treatment. Clark's cognitive theory of panic proposes that individuals who experience panic attacks do so because they misinterpret benign bodily sensations as indications of physical or mental catastrophe (e.g., perceiving palpitations as an impending heart attack). Evidence for the theory includes the following empirically determined facts: 1) panic disorder patients are more likely than other anxiety disorder patients or nonpsychiatric control subjects to misinterpret bodily sensations; 2) activating these negative interpretations produces panic attacks in panic disorder patients; and 3) cognitive procedures that prevent panic disorder patients from misinterpreting the sensations induced by pharmacological challenge tests, such as those using carbon dioxide and lactate, block laboratory-induced panic attacks. Clark also reports case series data from clinical researchers in England, Hungary, and the United States as well as the data from three controlled studies showing that cognitive therapy is an effective treatment for a large majority of panic disorder patients (i.e., between 80% and 95% are panic-free after 3 months of treatment). Clark contends that cognitive change lies behind the efficacy of both psychological and pharmacological treatments. Of course, longer term follow-up of these dramatically improved patients is crucial. At the end of his chapter, Clark offers some tentative speculations regarding the possible mechanisms of action of psychological treatments with panic disorder patients.

It is left to Rachman in Chapter 11 to provide a fuller consideration of mechanisms by which psychosocial treatments produce change. The first part of Rachman's chapter includes a review of various hypothesized mechanisms, such as reciprocal inhibition, extinction, habituation, and self-efficacy. Rachman then turns his attention to Clark's cognitive theory of panic. Several deductions from the theory are made, followed by a review of the evidence that supports the theory. In general, the evidence shows a firm relationship between the reduction of negative cognitions during treatment and the maintenance of improvements.

Rachman correctly points out, however, that the decline in cognitions and in bodily sensations may be a cause, consequence, or correlate of the reduction in panic. After exploring the evidence for these alternative explanations, as well as noting some of the complexities involved in determining which cognitions seem related to panic, Rachman concludes that the cognitive explanation for the results of cognitive therapy is the one explanation best supported by the evidence to date. One of the interesting questions Rachman poses for future research is the extent to which the cognitive explanation can account for the therapeutic effects of exposure therapy and pharmacological treatments (e.g., see Rachman and Maser 1988). The first step would be to measure cognitive changes that occur with these other treatments.

The panel did not rush too quickly to accept this unidimensional explanation.

What had been overlooked by both camps was the impact of one modality on the variables routinely considered important by proponents of the other modality. Biomedical researchers rarely study the impact of biological treatments on psychological variables, and, conversely, psychosocial treatment researchers rarely study the effects that psychological treatments have on the biology of the patient. It is now time to include outcome variables typically measured by researchers from each perspective.

Chambless and Gillis's discussion in Chapter 12 of the psychological treatments for panic disorder provides a broad overview of the effects of cognitive and behavior treatments. These authors point to two major breakthroughs in the psychological treatment of panic disorder with agoraphobia. During the 1970s, the treatment focus was on the agoraphobic avoidance behavior. Exposure-based treatments developed during this era are now capable of producing meaningful change in a majority of patients with agoraphobia. But the associated panic attacks were not as effectively treated by in vivo exposure to feared external locations.

During the 1980s and early 1990s, a second breakthrough was the development of a cognitive-behavior treatment package that combines interoceptive exposure, breathing retraining, and cognitive therapy. As mentioned above, the typical finding in controlled studies of the efficacy of this form of treatment is that over 80% of patients are panic-free by the end of treatment, and a similar percentage of patients remain panic-free at 1 and 2 years posttreatment.

Although definite strides have been made in developing a comprehensively effective treatment for panic disorder with agoraphobia, Chambless and Gillis caution against complacency. Additional research into the psychosocial treatment of panic disorder should focus on increasing the global effectiveness of treatment, including panic, phobia, generalized anxiety, depression, fear of panic, and social and occupational functioning. Research also needs to investigate the efficacy of treatment with panic disorder patients who present with comorbid disorders. Finally, Chambless and Gillis recommend research on the dissemination of the available treatments, as this is a perennial problem for psychological treatments.

Combined Treatments

There are many rationales for combining pharmacological and psychological treatments. In fact, the modal clinical practice is to administer a combined treatment regimen to panic disorder patients, although the psychosocial treatment most often co-administered with medication is not the empirically tested cognitive-behavior therapies. Moreover, there is a pervasive belief—with little empirical data to support it—that combined treatment regimens are superior to other treatments administered alone. Third, the investigation of combined treatments may serve as a political vehicle for the ongoing depolarization of biological and psychological treatment investigators.

Telch and Lucas have organized their review of this literature in Chapter 13 around five issues: 1) the rationale for investigating combined treatments for panic disorder, 2) the current scientific knowledge base, 3) the clinical efficacy of combined treatments, 4) the implications of research findings for clinical practice, and 5) future research priorities. Their review of the short-term efficacy literature leads them to conclude that 66%–75% of patients with panic disorder with agoraphobia achieve marked improvement with a combination of imipramine plus exposure or alprazolam plus exposure, and that the combined treatment regimen offers some advantage over either treatment administered by itself.

With respect to the long-term efficacy of combined treatment, the findings depart somewhat from those for the short-term efficacy. Between one-half to two-thirds of patients show marked improvement at 12- to 24-month follow-up. But for patients displaying panic disorder with agoraphobia, the combination of imipramine and exposure is no more effective than exposure administered alone. The use of alprazolam in combination with exposure produces higher relapse and poorer long-term outcome than exposure alone. The most optimistic finding for Telch and Lucas, however, is the fact that a number of multicenter investigations involving collaborations between biological and psychological treatment investigators are now under way. As the authors conclude, "Demonstration of such cooperation provides hope that in the years to come depolarization between the two disciplines will occur and with it a deeper understanding of combined treatments."

In Klerman's discussion (Chapter 14),[1] methodological and research design issues in the conduct of combined treatment research are scrutinized. For the proper evaluation of combined treatment regimens, Klerman recommends the randomized, placebo-controlled, parallel group designs that have been so successful in evaluating single, new treatments. Combined treatments within this framework may be administered concurrently and sequentially. Klerman spells out some of the differing research considerations when employing concurrent and sequential designs. Finally, he remarks on the role of conflicting ideologies that have produced the polarization between biological and psychological treatment investigators. He, like Telch and Lucas, is hopeful that the impartial eye of science will help encourage the rapprochement between the two camps.

---

[1] We note with sadness the passing of Dr. Gerald Klerman in April 1992. He died before completing his paper for this publication. The editors have decided to publish the abstract to give the reader a sense of the direction of his thinking.

Risk-Benefit Issues

Potent treatments are likely to present some risk of adverse effects. In this section, risk-benefit analyses for pharmacological and psychological treatments are given. In Chapter 15, Rickels and Schweizer cover the psychopharmacological agents. They present, in turn, the benefits and risks of the three major classes of medications for which clinical efficacy has been determined: the tricyclic antidepressants, the monoamine oxidase inhibitors, and the high-potency benzodiazepines. The benefits of the latter class of medications include early onset of panic relief and, to some extent, reductions in the concurrent symptoms of phobia and anxiety. Imipramine and phenelzine appear to be better antiphobic agents, and discontinuation of these medications does not produce any clinically significant withdrawal problems.

The major risks of benzodiazepines include some disturbing side effects, the potential for withdrawal problems, a high relapse rate once medication is discontinued, and the development of physical dependence. The major problem with the other two classes of drugs is their disturbing potential for side effects. Rickels and Schweizer do not include a risk-benefit analysis of the newer serotonin reuptake blockers because of the paucity of efficacy data on these drugs. Some of the problems with benzodiazepines can be minimized by careful attention to dosing and length of administration.

In Chapter 16, Michelson covers similar ground for the psychological treatments. He presents us with 100 hypothetical panic disorder patients with agoraphobia who are assumed to have received alternative psychosocial and pharmacological treatments. He then constructs a table that delineates the percentages of patients who drop out, achieve clinically significant improvement, and relapse. These data represent estimates based on literature reviews, recent meta-analyses, and current clinical research. Michelson arrives at an overall efficacy index for each treatment reviewed. On the basis of this analysis, Michelson concludes that the treatment of choice for panic disorder with no or mild phobic avoidance is cognitive-behavior therapy aimed at panic cessation. For patients experiencing panic disorder with agoraphobia, more multimodal treatments are needed, such as cognitive-behavior therapy plus programmed practice and therapist-assisted graded exposure. He also recommends an in-depth cognitive therapy to address the implicit core beliefs that maintain the disorder.

In terms of risks, Michelson cites a problem common to all treatments—failure to address comorbid disorders and dysfunctions often found in panic disorder patients. A second issue is the lack of attention to the thorough emotional processing of phobic cues that appears to be necessary for the successful resolution of the disorder. His final two concerns relate to the sparse and haphazard dissemination of efficacious psychological treatments. Michelson recommends that therapists should avail themselves of training workshops in cognitive-behavior treatments, and that such treatments should be included in advanced degree training programs in psychology, psychiatry, and social work. It seems likely to us, however, that dissemination of this methodology must be done with care because, once out of the skilled hands of those responsible for its development, administration may become both careless and unsystematic. Efficacy is likely to decline. The same argument already holds for pharmacotherapy, as conservative practitioners tend to undermedicate. Consequently, the level of symptom relief often is less than optimal.

Future Issues

The final chapter focuses on future research issues in the treatment of panic disorder. Shear, Leon, and Spielman, after acknowledging the genuine progress that has been made in the treatment of this disorder, present a sobering list of issues for future research. They enumerate four major deficiencies with the current research: 1) lack of standardized methodology for assessing treatment outcome; 2) lack of data on optimal treatment, despite the existence of effective treatments as determined by controlled investigations; 3) lack of data on cognitive-behavior treatments that simultaneously focus on phobic avoidance and panic reduction; and 4) the lack of data on the origins and vicissitudes of comorbidity. A review of these problems leads Shear et al. to conclude that there is a need to broaden our working model of the panic-agoraphobic syndrome to incorporate data that address residual symptoms, the discontinuity between panic and phobic avoidance, and the prevalence and impact of comorbidity (see Maser and Cloninger 1990).

Summary

In summary, we have come far in demonstrating the efficacy of specific interventions with panic disorder, but the direct translation of these results into recommendations for optimal clinical practice is fraught with difficulties. The editors resonate to Shear et al.'s conclusion: "We should be particularly wary of drawing premature conclusions about relative effectiveness of treatments that have not yet been properly compared, and in patient populations that may not have been fully characterized."

References

American Psychiatric Association: Diagnostic and Statistical Manual of Mental Disorders, 3rd Edition. Washington, DC, American Psychiatric Association, 1980

American Psychiatric Association: Diagnostic and Statistical Manual of Mental Disorders, 3rd Edition, Revised. Washington, DC, American Psychiatric Association, 1987

Maser JD, Cloninger CR: Comorbidity of Mood and Anxiety Disorders. Washington, DC, American Psychiatric Press, 1990

Rachman S, Maser JD: Panic: Psychological Perspectives. Hillsdale, NJ, Lawrence Erlbaum, 1988

Robins LN, Regier DA: Psychiatric Disorders in America: The Epidemiologic Catchment Area Study. New York, Free Press, 1991

Overview of Panic Disorder

Chapter 2

Diagnosis and Clinical Course of Panic Disorder With and Without Agoraphobia

Michael R. Liebowitz, M.D.,
and Abby J. Fyer, M.D.

I n this chapter we focus on the following issues:

1. The criteria by which panic disorder with and without agoraphobia are diagnosed, and the changes in diagnostic criteria contemplated for the American Psychiatric Association's *Diagnostic and Statistical Manual of Mental Disorders,* Fourth Edition (DSM-IV)[1]
2. Typical instruments, methods, and procedures for assessing and diagnosing panic disorder with and without agoraphobia
3. The clinical course of panic disorder with and without agoraphobia

---

[1] It is important to note that, in addition to ourselves, a number of individuals have contributed to the revisions proposed for panic disorder in DSM-IV: James Ballenger, M.D.; David Barlow, Ph.D.; Jonathan Davidson, M.D.; and Edna Foa, Ph.D.

Current and Proposed Criteria for Diagnosing Panic Disorder

Three types of issues are identified as problems with panic disorder as defined in DSM-III-R (American Psychiatric Association 1987): threshold issues, cognitive issues, and boundary issues.

Threshold Issues

The threshold issues for panic disorder involve two questions: How many symptoms should be required to define a panic attack? and How many panic attacks should be required to define panic disorder?

Researchers are attempting to find the minimum levels of symptomatology required for making a diagnosis of panic attacks or panic disorder while trying to maximize specificity and sensitivity. If the threshold is set too low, although all affected individuals will be included, many individuals who really do not merit a diagnosis will also be included. On the other hand, if the threshold is set too high, although only individuals who have the disorder will be included, some individuals who really have the disorder will not be. The lower thresholds listed for panic disorder and for a number of other psychiatric disorders in DSM-III (American Psychiatric Association 1980) and DSM-III-R were based on expert opinion rather than on empirical validation. The criteria for panic disorder listed in DSM-III required four or more symptoms during at least one panic attack as well as three panic attacks in 3 weeks and at least one nonsituational panic attack. DSM-III-R also used four or more symptoms to define a panic attack.

Leon et al. (1992) recently reanalyzed the Epidemiologic Catchment Area (ECA) study (Myers et al. 1984) data to assess the validity of the four-symptom threshold for defining a panic attack. Two parameters were used as validating measures: use of an emergency room for emotional problems and psychiatric hospitalization. Leon and co-workers then plotted the specificity and sensitivity of different numbers of symptoms for defining a panic attack, using first emergency room visits and then psychiatric hospitalizations as the validating measure. Using either measure, three or four symptoms gave the best separation from the random curve (i.e., the maximal specificity and sensitivity). These data provide empirical support for requiring three or four symptoms to define a panic attack.

Another question addressed by Leon et al. was, Which component of the panic disorder criteria contributed most to defining a case? Was it the number of panic symptoms or the frequency of panic attacks? One validating measure might be the percentage of patients seeking emergency room visits, figures for which are found in the ECA data. In the ECA study, 28% of the individuals who met criteria for a full panic disorder visited the emergency room. If the impairment criteria were discounted, less than 6% sought emergency room care. If the four-symptom requirement was removed, only 2.4% visited the emergency room. If the three-attacks-in-3-weeks criterion for frequency was deleted, 19% still sought visits, and if the criteria that panic attacks be spontaneous were removed, the number was also 19%. Therefore, in terms of defining a case, requiring four symptoms was very important, but requiring a patient to have three panic attacks in 3 weeks was less important. Using psychiatric hospitalization as a validating measure demonstrated the same pattern. The biggest loss in severity, measured by a drop in the percentage of patients seeking psychiatric hospitalization, occurred when Leon et al. departed from the four-symptom criterion, which then also validated that criterion for defining a panic attack. The proposal for DSM-IV is still to require four symptoms for a panic attack.

The second threshold issue is, What frequency of panic attacks should be required for the diagnosis of panic disorder? To recapitulate briefly, the Research Diagnostic Criteria (RDC) (Spitzer et al. 1978) originally required six panic attacks in 6 weeks, DSM-III required three panic attacks in 3 weeks, and DSM-III-R requires four or more panic attacks in 4 weeks. DSM-III-R also includes a "back door" criterion in that an individual can be diagnosed with panic disorder after having one or more panic attacks followed by a period of at least 1 month of persistent fear of having another attack. In DSM-III-R, the diagnosis of panic disorder can be based on retrospective report of only one spontaneous panic attack if worry is also present, but individuals who do not worry about recurrent panic attacks are excluded if they report fewer than four spontaneous attacks in 4 weeks.

Epidemiological and clinical investigations have demonstrated that a substantial number of patients have infrequent panic attacks. Angst et al.'s (1990) epidemiological study found a prevalence of panic of 1.9% and of infrequent panic of 3.1%. Von Korff and Eaton (1989) reported a prevalence of 1.4% for panic disorder and 2.1% for infrequent panic. Wittchen (1988) found a 2.4% prevalence of panic and a 1.8% prevalence of infrequent panic. In all of these studies, infrequent panic was defined as at least one but less than three panic attacks in 3 weeks; in addition, the individuals with infrequent panic had sought treatment, although not with the same frequency that individuals with panic disorder had. Up to 60% of the panic disorder group sought treatment, depending on the study, whereas 21%–23% of infrequent panickers sought treatment. However, infrequent panic was still associated with real clinical morbidity.

In the diagnostic criteria for panic disorder, the minimum frequency of unexpected panic attacks is one issue and the duration and content of the intercurrent anxiety is another issue. DSM-IV is moving to clarify the subtypes of panic, including unexpected attacks, situationally bound attacks, and an intermediate category of situationally predisposed attacks. *Unexpected panic attacks,* which are really characteristic of panic disorder, come out of the blue without any known precipitation at all. *Situationally bound attacks* are characteristic of simple and social phobia in the sense that they are always tied to particular kinds of stimuli. *Situationally predisposed attacks* are those in which an individual entering a particular situation is more likely, but not guaranteed, to have a panic attack; in addition, the attack may occur sometime later. An example would be individuals with panic and agoraphobia who are afraid to go to a shopping mall because they are likely to have a panic attack. DSM-IV will require at least some unexpected panic attacks for panic disorder, defining these as "not occurring immediately before an exposure to a situation that almost always provoked anxiety." Panic attacks, except recurrent unexpected attacks, will be allowed in simple and social phobia. Individuals with these disorders have crescendo-like panic experiences that fit the panic attack definition except for the fact that the attacks are not unexpected.

A number of options are being considered for the threshold definition for panic disorder in DSM-IV:

▮ Retain the DSM-III-R thresholds of four panic attacks in 4 weeks with no requirement of intercurrent anxiety or one unexpected attack with at least 1 month of worry about panic recurrence.

▮ Require an unexpected panic attack and 1 month of persistent worry about the next panic, which would follow the liberal threshold from DSM-III-R.

▮ Require recurrent unexpected panic attacks and 1 month of persistent worry about the next panic.

▮ Require one unexpected attack and 1 month of persistent worry about the next panic or its implications in terms of health worries and loss of control (i.e., a broader worry definition, which is more typical of what patients with panic attacks experience). A broadened worry definition would be the following: "Between episodes of panic, persistent anxiety or worry develops, often concerning recurrence of panic attacks, fear of episodes of loss of control, or worry that the anxiety symptoms reflect underlying medical or psychiatric illness."

▮ Require recurrent unexpected panic attacks and a month of worry about the next panic or implications (i.e., recurrent panic and the broader worry criterion).

▮ Simply require recurrent unexpected panic attacks.

Cognitive Issues

If only unexpected panic attacks were required and no worry criteria were speci-
fied, the cognitive aspects of panic in the definition of panic disorder would be left
out. The contribution of cognitive features to the definition has been debated.
More cognitively oriented researchers, such as Clark (1986) and Telch et al.
(1989), have agreed that worries should be part of the definition. They believe that
fears of physical catastrophe (e.g., serious illness or heart attack), loss of control
(e.g., going crazy or doing something uncontrolled), and social embarrassment
(e.g., that others will perceive the panic) should be part of the definition of panic
attacks and also part of the definition of panic disorder. At the other extreme,
Beitman et al. (1990) stated that the emphasis should be on autonomic symptomatology. They argued that some patients have nonfearful panic disorder, which
involves paroxysms of autonomic symptomatology not accompanied by any particular kind of catastrophic thinking. Such patients are reported to be frequently
found in cardiac or other medical clinics. If this kind of a definition were used, a
panic attack would be described as a discrete period of intense fear or discomfort,
a definition that would then include the nonfearful types of panic.

Boundary Issues

Boundary issues involve the distinctions between panic disorder and other psychiatric disorders. The boundaries between panic disorder with agoraphobia and
social phobia have proven to be more difficult to articulate than previously
thought. In DSM-III-R, part of the definition of social phobia included a criterion
B: " if an Axis III or another Axis I disorder is present, the fear (in A) that is part of
social phobia is unrelated to it, e.g., the fear is not of having a panic attack (this is
panic disorder)." What really was meant, but not stated explicitly enough, was that
the fear is not one of having an unexpected panic attack. Individuals with social
phobia characteristically have panic attacks in social, interpersonal, or performance situations. In addition, even with that clarification, there are still several
kinds of ambiguous situations. For example, an individual might meet criteria for
panic disorder with agoraphobia, but avoid public speaking due to the fear of both
panic and humiliation over inept behavior. Should such a patient be said to have
social phobia as well as panic disorder? As another example, consider the individual who begins with recurrent, unexpected panic attacks, thus meeting the criteria
for panic disorder, and who avoids public speaking because of a fear of panic. But
then, although the unexpected panic attacks stop, the individual continues to
avoid the social or performance situation. Does the individual then have panic
disorder, or is it now social phobia? According to the DSM-III-R approach, with

its emphasis on a historical perspective, the latter patient would still meet panic disorder criteria. However, if one took a cross-sectional approach, in the second stage the individual would look more like someone with social phobia.

In DSM-IV, as part of the criteria for social phobia, a criterion B may be added, stating that "exposure to the specific phobic stimulus almost invariably provokes an immediate anxiety response that may take the form of a panic attack," and a criterion F, stating that "the fear and avoidance is not better accounted for by panic disorder with agoraphobia." These additions would leave ambiguous cases to clinical judgment. To help guide clinical judgment further, a statement may be placed in the criteria for panic disorder with agoraphobia such as, "Consider a simple or social phobia diagnosis when 1) avoidance is limited to one or two situations and 2) the current panic attacks are situationally bound or predisposed." Situationally predisposed panics can also be ambiguous, but situationally bound panics should certainly lead one's thinking toward simple or social phobia.

Part of the difficulty in specifying the boundary between a panic and a phobic disorder is the limited data available about diagnostic validity and the reliability of descriptive categories. Controversy about the importance of historical versus current presentation and the frequent occurrence of cases that do not fit the prototype are also factors to be considered.

A second boundary issue is the distinction between panic disorder with agoraphobia and the specific phobias. DSM-III-R criterion A for simple phobia reads "a persistent fear of a circumscribed stimulus other than the fear of having a panic attack (as in panic disorder) or of humiliation or embarrassment in certain social situations (as in social phobia)" (p. 244). What is meant, but not explicitly stated, in that statement is again that unexpected panic attacks should lead to a diagnosis of panic disorder, not simple phobia. Even if this understanding were made explicit, however, there would still be some ambiguous situations. Consider, for example, an individual who has an unexpected panic attack in a specific situation, such as an elevator. That individual then begins to avoid elevators, fearing the onset of panic. All subsequent anxiety, avoidance, or panic attacks are limited to exposure or anticipation of exposure to elevators. Is this panic disorder or simple phobia? To further clarify this boundary issue in DSM-IV, it is proposed that an addition be made to the criteria for simple phobia that would state that "the anxiety or avoidance is not better accounted for by panic disorder with agoraphobia (i.e., a fear of having unexpected or situationally predisposed panic attacks)"; again, the clinician would be left to rely on his or her judgment. Raters would be instructed to consider simple or social phobia when the avoidance is limited to one or two situations and the current panic attacks are situationally bound or predisposed.

The boundaries between panic and the phobic disorders have been explored in the DSM-IV panic disorder field trial. The field trial assessed reliability, coverage, and descriptive features of the various panic and phobic disorders criteria proposed for DSM-IV and also those from DSM-III-R and the *International Classification of Diseases,* 10th Edition (ICD-10; World Health Organization 1992). However, any solution is still a problem because external validators are not currently available.

Methods for Diagnosis and Assessment

The most effective method for diagnosing panic disorder is a clinical interview that includes both careful definition and assessment of panic attacks and the commonly associated symptoms of avoidance and worry about recurrent panic or its implications. Excellent test-retest reliability for the DSM-III-R categories of panic disorder with and without agoraphobia has been demonstrated with several widely available, semistructured interview schedules, including the Anxiety Disorders Interview Schedule—Revised for DSM-III-R (ADIS-R; DiNardo and Barlow 1988), the Schedule for Affective Disorders and Schizophrenia—Lifetime Anxiety Disorders Version (SADS-LA; Fyer et al. 1989; Mannuzza et al. 1989), and the Structured Clinical Interview for DSM-III-R (SCID; Spitzer and Williams 1992).

As the clinical presentation of panic disorder can vary considerably, a systematic review of all components of the illness (i.e., panic attacks, avoidance, and anticipatory and generalized anxiety) is important. Some patients present with a clear history of recurrent, unexpected attacks and concern about the disruption and fear that these have produced. In other patients, particularly those who present in nonpsychiatric settings (e.g., primary care clinics, epidemiologically drawn community samples) or whose illness is long-standing and undiagnosed, the distinction between panic and other anxiety is lost, and the presenting complaint may simply be one of constant unreasonable worry and demoralization about an inability to carry out routine responsibilities. A completely somatic presentation (e.g., palpitations and chest pains, episodic gastrointestinal or neurological symptoms) with a focus on the health implications of these "unexplained" physical symptoms is also common (Katon 1991).

Although a number of biological challenges reliably elicit panic in a subset of clinically diagnosed patients, none has as yet been shown to be sufficiently sensitive and specific for use as a diagnostic test (Gorman et al. 1990). For example, intravenous sodium lactate, one of the most widely studied panicogens, is relatively specific. It provokes panic in 50%–75% of patients with DSM-III-R panic disorder, but not in subjects with other anxiety disorders or depression who do not also have a history of unexpected panic. However, if used for diagnosis, the lactate challenge would miss the 25%–50% of clinically diagnosed patients who are lactate nonpanickers and who, on further study, do not appear to differ from lactate panickers with respect to either treatment response or clinical features. Other biological measures (e.g., growth hormone blunting, anxiety response to yohimbine, carbon dioxide sensitivity) may have greater sensitivity; however, their specificity is not yet well studied.

Self-report questionnaires, although useful as initial screening tools, have shown similar limitations. Studies (e.g., Fyer and Rassnick, in press) contrasting self-report to clinician diagnoses in nonclinical samples have indicated a high degree of sensitivity (i.e., low false-negative rates) but poor specificity (i.e., many false positives).

With respect to assessment of change and treatment outcome, four major variables have been identified as important and useful: frequency of panic attacks, phobic avoidance, nonpanic anxiety, and global clinical condition. The frequency of panic attacks is most accurately measured with the help of a daily, patient-recorded "anxiety diary" that incorporates the DSM-III-R panic definition and simplifies recording of symptoms and the context of attacks. The diary is then jointly reviewed by patient and clinician to clarify symptom classification and arrive at a final assessment of panic frequency. Daily recording of panic or anxiety symptoms by the patient and joint patient-clinician review of the diary are particularly important for several reasons. The distinction between partially treated panic attack symptoms and nonpanic anxiety, which is often critical in choices concerning medication dosage or psychotherapy strategy, is one of the most difficult areas in the assessment of panic disorder treatment outcome. Clinician inexperience or inadequate patient education can often result in misdiagnosis of limited-symptom panic as anticipatory anxiety or somatization. Contrarily, anticipatory surges before entering phobic situations, intense or dramatically reported responses to interpersonal conflicts, or even nonanxious episodic disturbances such as seizures may be mistakenly assessed as panic attacks. The development of a shared, operational definition of panic, which is made possible by repeated joint patient-clinician diary review, greatly facilitates this task.

Contrasts between in vivo monitoring and unstructured, retrospective self-report of panic symptoms also suggest that the latter can be associated with both forgetfulness and symptom distortion. Moreover, although good reliability has been obtained for lifetime history of ever having had a spontaneous panic attack, reliability for retrospective assessment of frequency of panic attacks within a specific time period is mixed (Ballenger et al. 1988; Fyer and Rassnick, in press).

A number of self-report and clinician-administered questionnaires and behavioral assessment tests provide reliable and treatment-responsive measurement of phobic avoidance. Two main approaches have been used. In the first, all subjects are routinely assessed for level of fear or avoidance on a standardized set of situations for which phobic fears have been commonly reported. In the second, subjects are asked to identify one or two main (i.e., most disturbing and functionally impairing) phobias, whose progress is charted throughout the study (Marks 1987). However, although both techniques are clinically useful, their correspondence to the patient's actual functioning in daily life is not known. Use of continuous, in vivo, computer-assisted monitoring systems may be helpful. However, at present this methodology is neither widely available nor feasible from a cost-benefit perspective.

Assessment of nonpanic anxiety has included the use of both standard generalized anxiety scales (e.g., Hamilton Anxiety Scale [Hamilton 1959]) and newer instruments that address characteristic cognitions and worries in this illness. Examples of these more specific scales are the Anxiety Sensitivity Index (Reiss et al. 1986), which measures a subject's tendency toward catastrophic interpretation of events, and the Fear of Autonomic Sensations Questionnaire (Van den Hout and Griez 1986), which measures a subject's somatic symptoms.

Global condition is measured using a standard 7- or 10-point scale (0 = worst among patients in this population, highest score = not ill). A useful and frequent strategy in making this type of global rating is to rate subjects first on a similar 7- or 10-point scale with respect to the different components of the illness (i.e., panic, avoidance, anticipatory anxiety, functional impairment) and to base the overall global rating on clinician integration of these components.

Clinical Course of Panic Disorder
With and Without Agoraphobia

Empirical data concerning the long-term natural history and posttreatment course of panic disorder are limited and methodologically uneven. The large-scale prospective studies in epidemiological samples needed to definitively answer these questions have not been done. Currently available information, which is summarized here, is derived almost exclusively from studies using the methodologically limited, retrospective life history or naturalistic patient follow-up designs.

The usual age at onset of panic disorder is late adolescence or early adulthood (ages 18–35). However, panic disorder in childhood, although not common, is now well documented. Since the latter is readily treatable, it is an important consideration in the differential diagnosis of this age group (Ballenger et al. 1988; Black and Robbins 1990; Klein and Klein 1990).

In the majority of clinical cases, the disorder begins with an episode of recurrent, unpredictable panic attacks followed by development of worry about the implications of the attacks (e.g., medical illness) and efforts to avoid or explain them (Breier et al. 1986; Schneier et al. 1991; Uhde et al. 1985). Approximately 70%–90% of panickers who seek treatment report some degree of panic-related phobic avoidance, and one-third to one-half meet criteria for agoraphobia, although the reasons for this variation in severity are not known.

Comorbidity for depression, other anxiety disorders, and substance abuse is also common. A lifetime history of depression is reported in as many as 30%–80% of patients diagnosed with panic disorder in both clinical and epidemiological samples. Clinical studies have indicated a 20%–30% rate of lifetime comorbidity for social phobia and for obsessive-compulsive disorder (Barlow 1988; Robins and Regier 1990; Stein et al. 1989) and a 15%–25% rate for alcohol abuse (Cox et al. 1990).

The currently available data suggest that, although panic disorder in the majority of affected individuals is a chronic waxing and waning illness, the overall prognosis can be favorable (Hirschfeld 1992). Although untreated prognosis is unknown, long-term prospective, naturalistic studies of clinically identified individuals have consistently found that at follow-up approximately 35%–50% are well or only mildly symptomatic, 35% have significant symptoms but are improved from their baseline, and the remaining 15%–30% are unchanged or worse. Baseline correlates of poor outcome include significant personality disorder, severity of anxiety and phobic symptoms, and depression and poor social adjustment (Hirschfeld, in press; Noyes et al. 1990; Pollack et al. 1990).

Relapse rates following treatment discontinuation vary widely among studies and are difficult to interpret given differences in definitions of illness recurrence and remission and in the length and types of treatment (Fyer 1988). Further studies with uniform criteria as well as designs that systematically compare the several treatment options are needed to clarify this issue.

References

American Psychiatric Association: Diagnostic and Statistical Manual of Mental Disorders, 3rd Edition. Washington, DC, American Psychiatric Association, 1980

American Psychiatric Association: Diagnostic and Statistical Manual of Mental Disorders, 3rd Edition, Revised. Washington, DC, American Psychiatric Association, 1987

Angst J, Vollrath M, Merikangas KR, et al: Comorbidity of anxiety and depression in the Zurich cohort study of young adults, in Comorbidity of Mood and Anxiety Disorders. Edited by Maser JD, Cloninger CR. Washington, DC, American Psychiatric Press, 1990, pp 123–137

Ballenger JC, Burrows GD, DuPont RL, et al: Alprazolam in panic disorder and agoraphobia: results from a multicenter trial. Arch Gen Psychiatry 45:413–422, 1988

Barlow DH: Anxiety and Its Disorders: The Nature and Treatment of Anxiety and Panic. New York, Guilford, 1988

Beitman BD, Kushner M, Lamberti JW, et al: Panic disorder without fear in patients with angiographically normal coronary arteries and panic disorder. J Nerv Ment Dis 178(5):307–312, 1990

Black B, Robbins DR: Panic disorder in children and adolescents. J Am Acad Child Adolesc Psychiatry 29:36–44, 1990

Brier A, Charney DS, Heninger GR: Agoraphobia with panic attacks: development, diagnostic stability, and course of illness. Arch Gen Psychiatry 43:1029–1036, 1986

Clark DM: A cognitive approach to panic. Behav Res Ther 24(4):461–470, 1986

Cox BJ, Norton GR, Swinson RP, et al: Substance abuse and panic-related anxiety: a critical review. Behav Res Ther 28(5):385–393, 1990

DiNardo PA, Barlow DH: Anxiety Disorders Interview Schedule—Revised (ACIS-R). Albany, NY, Center for Stress and Anxiety Disorders, University at Albany, State University of New York, 1988

Fyer AJ: Effects of discontinuation of antipanic medication, in Panic and Phobias 2: Treatments and Variables Affecting Course and Outcome. Edited by Hand I, Wittchen HU. New York, Springer-Verlag, 1988, pp 47–53

Fyer AJ, Rassnick H: Frequency and symptom thresholds for panic disorder, in DSM-IV Sourcebook, Vol 2. Washington, DC, American Psychiatric Press (in press)

Fyer AJ, Endicott J, Mannuzza S, et al: Schedule for Affective Disorders and Schizophrenia— Lifetime Version, Modified for the Study of Anxiety Disorders (SADS-LA). New York, Anxiety Disorders Clinic, New York State Psychiatric Institute, 1985

Fyer AJ, Mannuzza S, Martin LY, et al: Reliability of anxiety assessment, II: symptom agreement. Arch Gen Psychiatry 46:1102–1110, 1989

Gorman JM, Papp LA, Martinez J, et al: High-dose carbon dioxide challenge test in anxiety disorder patients. Biol Psychiatry 28(9): 743–757, 1990

Hamilton M: The assessment of anxiety states by rating. Br J Med Psychol 32:50–55, 1959

Hirschfeld RMA: The clinical course of panic disorder and agoraphobia, in Handbook of Anxiety, Vol 5. Edited by Burrows GD, Roth M, Noyes RJ Jr. Elsevier, 1992, pp 105–119

Katon WJ: Panic Disorder in the Medical Setting. Washington, DC, American Psychiatric Press, 1991

Klein DF, Klein RG: Does panic disorder exist in childhood? (letter). J Am Acad Child Adolesc Psychiatry 29:834, 1990

Leon AC, Klerman GL, Weissman MM, et al: Evaluating the diagnostic criteria for panic disorder: measures of social morbidity as criteria. Soc Psychiatry Psychiatr Epidemiol 27(4):180–184, 1992

Mannuzza S, Fyer AJ, Martin LY, et al: Reliability of anxiety assessment, I: diagnostic agreement. Arch Gen Psychiatry 46:1093–1101, 1989

Marks IM: Fears, Phobias and Rituals: Panic, Anxiety and Their Disorders. New York, Oxford University Press, 1987

Myers JK, Weissman MM, Tischler GL, et al: Six-month prevalence of psychiatric disorders in three communities: 1980–1982. Arch Gen Psychiatry 41:959–967, 1984

Noyes R, Reich J, Christiansen J, et al: Outcome of panic disorder: relationship to diagnostic subtypes and comorbidity. Arch Gen Psychiatry 47:809–818, 1990

Pollack MH, Otto MW, Rosenbaum JF, et al: Longitudinal course of panic disorder: findings from the Massachusetts General Hospital Naturalistic Study. Paper presented at the annual meeting of the American Psychiatric Association, New York, May 1990

Reiss S, Peterson RA, Gursky DM, et al: Anxiety sensitivity, anxiety frequency, and the prediction of fearfulness. Behav Res Ther 24:1–8, 1986

Robins LN, Regier DA: Psychiatric Disorders in America. New York, Free Press, 1990

Schneier FR, Fyer AJ, Martin LY, et al: A comparison of phobic subtypes within panic disorder. Journal of Anxiety Disorders 5:65–75, 1991

Spitzer RL, Williams JBW: Structured Clinical Interview for DSM-III-R (SCID): User's Guide. Washington, DC, American Psychiatric Press, 1992

Spitzer R, Endicott J, Robins E: Research Diagnostic Criteria: rationale and reliability. Arch Gen Psychiatry 35:773–782, 1978

Stein MB, Shea CA, Uhde TW: Social phobic symptoms in patients with panic disorder: practical and theoretical implications. Am J Psychiatry 146(2):235–238, 1989

Telch MJ, Brovillard M, Telch CF: Role of cognitive appraisal in panic-related avoidance. Behav Res Ther 27:373–383, 1989

Uhde TW, Boulenger JP, Roy-Byrne PP, et al: Longitudinal course of panic disorder: clinical and biological consideration. Prog Neuropsychopharmacol Biol Psychiatry 9:39–51, 1985

Van den Hout MA, Griez E: Experimental panic: biobehavioral notes on empirical findings, in Panic and Phobias: Empirical Evidence of Theoretical Models and Long-Term Effects of Behavioral Treatments. Edited by Hand I, Wittchen HU. New York, Springer-Verlag, 1986

Von Korff M, Eaton WW: Epidemiologic findings on panic, in Panic Disorder: Theory, Research and Therapy. Edited by Baker R. New York, Wiley, 1989

Wittchen HU: Natural course and spontaneous remissions of untreated anxiety disorders: results of the Munich follow-up study (MFS), in Panic and Phobias 2: Treatments and Variables Affecting Course and Outcome. Edited by Hand I, Wittchen HU. New York, Springer-Verlag, 1988

World Health Organization: International Classification of Diseases, 10th Edition. Geneva, World Health Organization, 1992

Chapter 3

Panic Disorder: Epidemiology and Genetics

Myrna M. Weissman, Ph.D.

Although the etiology of panic disorder is unclear, there is now considerable information on its epidemiology, comorbidity, and familial aggregation based on large probability samples drawn from the community, both in the United States and cross-nationally, and from family studies independently undertaken in several centers. In this chapter I review our current understanding of the epidemiology and family genetics of panic disorder.

Epidemiology

The information on the epidemiology of panic disorder in the United States comes from the Epidemiologic Catchment Area (ECA) study (Robins and Regier 1991), a community survey of over 18,000 adults, 18 years old or older, living in five United States communities (New Haven, Connecticut; Baltimore, Maryland; St. Louis, Missouri; Durham, North Carolina; and Los Angeles, California). These studies were conducted in the early 1980s. Although they were conducted independently, they used similar methodology and identical diagnostic procedures.

These studies found that, over a lifetime, about 25% of the subjects felt that they were nervous people; 9.3% had isolated panic attacks; 3.6% had experienced panic attacks not meeting the full criteria for panic disorder because of insufficient symptoms, duration, or frequency of attacks; and about 1.5% met the DSM-III (American Psychiatric Association 1980) criteria for panic disorder at some time in their life (Table 3–1). About one-third of the subjects with panic disorder and

31

one-half with panic attacks also met the criteria for agoraphobia. This proportion was consistent across sexes. Cross-sectionally, the rates of panic disorder were highest in persons ages 25–44 years and lowest in older persons ages 65 years or older. Panic disorder had a peak age at onset in young adulthood (mid-20s); however, many onsets first occurred in adolescence and a small number were reported to occur before puberty.

Blacks and whites were the predominant races in the five sites; there was a large sample of Mexican-Americans in the Los Angeles site. There were no significant variations in rates among the races studied, and these rates also did not vary in the Mexican-Americans by whether they were born in the United States or in Mexico.

The lifetime prevalence rates of panic disorder were similar in epidemiological studies conducted in Edmonton, Canada; Florence, Italy; Puerto Rico; Seoul, Korea; New Zealand; and Munich, Germany. The one exception was Taiwan, where rates for most psychiatric disorders, including panic disorder, were considerably lower (Table 3–2).

A comparison of the ECA subjects with panic disorder, major depression, or neither disorder showed that panic disorder had a serious impact on the quality of life. Panic disorder, like major depression, was associated with a self-perception of poor physical or emotional health, increased alcohol abuse, marital and financial problems, increased medication and emergency room use, and suicide attempts (Johnson et al. 1990; Markowitz et al. 1989; Weissman et al. 1989).

The association between panic disorder and suicide attempts was unexpected and was examined further to determine whether comorbidity with other psychiatric disorders might account for the finding. Johnson et al. (1990) found, in fact, that in only a small proportion (about 33%) of subjects with either panic disorder

Table 3–1.   Lifetime rate (per 100) of panic disorder and panic attacks

Site of study	Panic disorder	Panic attacks
New Haven	1.5	4.5
Baltimore	1.5	3.8
St. Louis	1.5	2.3
Durham	1.6	3.6
Los Angeles	1.5	3.7
Total	1.5	3.6

Note. Disorders are as defined by DSM-III criteria.
Source. Data based on the National Institute of Mental Health's Epidemiologic Catchment Area Community Survey, compiled by Weissman et al. 1989.

or major depression was their disorder uncomplicated (i.e., those subjects had had no other psychiatric disorders over their lifetime). However, when the authors examined the suicide-attempt rates in both the uncomplicated and the comorbid forms of panic disorder and major depression, they found that both panic disorder and major depression in their uncomplicated or comorbid forms were associated with a significantly increased risk of suicide attempt (Table 3–3). The rates of suicide attempts were significantly higher in subjects with comorbid panic disorder or comorbid major depression— 23.6% and 19.8%, respectively. However, the rates of suicide attempts in subjects with uncomplicated panic disorder (7%) and uncomplicated major depression (7.9%) were significantly higher than the rate of suicide attempts in subjects with no psychiatric disorders (1%). Johnson et al. concluded, therefore, that panic disorder, in both its uncomplicated and comorbid forms, like major depression, was substantially associated with suicide attempts.

These findings were replicated by Katschnig in a 4-year follow-up of 314 patients who had undergone treatment for panic disorder. Over the 4 years, six suicide attempts were found (H. Katschnig, personal communication, June 1990). This number would yield a suicide attempt rate of 9.8/100, assuming a 20-year lifetime risk period. In another longitudinal community study of young adults, Angst also found that the rate of suicide attempts in subjects with panic disorder but no major depression was 5%, with major depression but no panic disorder was 13%, and in subjects with both major depression and panic was 29% (J. Angst, personal communication, June 1990). These rates were substantially higher than those for other disorders. In a study of 100 consecutive panic patients in a hospital in Paris, Lepine et al. (1991) found a 42% prevalence rate of suicide attempts, 90%

Table 3–2.   Lifetime rate (per 100) of panic disorder

Site of study	Rate	Study
Taiwan	0.2	Hwu et al. 1989
Edmonton, Canada	1.2	Bland et al. 1988
Florence, Italy	1.3	Faravelli and Incerpi 1989
United States (five communities)	1.5	Weissman et al. 1989
Puerto Rico	1.7	Canino et al. 1987
Seoul, Korea	1.7	Lee et al. 1987
New Zealand	2.2	Joyce et al. 1989
Munich, Germany	2.4	Wittchen 1986

Note. Panic disorder as defined by DSM-III criteria.

of the attempts being medically attended and 43% requiring medical care or hospitalization for more than 24 hours.

The findings on the association between panic and suicide attempts have generated discussion. Most recently, Beck et al. (1991), based on a study of patients referred to a clinic for cognitive therapy, did not find any indication of any increased association between panic disorder and suicide attempts and questioned whether our findings (Weissman et al. 1989) were anomalous.

However, several aspects of the Beck et al. (1991) report challenged those investigators' own conclusions:

1. The accumulating reports from other distinguished investigators replicating the association between panic disorder and suicidal behavior, to which Beck et al. made no reference (Allgulander and Lavori 1991; Anthony and Petronis 1991; Coryell 1988; Fawcett et al. 1990; Lepine et al. 1991; Noyes 1991; Noyes et al. 1991).
2. Beck et al.'s use of current, not lifetime, diagnoses, which may have missed patients with a current diagnosis of major depression but with a history of panic disorder or panic attacks.
3. The probability of bias in Beck et al.'s own sampling. For example, patients with a history of suicidal behavior are probably less likely to be referred for treatment to a center for cognitive therapy.

The association between panic disorder and suicide attempts has been confirmed in several studies of persons with panic disorder. The specific etiologic model(s) explaining this association certainly requires further investigation.

Table 3–3. Lifetime rate (per 100) of suicide attempts by psychiatric diagnosis and comorbidity

Diagnosis	Rate
Panic disorder	
Uncomplicated	7.0
Comorbid	23.6
Major depression	
Uncomplicated	7.9
Comorbid	19.8
Panic disorder plus major depression	19.5
No psychiatric disorder	1.0

Source. Adapted from Johnson et al. 1990.

To understand the consequences of panic attacks not meeting full criteria for disorders, Klerman et al. (1991) examined the impact of panic attacks on perception of physical and emotional health, alcohol abuse, marital and financial problems, emergency room use, and suicide attempts. The authors concluded that panic attacks, like panic disorder, were associated with significant impairment in the quality of life that was intermediate in severity between panic disorder and other psychiatric disorders. These findings also could not be explained by comorbidity with other psychiatric disorders. Klerman et al.'s conclusion was that panic attacks also have clinical significance.

Genetics

Evidence for the genetic etiology of any disorder develops from different strategies, including family, twin, adoption, and linkage studies. In a family study, the aggregation of an illness within first-degree relatives is examined and compared with rates in a control group. In a twin study, the concordance rate of an illness among monozygotic (MZ) versus dizygotic (DZ) twins is examined, with a higher concordance among MZ twins suggesting a genetic etiology. Adoption studies can be conducted in different ways, but basically a higher rate of illness is expected among the biological as compared with the adoptive relatives of an ill person. In a linkage study, genetic linkage of an illness with an identifiable allele to a marker locus on a chromosome is sought.

For panic disorder, there are at least nine family studies, eight of which have been completed (see Table 3–4). There is one twin study completed (see Table 3–5) and one under way. There are no adoption studies, and there are at least four linkage studies under way, with no definitive results as yet.

The most recent family studies that used DSM-III criteria or the Research Diagnostic Criteria (RDC; Spitzer et al. 1978) showed the highly familial nature of panic disorder (Table 3–4). Whereas the population lifetime rates of panic disorder range between 1% and 2%, the lifetime rates of panic disorder in the first-degree relatives of patients with panic disorder range between 7% and 20%. The absolute rates vary by the strictness of the diagnostic criteria used. In all cases, the rates of panic in the relatives of the panic patients as compared with the relatives of control subjects were significantly higher. The variability in the rates of panic in the relatives of control subjects has to do with the different types of control groups used.

There is also evidence from family studies for the separation of panic disorder and generalized anxiety disorder (GAD) (Table 3–5). In three studies where the rates of panic disorder were significantly higher in the relatives of patients with panic disorder, there was no increased risk of GAD in those relatives. Alternately, the relatives of patients with GAD show increased risks of GAD, but not panic disorder (see Weissman 1990). This suggests, but does not firmly establish, that there is a separation between these disorders. The evidence for the relationship between panic disorder and major depression based on family studies is under investigation.

The twin study published by Torgersen (1983) had very small samples. Although his study suggested a higher rate of anxiety disorder with panic disorder in the MZ as opposed to the DZ co-twins of panic probands, Torgersen did not find a similar association in the co-twins with regard to anxiety disorder without panic disorder (Table 3–6). A considerably larger twin study under way by Kendler in Virginia has not yet been published.

Summary

Although the mode of transmission is unclear, the high lifetime rates of panic disorder, the strong evidence for vertical transmission, and the potential biological markers have increased interest in the application of modern linkage techniques to the study of large pedigrees with panic disorder. Several genetic linkage studies of

Table 3–4.   Lifetime rate (per 100) of panic disorder in first-degree relatives in family studies

Study	Panic disorder subjects	Control subjects
Direct interview studies		
Harris et al. 1983	20.5	4.2
Crowe et al. 1983	17.3	1.8
Noyes et al. 1986	14.9	3.5
Weissman et al., in press	14.2	0.8
Mendlewicz et al., in press	13.2	0.9
Maier et al., in press	7.9	2.3
Family history studies		
Moran and Andrews 1985	12.5	—
Hopper et al. 1987	11.6	—

Note. Panic disorder as defined by DSM-III criteria or Research Diagnostic Criteria (Spitzer et al. 1978).

panic disorder are ongoing: at Columbia University, in Iowa, at the National Institute of Mental Health, and in Belgium. The approach that is being used in these studies is to identify a chromosomal location of a suspected gene.

Linkage of a disease to a marker on a chromosome, of course, is only the first step in understanding its etiology. The linked region may be large, the actual gene must be identified, the pathophysiology must be understood, and the other factors, both genetic and nongenetic, that identify the expression of the disorder must be isolated. The genetic linkage studies on panic have just begun, and there are no definitive results. However, large pedigrees in which panic disorder occurs across multiple generations can be located. Results will be forthcoming over the next 5 years.

Table 3–5. Evidence for the separation between panic disorder and generalized anxiety disorder based on family studies

Study	Proband	Lifetime rate (per 100) in first-degree relatives	
		Panic disorder	Generalized anxiety disorder
Harris et al. 1983	Panic disorder patients	20.5	6.5
	Control subjects	4.2	5.3
Crowe et al. 1983	Panic disorder patients	17.3	4.8
	Control subjects	1.8	3.6
Noyes et al. 1987	Generalized anxiety disorder patients	4.1	19.5
	Panic disorder patients	14.9	5.4
	Control subjects	3.5	3.5

Table 3–6. Results of twin study of panic disorder

Proband diagnosis	n	Co-twin diagnosis		
		Anxiety disorder with panic (%)	Anxiety disorder without panic (%)	Other psychiatric disorder (%)
Panic disorder				
Monozygotic	13	31	15	8
Dizygotic	16	0	25	6

Source. Adapted from Torgersen 1983.

References

Allgulander E, Lavori PW: Excess mortality among 3,302 patients with "pure" anxiety neurosis. Arch Gen Psychiatry 48:599–602, 1991

American Psychiatric Association: Diagnostic and Statistical Manual of Mental Disorders, 3rd Edition. Washington, DC, American Psychiatric Association, 1980

Anthony JC, Petronis KR: Panic attacks and suicide attempts (letter). Arch Gen Psychiatry 48:1114, 1991

Beck AT, Steer RA, Sanderson WC, et al: Panic disorder and suicidal ideation and behavior: discrepant findings in psychiatric outpatients. Am J Psychiatry 148:1195–1199, 1991

Bland RC, Orn H, Newman SC: Lifetime prevalence of psychiatric disorders in Edmonton. Acta Psychiatr Scand 77:24–32, 1988

Canino GJ, Bird HR, Shrout PE, et al: The prevalence of specific psychiatric disorders in Puerto Rico. Arch Gen Psychiatry 44:727–735, 1987

Coryell W: Panic disorder and mortality. Psychiatr Clin North Am 11:433–440, 1988

Crowe RR, Noyes R, Pauls D, et al: A family study of panic disorder. Arch Gen Psychiatry 40:1065–1069, 1983

Faravelli C, Incerpi G: Epidemiology of anxiety disorders in Florence. Acta Psychiatr Scand 79:308–312, 1989

Fawcett J, Scheftner WA, Fogg L, et al: Time-related predictors of suicide in major affective disorder. Am J Psychiatry 147(9):1189–1194, 1990

Harris EL, Noyes R, Crowe RR, et al: Family study of agoraphobia. Arch Gen Psychiatry 40:1061–1064, 1983

Hopper JL, Judd FK, Derrick PL, et al: A family study of panic disorder. Genet Epidemiol 4:33–41, 1987

Hwu HG, Yeh EK, Chang LY: Prevalence of psychiatric disorders in Taiwan defined by the Chinese Diagnostic Interview Schedule. Acta Psychiatr Scand 79:136–147, 1989

Johnson J, Weissman MM, Klerman GL: Panic disorder, comorbidity, and suicide attempts. Arch Gen Psychiatry 47:805–808, 1990

Joyce PR, Bushnell JA, Oakley-Brown MA, et al: The epidemiology of panic symptomatology and agoraphobic avoidance. Compr Psychiatry 30(4):303–312, 1989

Klerman GL, Weissman MM, Ouellette R, et al: Panic attacks in the community: social morbidity and health care utilization. JAMA 265(6):742–746, 1991

Lee CK, Han JH, Choi JO: The epidemiological study of mental disorders in Korea, (IX): alcoholism, anxiety and depression. Seoul Journal of Psychiatry 12:183–191, 1987

Lepine JP, Chignon JM, Teherani M: Suicidal behavior and onset of panic disorder. Arch Gen Psychiatry 32:261–267, 1991

Maier W, Lichtermann D, Meyer A, et al: A controlled family study in panic disorder. J Psychiatr Res (in press)

Markowitz JS, Weissman MM, Ouellette R, et al: Quality of life in panic disorder. Arch Gen Psychiatry 46:984–992, 1989

Mendlewicz J, Papadimitriou G, Wilmotte J: Family study of panic disorder: comparison with generalized anxiety disorder, major depression, and normal subjects. Psychiatric Genetics (in press)

Moran C, Andrews G: A familial occurrence of agoraphobia. Br J Psychiatry 146:262–267, 1985

Noyes R Jr: Suicide and panic disorder: a review. J Affect Disord 22:1011, 1991

Noyes R Jr, Crowe RR, Harris EL, et al: Relationship between panic disorder and agoraphobia. Arch Gen Psychiatry 43:227–232, 1986

Noyes R Jr, Clarkson C, Crowe RR, et al: A family study of generalized anxiety disorder. Am J Psychiatry 144(8):1019–1924, 1987

Noyes R, Christiansen J, Clancy J, et al: Predictors of serious suicide attempts among patients with panic disorder. Compr Psychiatry 32:261–267, 1991

Robins LN, Regier DA (eds): Psychiatric Disorders in America. New York, Free Press, 1991

Spitzer RL, Endicott J, Robins E: Research Diagnostic Criteria: rationale and reliability. Arch Gen Psychiatry 35:773–782, 1978

Torgersen S: Genetic factors in anxiety disorders. Arch Gen Psychiatry 40:1085–1089, 1983

Weissman M: Panic and generalized anxiety: are they separate disorders? J Psychiatr Res 24:157–163, 1990

Weissman MM: Family genetic studies of panic disorder. J Psychiatr Res (in press)

Weissman MM, Klerman GL, Markowitz JS, et al: Suicidal ideation and suicide attempts in panic disorder and attacks. N Engl J Med 321:1209–1214, 1989

Weissman MM, Adams P, Lish JD, et al: The relationship between panic disorder and major depression: a new family study. Arch Gen Psychiatry (in press)

Wittchen HU: Epidemiology of panic attacks and panic disorders, in Panic and Phobias: Empirical Evidence of Theoretical Models and Long-Term Effects of Behavioral Treatments. Edited by Hand I, Wittchen HU. New York, Springer-Verlag, 1986, pp 18–28

Chapter 4

Primary Care–Psychiatry Panic Disorder Management Module

Wayne Katon, M.D.

My purpose in this chapter is to describe a primary care–psychiatry management module of panic disorder. There are four essential steps in this management module: 1) case identification, 2) clinical history and assessment, 3) patient treatment planning, and 4) specific treatment modalities.

Epidemiological studies of panic disorder in community and primary care settings have shown this type of severe anxiety to be a very common disorder. Investigators in four studies have estimated that between 1.6% and 2.9% of women and between 0.4% and 1.7% of men in the general population have panic disorder (Angst et al. 1990; Crowe et al. 1983; Myers et al. 1984; Weissman et al. 1978). Moreover, a larger percentage of people in the community (3.6%–10%) experience infrequent panic attacks (Klerman et al. 1991). Panic attacks have been found to occur in 0.4%–8% of primary care patients (Finlay-Jones and Brown 1981; Katon et al. 1986; Taylor et al., in press; Von Korff et al. 1987). These prevalence rates of panic disorder in primary care are very similar to those for other common medical disorders, such as hypertension, which occurs in approximately 4%–5% of patients and is routinely screened for in primary care settings.

Case Identification

Because of the current lack of routine screening for panic disorder in primary care, it is essential that physicians recognize and evaluate patients who are at a high risk for panic disorder. Four groups of patients are found in the primary care setting

41

who probably have an increased risk for panic disorder. These include patients who present with 1) complaints of anxiety and tension; 2) recent increased hypochondriacal concerns and increased medical clinic and emergency room utilization; 3) cardiological (tachycardia, chest pain), gastrointestinal (epigastric pain and irritable symptoms), or neurological symptoms (headache, faintness, or syncope); and 4) specific medical problems, such as labile hypertension, mitral valve prolapse, and migraine headaches.

■ **Complaints of anxiety and tension.**   Of primary care visits, 11% are associated with a primary or chief complaint of anxiety or nervousness (Schurman et al. 1985). Other physiological complaints often associated with severe anxiety were also reported frequently in Schurman et al.'s study, such as headache and dizziness (11.2%) and abdominal or stomach pain (7.5%). It is likely that patients complaining of anxiety and tension are at high risk for panic disorder and affective illness.

■ **Increased hypochondriacal concerns and emergency room utilization.**   Patients with increased hypochondriacal concerns and increased medical and emergency room utilization have also been found to have a high prevalence of panic disorder (Katon et al. 1990; Klein et al., in press; Klerman et al. 1991; Simon 1992). In the Epidemiologic Catchment Area (ECA) study, persons with either panic disorder or infrequent panic attacks were found to be significantly higher users of emergency medical services and were more likely to be hospitalized for physical problems than people without panic disorder (Klerman et al. 1991). Panic disorder patients often misattribute their autonomic symptoms to cardiac disease (heart attack) or a neurological illness (stroke or seizure) and therefore frequently visit emergency services (Katon 1989). In a recent study of 100 patients who visited the emergency room for a medically unexplained somatic complaint, Klein et al. (in press) found that the prevalence of panic disorder and generalized anxiety disorder was six times that of an emergency room control group. A study by Wulsin et al. (1988) of emergency room patients who presented with chest pains but had negative workups also indicated an extremely high prevalence of panic disorder.

■ **Increased use of general medical services.**   Data from the ECA study showed that patients with panic disorder had the highest odds ratio for high use of general medical services (six or more visits over a 1-year period) (Simon and Von Korff 1991). Patients with panic disorder had odds ratios of being high medical service users (8.2 in males and 5.2 in females), which can be compared with the odds ratios for major depression (1.5 in males and 3.4 in females). Most studies have found major depression to be associated with two to three times the normal usage rate of medical services, and yet panic disorder seems to be even more strongly associated with high medical utilization. In a recent study (Katon et al. 1990) of 767 distressed, high users of primary care, 11.8% met diagnostic criteria for current panic disorder and 30.2% met criteria for lifetime panic disorder. These high users of primary care were among the top 10% of users from two primary care clinics. They were responsible for 29% of all ambulatory visits, 52% of all inpatient unit stays, 26% of all prescriptions, and 52% of all outpatient specialty visits over a 1-year period. Moreover, 39% of these patients continued as high users of ambulatory care over the next 1-year period and only 15% dropped below the mean of utilization.

Klerman et al. (1991) reported that people in the community with panic disorder as well as panic attacks viewed their physical as well as emotional health as significantly poorer than patients without psychiatric disorders. In addition, panic disorder was found in the ECA data base to have the highest odds ratio (204) of being associated with five or more current medically unexplained physical symptoms (Katon, in press), with almost one-fifth of the patients with panic disorder having had five or more of such symptoms during the previous 6 months. This high association between panic disorder and medically unexplained symptoms can be compared with the lower odds ratio of major depression (16.9) being associated with five or more medically unexplained symptoms, a disorder that has also been linked in multiple studies with somatization.

Many patients with panic disorder select one of the most frightening autonomic symptoms of panic disorder (e.g., chest pain or a symptom that is a sequela to the anxiety attack, such as diarrhea or headache) and present to their physician with that complaint (Katon 1989). Prior studies have determined that three types of physical symptoms are the most common presentation in primary care patients with panic disorder: cardiological complaints (chest pain or rapid heart beat), gastrointestinal complaints (epigastric pain or symptoms of irritable bowel syndrome), and neurological complaints (headache or dizziness) (Katon 1989). Other less common presentations include breathlessness, choking sensations, and syncope.

Recent studies of patients with chest pain and negative angiograms (Bass and Wade 1984; Beitman et al. 1987; Katon et al. 1988), rapid or irregular heart beat and normal Holter monitor examinations (Barsky 1992; Savage et al. 1983), irritable bowel syndrome (Fossey et al. 1990; Walker et al. 1990), medically unexplained dizziness (Linzer et al. 1990), migraine headaches (Merikangas et al. 1990; Stewart et al. 1989), and chronic fatigue (Katon et al. 1991; Manu et al. 1991) have all found high rates of panic disorder among their subjects. Generalized anxiety disorder and affective disorders are also common in patients with these somatic complaints. Many of the patients with symptoms such as chest pain tachycardia and irritable bowel syndrome receive costly and often invasive diagnostic procedures before the correct psychiatric diagnosis is made.

∎ **Increased reporting of specific medical problems.** A final high-risk group includes patients with several specific medical problems, including labile hypertension, mitral valve prolapse, peptic ulcer disease, and migraine headaches (Katon 1989). One prospective longitudinal study of patients with panic disorder found a higher prevalence of the development of hypertension and peptic ulcer disease in patients with panic than in a surgical control group over a 5-year period (Noyes and Clancy 1976). Approximately 30%–40% of patients with panic disorder also have mitral valve prolapse, although this is believed to be a benign type of prolapse. Clinical experience suggests that treatment of the panic disorder leads to amelioration of the cardiac symptoms, such as chest pain and tachycardia, that may have been misattributed to the mitral valve prolapse. Also, patients with mitral valve prolapse (diagnosed by echocardiogram) have no more cardiac symptoms than do control subjects without mitral valve prolapse (Savage et al. 1983).

Inquiring About Symptoms of Panic Disorder

To screen for panic disorder, the primary care physician will need to ask at least two screening questions. The first recommended question to be asked is, "Have you ever had sudden episodes of rapid heart beat, chest tightness, shortness of breath, trembling, or feeling sweaty or hot?" Second, if the patient presents with a specific symptom, such as chest pain or faintness, then the clinician should ask, "When you have your episode of chest pain, what other physical sensations do you get?" If the patient does not remember any other sensations, then the physician should specifically inquire, "When you have your episodes of chest pain, do you also experience rapid heart rate, shortness of breath, dizziness or faintness, trembling or shaking?" and so on. It is also helpful for the clinician to advise the patient that, although everyone has stress-related anxiety difficulties and times of feeling keyed up or tense, the clinician is inquiring about a specific type of disorder associated with a burst of autonomic symptoms that occur over several minutes, peak in intensity, and then decrease over several minutes.

Clinical History and Assessment

To assess treatment needs fully, the physician should inquire about specific etiologic agents in panic disorder as well as the severity and impact of the disorder.

Important historical items to screen include 1) family history of panic disorder, hypochondriasis, depression, or substance abuse; 2) stressful life events and daily life problems; 3) developmental vulnerability; and 4) health concerns and the patient's explanatory model.

▋ **Family history and genetic factors.** There is excellent evidence that there is a genetic input in panic disorder (Katon 1989). Family studies have found an increased morbidity risk of panic disorder among first-degree relatives of patients with panic disorder compared with first-degree relatives of control families. The highest risk of first-degree relatives of patients with panic disorder was found by Crowe et al. (1983) in a study in which panic disorder patients and family members were interviewed with a structured psychiatric interview. The investigators found a 41% morbidity risk of panic disorder among first-degree relatives compared with 4% among control subjects. Torgerson (1983) found that there is a higher concordance rate of panic disorder in monozygotic twins than in dizygotic twins, noting that, overall, anxiety disorders with panic attacks were more than five times as frequent in monozygotic as in dizygotic twins.

The diathesis for anxiety disorders such as panic disorder may be a temperamental trait characterized by behavioral inhibition to novel or unfamiliar stimuli (Biederman et al. 1990; Rosenbaum et al. 1988). Investigators in recent studies found an increased prevalence rate of this temperamental trait in offspring of patients with panic disorder (Rosenbaum et al. 1988) and increased anxiety disorders in children with this form of behavioral inhibition (Biederman et al. 1990).

▋ **Stressful life events and daily life problems.** In four controlled studies of patients with panic disorder (Brown et al., in press; Faravelli 1985; Finlay-Jones and Brown 1981; Roy-Byrne et al. 1986), the authors determined that patients with panic disorder experienced significantly more stressful life events and had a higher proportion of events viewed as extremely dangerous, uncontrollable, undesirable, and potentially causing lowering of self-esteem. Brown and colleagues (in press) found that stressful life events associated with danger and lack of security were significantly more common in patients with panic disorder compared with control subjects in the 6 months prior to the development of this severe anxiety disorder. Sixty percent of these stressful life events in patients with panic disorder occurred within 2 months of the development of their disorder.

▋ **Developmental vulnerability.** In addition to family history, temperamental factors, and stressful life events, it is important to assess the patient's history of developmental vulnerability. Panic disorder can occur in patients who have had either normal childhood environments and adult adjustment or a chaotic family upbringing with, perhaps, abuse and neglect. The developmental history may enable the physician to judge the patient's strengths and how well he or she can cope with panic disorder. These developmental factors may influence the course and severity of panic disorder as well as influence how the patient copes with panic attacks. Joyce et al. (1989) found that patients with panic disorder and moderate-to-severe phobic avoidance were more likely to have grown up in a family with parental conflict, to have had symptoms of a childhood conduct disorder, and to have left school at a younger age than did patients with panic disorder and no or mild phobic problems. In a large epidemiological study, Brown and Harris (in press) recently found that panic disorder, agoraphobia, generalized anxiety disorder, and social phobia were all highly related to negative early developmental experiences. Panic disorder had the greatest association with early negative experience. Patients with panic disorder had an odds ratio of having had an early negative experience of 7.7 when compared with patients without anxiety. Parental indifference, the patient's experience of violence within the family, and separation from a parent for 1 year or death of a parent were the adverse early experiences most associated with adult panic disorder.

∎ **Patient's health concerns and explanatory model.**   The final important aspect of assessment includes the patient's health concerns and explanatory model. As reviewed above, many patients with panic disorder have hypochondriacal concerns that something is wrong with their body. They may have questions about whether their symptoms suggest heart disease or strokes, and these will need to be dealt with forthrightly. Often, only after some degree of history, physical examination, and medical testing will the patient accept the physician's diagnosis of panic disorder.

It is essential for the patient that the physician inquire about the patient's explanatory model of illness (Kleinman et al. 1978). This should include questions about the patient's ideas, fears, and concerns about what disorder he or she may have, what treatment is expected, and his or her understanding of the pathophysiology and etiology of the symptoms. Understanding the patient's model will allow the physician to present a model of illness that is credible and palatable to the patient. Thus, education about this disorder should begin only after a full exploration of the patient's fears, concerns, and ideas.

∎ **Other issues to be addressed in assessment.**   Assessment should also include inquiries into the panic disorder's severity and its impact on patient functioning. The inquiries should include questions on severity and frequency of panic symptoms, impact on daily functioning, suicidal potential, possible comorbid psychiatric and medical disorders, and other factors that may be complicating the disorder.

It is helpful to find out how much avoidance and phobic behavior the patient has developed since the symptoms began. A simple inquiry about whether the current symptoms are leading to avoidance of work, family, or social responsibilities will help determine agoraphobic tendencies. Also, specific questions should be asked about whether the patient is more uncomfortable in crowds and social situations. The patient should also be asked about sick leave from work, medical leave of absence, or medical bills he or she may have incurred since the development of the disorder.

The data from the ECA study indicated that panic disorder and panic attacks were associated with both suicidal ideation and suicide attempts (Weissman et al. 1989). Subjects with panic disorder had an adjusted odds ratio for suicide attempts of 2.62 compared with subjects with other psychiatric disorders, and an adjusted odds ratio of 17.99 compared with subjects without a psychiatric disorder. Approximately one in five patients with panic disorder and one in nine with panic attacks had made suicide attempts. These data emphasize the need to ask about hopelessness and suicidal ideation.

It is also important to screen for comorbid psychiatric and medical disorders. In the ECA study, patients with panic disorder were found to have an increased prevalence of agoraphobia, major depression, alcohol abuse, and drug abuse (Klerman et al. 1991). Approximately 33% of patients with panic disorder were found to have had a lifetime episode of agoraphobia; 33%, a lifetime episode of major depression; 26%, a lifetime episode of alcohol abuse; and 18%, a lifetime episode of drug abuse. In addition, approximately 40% of patients with panic disorder have been shown to have a comorbid personality disorder, with about 25% of patients having a cluster B or cluster C personality disorder (Pollack et al. 1990). These disorders can all complicate the management of panic disorder, and probably are associated with significantly more treatment resistance to the usual psychopharmacological and psychotherapeutic modalities (Katon 1989).

Pharmacological agents that may have provoked or worsened the panic disorder should also be assessed. For example, treatment of chronic asthma with theophylline can cause significant anxiety symptoms or worsening of a preexisting anxiety disorder. The frequent intake of beverages with a high caffeine content may also provoke severe anxiety and panic disorder (Katon 1989). Many patients with panic disorder who have a comorbid medical disorder will also find that their medical disorder is significantly more symptomatic when they are having panic attacks (Katon 1989). Thus, if a patient has coronary artery disease and develops panic disorder, he or she will have more episodes of chest pains. This is probably due both to a physiological worsening of the illness stemming from the severe autonomic nervous system activation and to the amplification of pain that severe anxiety seems to cause. Finally, medically unexplained symptoms, such as symptoms of irritable bowel syndrome, may complicate panic disorder and necessitate separate treatment. Thus an increase in fiber and water intake and exercise may help a patient with irritable bowel and panic disorder.

Treatment Planning

In the stages of treatment planning, it is essential to inquire about past episodes of panic disorder, which will include 1) the number of episodes of panic disorder the patient has experienced; 2) comorbid psychiatric disorders and symptoms with these episodes (i.e., agoraphobia, major depression, suicidality, substance abuse); 3) the types of treatments received; and 4) the perceived value of those treatments. Also, it is especially important to inquire again about the patient's desires for specific types of intervention, including medical tests, medication, and psychotherapy. This history may be invaluable in allowing the choice of an agent that is credible and palatable to the patient. For example, if the patient has been treated with a specific antidepressant and had a severe side effect, an attempt to prescribe that antidepressant again may lead to noncompliance with the medication. Alternatively, if a prior episode was treated effectively with imipramine, this antidepressant might be prescribed for the current episode.

Specific Treatment Modalities in Primary Care–Psychiatry

The first step in the treatment is understanding the patient's health concerns and beliefs and providing reassurance and education to the patient. Patients with panic disorder are often convinced they have a cardiac or neurological disorder and that their anxiety or nervousness is secondary to their physical symptoms. Studies that support the patient's perception of the primacy of physical symptoms in panic attacks (Katerndahl 1988) have shown that, during a panic attack, fear and anxiety are late symptoms following autonomic symptoms of dyspnea, palpitations, chest pains, and hot or cold flashes.

When the physician informs the patient with panic attacks that he or she has a severe anxiety disorder, the patient may feel that the physician does not believe that he or she has real physical symptoms. It is helpful to educate these patients about the biological research on panic disorder. It is useful to explain that panic

dyspnea

disorder is thought to result from dysfunction of the sympathetic nervous system, in which bursts of catecholamines are released into the peripheral circulation, causing symptoms such as tachycardia, chest pain, dyspnea, and hot and cold flashes. A further analogy about panic attacks being very similar to the fight-or-flight response may also be helpful. The patient can be provided with this explanation: "If you were walking down a dark street and heard a sudden sound behind you, your heart might begin to race; your respiratory rate would increase; you would feel warm, shaky, and sweaty; and you would be prepared to either flee or fight for your life. The current attacks you are having are set off by dysregulation of the same part of the brain that controls this fight-or-flight response; however, you are having this alarm or danger response at times when there is no actual danger. Therefore, these attacks are very frightening." Because the clinician has already taken a complete history about current stressful life events, the physician can further state that stressful events in the patient's life may lead to expression of a genetic potential toward these attacks and lead to bursts of catecholamines like epinephrine or norepinephrine being released into the peripheral circulation.

The second important step is to provide patients with reading materials that will allow them to understand their disorder further. Patients with panic disorder are usually quite obsessed with and hypervigilant to bodily symptoms. They often interpret bodily symptoms in a catastrophic manner, assuming that they mean something is dreadfully wrong with their heart or gastrointestinal or respiratory systems. The proper reading materials will help them objectively see their symptoms as part of a bodily process that is uncomfortable but not dangerous. There are several fine books written for the layperson as well as articles that can be provided to patients with panic disorder (Katon 1989; Sheehan 1986; Wender and Klein 1981).

Medication

There are four types of medication that have been demonstrated in double-blind trials to be effective in the psychopharmacological treatment of panic disorder: tricyclic antidepressants (TCAs), serotonin reuptake blockers, high-potency benzodiazepines, and monoamine oxidase inhibitors (MAOIs). There are three phases in the treatment of panic disorder: 1) acute blockade of the spontaneous panic attacks, 2) a continuation phase of treatment with a pharmacological agent to extend the gains of the first few months of treatment, and finally 3) a maintenance phase of prolonged treatment in patients with recurrent or severe panic disorder. A subset of patients may require lifelong medication treatment for effective prophylaxis (Kupfer 1991; Pollack et al. 1990; Roy-Byrne, in press).

Patients with panic disorder represent one of the most difficult groups of psychiatric patients to treat with medication. These patients already feel that they are having dangerous bodily symptoms that are out of their control, so they are hypervigilant to symptoms (Katon 1989). They also interpret minor symptoms, like increased heart rate after exercise, to be indicative of another catastrophic attack that could even lead to death. Therefore, they often view medications that are associated with minor side effects as dangerous because they make them feel more out of control. The following are several useful suggestions for starting medications in these patients:

1. Advise all patients that they will have minor side effects from the medications. It is helpful to list the common side effects and to point out that if the patient can tolerate 1–2 weeks of these side effects, the effects will gradually fade and that over about 2–4 weeks therapeutic effects will occur.
2. See these patients at least once a week and emphasize that it is important to call the physician if they have side effects, but that they should *not stop* the medication without talking to the doctor.
3. Continue to increase the dosage of medicine until the panic attacks are completely alleviated. A common mistake in primary care or psychiatry is to stop short of amelioration of all anxiety attacks.
4. Describe the approximate dosage that the physician would like to reach (e.g., 150–200 mg of a TCA), but give the patient control of the incremental increases of the medication.
5. Start at a very low dose of a medication (e.g., 10 mg of imipramine) and gradually increase the dose by small increments, rather than starting with a larger dose with the potential of causing jitteriness and other side effects.

∎ **Tricyclic antidepressants.**   The TCAs have been the best-studied medicines in the treatment of panic disorder. Specifically, imipramine has been found in 9 out of 10 double-blind, placebo-controlled studies to be significantly more effective than placebo (Katon 1989). Uncontrolled studies have also suggested that desipramine, nortriptyline, amitriptyline, and doxepin are effective agents. Trazodone and bupropion have not been found to be more effective than placebo in initial controlled trials. If a medication like imipramine, nortriptyline, or desipramine is chosen, it is useful to start the patient at 10 mg and gradually increase the medication by 10 mg every 2–3 days until the anxiety attacks are completely ameliorated. Perhaps 20% of patients will have a sensation of increased jitteriness during the first 1–2 weeks of treatment with imipramine. It is important to slow the rate of upward titration if this occurs and sometimes to decrease the dose until the patient becomes tolerant to this side effect. Available evidence suggests that perhaps one in five patients are not able to tolerate TCAs due to the side effects.

∎ **Serotonergic reuptake blockers.** Controlled trials support the effectiveness of clomipramine in the treatment of panic disorder (McTavish and Benfield 1990), and open studies suggest that fluoxetine also has antipanic actions (Katon 1989). Clomipramine can be used in dosages similar to those prescribed for other TCAs; however, care must be used in the dosing with fluoxetine. Fluoxetine, in our experience, must be started at a very low dose, often 2.5–5 mg, which can then be titrated upward every 3–4 days until the panic attacks have ceased. Starting the patient at 20 mg of fluoxetine will lead to severe jitteriness, anxiety, and increased frequency of anxiety attacks in a significant proportion of patients, therefore resulting in premature discontinuation of the medication.

∎ **Monoamine oxidase inhibitors.** MAOIs, particularly phenelzine, have proven to be effective in the treatment of panic disorder in double-blind, placebo-controlled trials (Sheehan et al. 1980). There is some evidence that they may be the most effective medication for the largest group of patients with panic disorder. However, the dietary prohibitions, which require patients to adhere to a low-tyramine diet, and the need to avoid medications that may interact with MAOIs frequently lead to these medications being regarded as second or third choices in the treatment of panic disorder. Also, the necessity to warn patients about potential hypertensive crises often leads them to be wary of these agents.

Ironically, recent evidence has suggested that most patients do not adhere to the dietary restrictions, and yet hypertensive episodes are quite infrequent (Katon 1989). In my experience, the most dangerous interaction occurs with over-the-counter medicines (such as medication for respiratory tract infections); patients must be warned of these repeatedly.

Phenelzine can be started in dosages of 15 mg po bid without the worry of overstimulation and jitteriness that can occur with TCAs (Roy-Byrne, in press). To be effective in ameliorating panic, doses of phenelzine often have to be escalated to the range of 60–90 mg.

∎ **Benzodiazepines.** There are three high-potency benzodiazepines that have been well studied in double-blind, placebo-controlled trials: alprazolam (Klerman and Lavori, in press), clonazepam (Pollack et al. 1987), and lorazepam (Katon 1989). Dunner et al. (1986) also found that high-dosage diazepam (a mean of 30 mg/day) markedly decreases panic attacks, suggesting that older studies used too low a dosage as well as infrequent dosing. However, the necessity of using such high dosages of the lower potency benzodiazepines would probably lead to significant side effects such as sedation, and therefore these drugs are not as commonly used in panic disorder. Of the three agents, alprazolam has been found in double-blind, controlled trials to be as effective as imipramine and phenelzine. The high-potency benzodiazepines do ameliorate panic attacks and generalized anxiety at a faster rate than TCAs or MAOIs; however, it may be more difficult to withdraw patients from them after acute and maintenance treatment because of rebound anxiety as well as the recurrence of panic disorder.

There has been concern among the public and health professionals about the abuse potential of benzodiazepines. When patients are carefully selected for treatment, this does not prove to be a problem. However, psychiatrists often have 1 hour to evaluate a new patient with panic attacks, whereas primary care physicians may have only 10–15 minutes. It is essential to screen out and exclude most patients with prior histories of alcohol or substance abuse, chronic pain, personality disorders, and perhaps even family histories of alcoholism and substance abuse from benzodiazepine treatment. These are most likely to be high-risk patients who are more difficult to treat because of the abuse potential. Also, these groups of patients may be the most difficult to taper off of medication at the end of effective treatment.

Because a significant subset of patients will not tolerate antidepressant agents, benzodiazepines remain a viable treatment alternative that, in fact, acts more quickly than antidepressant agents. Alprazolam can be started in dosages of 0.25–0.5 po qid and increased gradually by 0.25- to 0.5-mg increments every 3–4 days until panic attacks are ameliorated. In primary care, most patients respond to doses of 1–2 mg; however, higher doses (4–6 mg) have been necessary in psychiatric trials. Alprazolam is associated in some patients with breakthrough anxiety and anxiety attacks within 3–5 hours of the last dose. This can lead to the patient waking up in the early morning with acute, severe anxiety and having to rush to take a dose of the medication. If this breakthrough anxiety occurs (probably because of a drop in serum benzodiazepine blood levels), then an agent such as clonazepam is often helpful because of its longer half-life.

The problem concerning most clinicians regarding the use of benzodiazepines for panic disorder is the apparent increased difficulty in tapering these medicines compared with TCAs and MAOIs at the end of maintenance treatment. Both withdrawal symptoms and reemergence of panic attacks can occur following taper of benzodiazepines, and it is often difficult to differentiate these two problems. Very slow tapering of these agents is necessary if this problem is to be prevented, usually at a rate of one-half tablet of alprazolam every 2–4 weeks. Alternatively, treating the patient with an antidepressant agent or carbamazepine (400–800 mg) prior to tapering may be helpful and may allow more symptom-free, gradual discontinuation of the medicine. Further trials are indicated to compare in a double-blind fashion the different mechanisms of tapering benzodiazepines.

Cognitive-Behavior Treatment

Investigators of multiple uncontrolled clinical series of cases have reported the effectiveness of cognitive-behavior treatments for panic disorder (Beck 1988; Clark et al. 1985; Gitlin et al. 1985; Öst 1988; Salkovskis et al. 1986). These reports have suggested that not only can agoraphobic avoidance be treated with cognitive-behavior treatments, but that panic attacks can also be eliminated with such treatments.

In a recent controlled trial of cognitive-behavior treatment, Barlow et al. (1989) found that groups receiving combined somatic exposure treatment and cognitive therapy did significantly better than a waiting-list control or relaxation treatment group. This type of therapy combines exposure to cues for anxiety and, indeed, provoking and desensitizing patients to somatic cues for anxiety (such as rapid heart rate or dizziness), with cognitive procedures aimed at decreasing fears of the consequences of anxiety. In another recent study, Klosko et al. (1990) found that a combined somatic exposure and cognitive therapy group and an al-prazolam-alone group were each significantly better on global clinical ratings than the waiting-list control group. However, there were no significant differences between the alprazolam group, cognitive-behavior and somatic exposure group, and placebo group on the global clinical rating. The therapy group had a significantly higher percentage of patients who were panic-free than the waiting-list control or placebo groups, but did not differ from the alprazolam.

References

Angst J, Vollrath M, Merikangas KR, et al: Comorbidity of anxiety and depression in the Zurich Cohort Study of Young Adults, in Comorbidity of Mood and Anxiety Disorders. Edited by Maser JD, Cloninger CR. Washington, DC, American Psychiatric Press, 1990, pp 123–137

Barlow DH, Craske MG, Cerney JA, et al: Behavioral treatment of panic disorder. Behav Res Ther 20:261–282, 1989

Barsky A: Palpitations, cardiac awareness and panic disorder. Am J Med 92 (suppl 1A):315–345, 1992

Bass C, Wade C: Chest pain with normal coronary arteries: a comparative study of psychiatric and social morbidity. Psychosom Med 14:51–64, 1984

Beck AT: Cognitive approaches to panic disorder: theory and therapy, in Panic: Psychological Perspectives. Edited by Rachman S, Maser JD. Hillsdale, NJ, Lawrence Erlbaum, 1988, pp 91–109

Beitman BD, Lamberti JW, Mukerji V, et al: Panic disorder in patients with angiographically normal coronary arteries. Psychosomatics 28:480–484, 1987

Biederman J, Rosenbaum JF, Hirshfeld DR, et al: Psychiatric correlates of behavioral inhibition in young children of parents with and without psychiatric disorders. Arch Gen Psychiatry 47:21–26, 1990

Brown GW, Harris TO: Etiology of anxiety and depressive disorders in an inner-city population, I: early adversity. Psychol Med 23:143–154, 1993

Brown GW, Lemyre L, Bifulco A: Social factors and recovery from anxiety disorders: a test of specificity. Br J Psychiatry 161:44–54, 1992

Clark DM, Salkovskis PM, Chalkley AJ: Respiratory control as a treatment for panic attacks. J Behav Ther Exp Psychiatry 16:23–30, 1985

Crowe RR, Noyes R, Pauls DL, et al: A family study of panic disorder. Arch Gen Psychiatry 40:1065–1069, 1983

Dunner DL, Ishiki D, Avery DH, et al: Effect of alprazolam and diazepam on anxiety and panic disorder: a controlled study. J Clin Psychiatry 47:458–460, 1986

Faravelli D: Life events preceding the onset of panic disorder. J Affect Disord 9:103–105, 1985

Finlay-Jones R, Brown GW: Types of stressful life events and the onset of anxiety and depressive disorders. Psychol Med 11:803–815, 1981

Fossey M, Lydiard RB, Harsh WH, et al: Psychiatric morbidity in irritable bowel syndrome. Paper presented at the annual meeting of the American Psychiatric Association, San Francisco, CA, May 6–11, 1989

Gitlin B, Martin M, Shear MK, et al: Behavioral therapy for panic disorder. J Nerv Ment Dis 173:742–743, 1985

Joyce PR, Bushnell JA, Oakley-Browne MA, et al: The epidemiology of panic symptomatology and agoraphobic avoidance. Compr Psychiatry 30:303–312, 1989

Katerndahl DA: The sequence of panic symptoms. J Fam Pract 26:49–52, 1988

Katon W: Panic disorder in the medical setting (DHHS Publ No ADM-89-1629). Washington, DC, National Institute of Mental Health, U.S. Government Printing Office, 1989

Katon W, Vitaliano PP, Russo J, et al: Panic disorder: epidemiology in primary care. J Fam Pract 23:233–239, 1986

Katon W, Hall ML, Russo J, et al: Chest pain: relationship of psychiatric illness to coronary arteriography results. Am J Med 84:1–9, 1988

Katon W, Von Korff M, Lin E, et al: Distressed high utilizers of medical care: DSM-III-R diagnoses and treatment needs. Gen Hosp Psychiatry 12:355–362, 1990

Katon W, Buchwald D, Russo J, et al: Psychiatric illness in patients with chronic fatigue and rheumatoid arthritis. J Gen Intern Med 6:277–285, 1991

Klein E, Linn S, Colin V, et al: The epidemiology of panic disorder and generalized anxiety disorder among emergency room patients: evidence for a group at risk (in press)

Kleinman AM, Eisenberg L, Good B: Culture, illness and care. Ann Intern Med 88:251–258, 1978

Klerman GL, Lavori P: Drug treatment of panic disorder: comparative efficacy of alprazolam, imipramine and placebo. Br J Psychiatry (in press)

Klerman GL, Weissman MM, Ouellette R, et al: Panic attacks in the community: social morbidity and health care utilization. JAMA 265:742–746, 1991

Klosko JS, Barlow DH, Tassinari R, et al: A comparison of alprazolam and behavioral therapy in treatment of panic disorder. J Consult Clin Psychol 58:77–84, 1990

Kupfer DJ: Lessons to be learned from long-term treatment of affective disorder: potential utility in panic disorder. J Clin Psychiatry 52:12–16, 1991

Linzer M, Felder A, Hackel A, et al: Psychiatry syncope: a new look at an old disease. Psychosomatics 31:181–188, 1990

Manu P, Matthews DA, Lane TJ: Panic disorder among patients with chronic fatigue. South Med J 84:451–456, 1991

McTavish D, Benfield P: Clomipramine: an overview of its pharmacologic properties and a review of its therapeutic use in obsessive-compulsive disorder and panic disorder. Drugs 39:136–153, 1990

Merikangas KR, Angst JA, Isler H: Migraine and psychopathology: results of the Zurich Cohort Study of Young Adults. Arch Gen Psychiatry 47:849–853, 1990

Myers JK, Weissman MM, Tischler GE, et al: Six-month prevalence of psychiatric disorder in three communities. Arch Gen Psychiatry 41:959–970, 1984

Noyes R, Clancy J: Anxiety neurosis: a five-year follow-up. J Nerv Ment Dis 162:200–205, 1976

Öst LG: Applied relaxation in the treatment of panic disorder. Behav Res Ther 26:13–22, 1988

Pollack MH, Rosenbaum JF, Tesar G, et al: Clonazepam in the treatment of panic disorder and agoraphobia. Psychopharmacol Bull 23:141–144, 1987

Pollack MH, Otto MW, Rosenbaum JF, et al: Longitudinal course of panic disorder: findings from the Massachusetts General Hospital longitudinal study. J Clin Psychiatry 51 (suppl 12):12–16, 1990

Rosenbaum JF, Biederman J, Gersten M, et al: Behavioral inhibition in children with panic disorder and agoraphobia: a controlled study. Arch Gen Psychiatry 45:463–470, 1988

Roy-Byrne P: Integrated treatment of panic disorder. Am J Med (in press)

Roy-Byrne PP, Geraci M, Uhde T: Life events and the onset of panic disorder. Am J Psychiatry 143:1424–1427, 1986

Salkovskis PM, Jones DRO, Clark DM: Respiratory control in treatment of panic attacks: replication and extension with concurrent measurement of behavior and pCO_2. Br J Psychiatry 148:526–532, 1986

Savage DD, Devereux RB, Garrison R, et al: Mitral valve prolapse in the general population, II: clinical features: the Framingham study. Am Heart J 106:577–581, 1983

Schurman RA, Kramer PD, Mitchel JB: The hidden mental health network: treatment of mental illness by non-psychiatrist physicians. Arch Gen Psychiatry 42:89–94, 1985

Sheehan DV: The Anxiety Disease. New York, Bantam Books, 1986

Sheehan DV, Ballenger J, Jacobson G: Treatment of endogenous anxiety with phobic, hysterical and hypochondriacal symptoms. Arch Gen Psychiatry 37:51–59, 1980

Simon G: Psychiatric disorder and functional somatic symptoms as predictors of health care use. Psychiatr Med 10:49–59, 1992

Simon G, Von Korff M: Somatization and psychiatric disorder in the Epidemiologic Catchment Area study. Am J Psychiatry 148:1494–1500, 1991

Stewart WF, Linet MS, Clentano DD: Migraine headaches and panic attacks. Psychosom Med 51:559–569, 1989

Taylor CB, Russiter EM, Agras WS: Utilization of health care services by patients with anxiety and anxiety disorders (in press)

Torgerson S: Genetic factors in anxiety disorders. Arch Gen Psychiatry 40:1085–1092, 1983

Von Korff M, Shapiro S, Burke JD, et al: Anxiety and depression in a primary care clinic: comparison of Diagnostic Interview Schedule, General Health Questionnaire and practitioner assessments. Arch Gen Psychiatry 44:452–456, 1987

Walker EA, Roy-Byrne PP, Katon WJ, et al: Psychiatric illness and irritable bowel disease. Am J Psychiatry 147:1656–1661, 1990

Weissman MM, Myers JK, Harding PS: Psychiatric disorders in a U.S. urban community: 1975–1976. Am J Psychiatry 135:459–462, 1978

Weissman MM, Klerman GL, Markowitz JS, et al: N Engl J Med 321:1209–1214, 1989

Wender P, Klein D: Mind, Mood and Medicine. New York, Farrar, Straus & Giroux, 1981

Wulsin LR, Hillard JR, Geier P, et al: Screening emergency room patients with atypical chest pain for depression and panic disorder. Int J Psychiatry Med 18:315–323, 1988

Pharmacological Treatments of Panic Disorder

Chapter 5

Overview of the Pharmacotherapy of Panic Disorder

James C. Ballenger, M.D.

It was not until the early 1980s that the treatment of panic disorder and agoraphobia generally involved specific pharmacological or behavior treatments. A survey of patients with panic disorder in the late 1970s (Doctor 1982) revealed that the majority of those patients were treated for long periods of time, with little or no benefit, irrespective of the type of practitioner seen. For example, 73% of the patients in the survey seen by psychiatrists were in treatment for more than 12 months, following which 65% of those patients were no better and 10% were worse.

Treatment During Acute Stage of Panic Disorder

The era of effective pharmacotherapeutic treatment of panic disorder was ushered in with the studies of imipramine by Klein and colleagues in the early 1960s (Klein 1964; Klein and Fink 1962), although replication of their results was not accomplished until the mid-1970s (Ballenger et al. 1977; Sheehan et al. 1980). Since that time, more than a dozen trials comparing imipramine with placebo have been completed, all demonstrating the significant superiority of imipramine (e.g., Lydiard and Ballenger 1987; Raskin 1990). There also have been five placebo-controlled trials with clomipramine (Amin et al. 1977; Escobar and Landbloom 1976; Johnston et al. 1988; Kahn et al. 1987; Karabanow 1977), the results of each again demonstrating the significant superiority of the drug over placebo. Placebo-controlled trials with other antidepressants, however, have been more limited. The results of a recently completed controlled trial showed desipramine to be significantly more effective than placebo (Lydiard et al. 1992a). In several controlled trials, fluvoxamine was shown to be effective when compared with other medications (e.g., Den Boer and Westenberg 1988; Den Boer et al. 1987). In one open trial, Gorman et al. (1987) demonstrated that fluoxetine is effective in treating panic disorder; furthermore, its clinical use has become increasingly popular. Also, clinical experience with other traditional antidepressants (e.g., maprotiline, amitriptyline, nortriptyline, doxepin) has suggested that all of these are effective in the treatment of panic disorder (Lydiard 1987; Lydiard and Ballenger 1987; Muskin and Fyer 1981). However, the study performed by Charney et al. (1986) indicated that trazodone was not as effective as imipramine or alprazolam. Another trial demonstrated that maprotiline was not as effective as fluvoxamine (Den Boer and Westenberg 1988), and an additional trial demonstrated that bupropion was ineffective in the treatment of panic disorder (Sheehan et al. 1983).

There are significantly fewer controlled trials with the monoamine oxidase inhibitor (MAOI) antidepressants, although the preponderance of evidence indicates that these are effective in the treatment of panic disorder. The largest controlled trial to date in the United States compared phenelzine with imipramine and placebo (Ballenger et al. 1977; Sheehan et al. 1980). In this study, phenelzine was, in fact, superior to imipramine on almost every outcome measure and was significantly superior on the two major clinical outcome scales. Clinical experience and one recent, large Brazilian trial (Versiani et al. 1987) demonstrated that tranylcypromine is probably at least as effective as phenelzine, and equal in efficacy to chlorimipramine and alprazolam. A recent open trial (Ballenger et al. 1987) again suggested that phenelzine was somewhat more effective than imipramine, lorazepam, and alprazolam.

Extensive clinical experience and the studies of Klein (1984) and Mavissakalian et al. (1984) have demonstrated that most patients require 150 mg/day of imipramine or its equivalent for a clinically significant response. If response is not obtained at this dosage, evidence suggests that dosages should be raised to 300 mg/day (Klein 1984).

It is unclear at this point whether serum levels of tricyclic antidepressants are useful in the management of panic disorder patients. Ballenger et al. (1984) compared two serum levels of imipramine (100–150 ng/ml and 200–250 ng/ml) for 3 months in combination with group therapy using behavioral exposure homework. They found essentially no difference in treatment response between the two levels, with some increase in side effects at the higher level. They concluded that the serum level of imipramine plus desipramine (combined) in the 150 ng/ml range appeared to represent a threshold for effective treatment of panic disorder. This result was replicated by Mavissakalian (1990a), who demonstrated that a threshold plasma level of imipramine (alone) of 125 ng/ml was associated with a significant clinical response, whereas two lower levels were not. Mavissakalian (1990a) was also able to demonstrate that lower imipramine levels were associated with a positive response in terms of panic attacks, but that higher serum levels (and oral doses) were required for significant antiphobic response, a result also reported for alprazolam (Ballenger et al. 1987).

Sheehan (1982) reported in early clinical trials that alprazolam, a triazolo-benzodiazepine, was also effective in the treatment of panic disorder. These early promising results led to the large Cross-National Collaborative Panic Study sponsored by the Upjohn Company in the 1980s. In Phase I of that trial, alprazolam was compared with placebo, and in Phase II, it was compared with imipramine and placebo.

In the Phase I study, 540 patients participated in eight centers in Canada, the United States, and Australia, and completed at least 3 weeks of treatment. This was a carefully conducted trial with rigorous methodological controls and certainly the largest panic disorder sample studied to date by almost tenfold. This was also the first extensive pharmacological trial in panic disorder to use medication alone (i.e., without any behavior treatment). The mean dosage of alprazolam was 5.4 mg/day at 4 weeks and 5.7 mg/day at 8 weeks (Ballenger et al. 1988).

In this trial, significant clinical effects were observed in the first week of alprazolam treatment in contrast to the usual 6–12 weeks required with the tricyclic antidepressants. There were significant drug-placebo differences on almost all of the outcome measures at almost every week of the 8-week trial. By the end of the first week, panic attacks were significantly reduced, with a significant drug-placebo difference favoring alprazolam. There were also reductions in anticipatory anxiety, phobic anxiety and behavior, and disability in occupational, social, and family roles. By the end of the fourth week, 30% of the alprazolam group versus 10% of the placebo group were in the markedly improved category on the Physician's Global Rating (Klerman et al. 1986). In addition, 52% of the alprazolam group (versus 33% of the placebo group) were rated moderately improved, making 82% of the alprazolam patients moderately improved or better at week 4. By week 8, 51% were markedly improved and 41% moderately improved, meaning that 92% of the alprazolam patients were at least moderately improved (Ballenger et al. 1988).

In a subsequent trial (Ballenger 1986; Lydiard et al. 1992b), 6 mg of alprazolam was compared with 2 mg of alprazolam and placebo in a 6-week trial. In this study, the 6-mg group showed greater improvement than the 2-mg or placebo groups on almost every outcome measure. The difference between the 2-mg and 6-mg groups reached statistical significance on only two major outcome measures: the percentage of patients who reached zero panic attacks and the reduction of phobic anxiety and avoidance. Therefore, this trial seems to offer at least partial replication of earlier trials, suggesting that panic attacks and background anxiety are significantly reduced with lower dosages of alprazolam (1–3 mg/day). However, in some proportion of patients, 3–6 mg per day or higher is required to maximally reduce panic attacks as well as reduce phobic avoidance.

In Phase II of the Cross-National Collaborative Panic Study, alprazolam was compared with placebo and imipramine (Cross-National Collaborative Panic Study, Second Phase Investigators 1992). This 8-week trial was conducted in 12 centers, with 1,168 patients divided into approximately equal cells of alprazolam, imipramine, and placebo treatment. The results from the Phase I alprazolam-placebo trial were almost immediately replicated. Again, alprazolam was demonstrated to be significantly more effective than placebo across the full range of psychopathological symptoms, including panic attacks, background anxiety, phobic avoidance, and secondary disability, with rapid clinical improvement and observation of significant effects in the first week. In the alprazolam group, significant clinical improvement was noted by week 1 and continued throughout the 8 weeks of the trial. In contrast, significant clinical effects in the imipramine cell were not observed until week 4, definitively replicating previous experience. However, by week 8, on most outcome measures, alprazolam and imipramine were roughly comparable in efficacy and both were superior to placebo. An additional clinical difference between the medications was that alprazolam was better tolerated by patients.

With the exception of the Phase II study just described, relatively few trials have allowed a comparison between effective medicines. As mentioned, Ballenger and colleagues (1987) reported on an open comparison trial of imipramine, alprazolam, phenelzine, and lorazepam. In that 8- to 12-week trial, alprazolam, phenelzine, and lorazepam were significantly effective by week 6, and all four agents had produced significant, roughly comparable effects by week 12. This was the first trial to demonstrate that lorazepam was also effective in the treatment of panic disorder in the average dosage range of 3–4 mg/day. Again, both benzodiazepines were effective in the first week or two. Subsequently, lorazepam was compared with alprazolam, and both drugs were demonstrated to be effective (Charney and Woods 1989.)

Versiani et al. (1987) reported a large comparative trial involving 434 panic disorder patients. In this trial, alprazolam, clomipramine, tranylcypromine, and imipramine were compared; at 2–3 months, 90% of the patients in all four groups were significantly improved. Again, in this trial, the efficacy of the four medications was roughly comparable although side effects and speed of onset differed, with significant effects observed in the first 1–2 weeks with only the benzodiazepine.

Recent clinical trials have reported that clonazepam is effective in treating panic disorder (Spier et al. 1986). In one double-blind comparison with alprazolam, Tesar et al. (1987) showed that clonazepam was equivalent in efficacy. Clonazepam's long half-life (greater than 24 hours) may afford certain advantages over the shorter half-life benzodiazepines, with the former having fewer interdose symptoms, once- or twice-per-day dosing, and fewer difficulties with withdrawal symptomatology.

Overall, then, the strategy adopted by most clinicians in the acute phase of panic disorder is to use one of the effective antidepressants—either a tricyclic or MAOI—or a benzodiazepine (alprazolam, clonazepam, or lorazepam) with the goals of rapidly reducing symptomatology and affording better control, if not resolution, of panic attacks. This phase can be accomplished in 4–6 weeks with benzodiazepines, but generally requires 2–3 months with antidepressants.

Treatment During Stabilization Stage of Panic Disorder

In the next phase, which I have called the *stabilization or continuation phase,* the major goal is to extend the acute response, particularly in terms of reduction in phobic avoidance. This phase generally occurs in months 2–6, and dosages are adjusted to maximize clinical response and minimize side effects. There are few controlled trials of length of treatment, but Curtis and colleagues (1990) recently reported a comparison of 8 months versus 2 months of treatment. In that trial, alprazolam, imipramine, and placebo responders were continued in double-blind treatment for 6 additional months after a 2-month acute trial. Gains in the two drug groups were extended by the end of the additional 6 months of treatment, essentially at the same dosage. However, there was some loss of efficacy in the placebo-responder group. Clinical experience has suggested that 6–12 months of treatment is superior to the usual 2 or 3 months of treatment in most controlled trials. The recent study by Mavissakalian and Perel (1992) supported these clinical findings. In their study, the group of patients who were treated with imipramine for 6 months and maintained at half-dose for an additional 12 months had no relapse or deterioration of clinical symptoms; in contrast, the patients who were totally discontinued from imipramine after 6 months of acute treatment had a high rate of relapse. These are among the first controlled data to document this anecdotal experience.

Treatment During Maintenance Stage of Panic Disorder

In the *maintenance phase* of treatment (months 3–12), the primary goals are to maintain symptomatic improvement and promote full social recovery. During this phase, patients often reestablish a normal life-style and talk about "feeling like themselves" again. Dosages can often be reduced during this period without loss of symptomatic improvement.

The principal difficulty in this phase of treatment is frequent side effects. In their follow-up of a large cohort ($N = 107$) of patients treated with long-term imipramine, Noyes et al. (1989) reported that at least 50% of patients had distressing (33%) or intolerable (17%) side effects, the most problematic of which was weight gain (see Table 5–1). The principal strategy for reducing side effects is reduction of dosage. Noyes and colleagues were able to successfully reduce dosage

Table 5–1. Side effects of long-term imipramine treatment reported by cohort ($N = 107$) of panic disorder patients

	Percentage reporting
Side effect	
Overstimulation	20
Palpitations	18
Sweating	17
Drowsiness	15
Light-headedness	36
Dry mouth	60
Weight gain	34
Degree of distress caused by side effects	
No side effects present	16
Present but not distressing	34
Distressing but tolerable	23
Very distressing	10
Intolerable	17

Source. Adapted from Noyes et al. 1989.

from a mean of 178 mg/day of imipramine in 25 of 33 patients. In this trial, the investigators reduced two-thirds of the patients to a dosage below 150 mg/day and one-third to below 100 mg/day, while still maintaining efficacy.

In a follow-up of a cohort of alprazolam patients from the Phase I trial, Burrows (1990) reported that initial improvement was maintained when dosages were reduced from 5 to 6 mg/day into the 2- to 3-mg range over a 12–24 month period of treatment. Nagy et al. (1989) reported similar findings in a 2.5-year follow-up. In another follow-up study (J. C. Ballenger, J. Stolk, unpublished data, 1989) 4–6 years after the Phase I trial, those patients on alprazolam at follow-up were generally in the 1- to 2-mg range. Although it has not been formally studied, most clinicians find that patients who respond to MAOIs in the 45- to 75-mg/day range generally maintain improvement if dosages are reduced to 30 mg/day, and even to 15 mg/day in some cases.

Discontinuing Pharmacotherapeutic Treatment

Generally, after 6–12 months of treatment, consideration should be given to discontinuing effective pharmacotherapy. The principal rationale for doing this is to determine whether patients can discontinue medication and still maintain their improvement. If so, they can be spared the expense, difficulty, and side effects of continued medication treatment. However, eventual discontinuation should be presented from the very beginning of treatment and subsequently accomplished with a careful, slow tapering of medication. This should involve the physician and patient choosing together an appropriate time to attempt discontinuation, as relapse is a distinct possibility. Both antidepressants and benzodiazepines should be discontinued quite slowly, over a period of at least 2–4 months. This type of very slow tapering reduces the benzodiazepine withdrawal symptomatology to a minimum, and, in one trial (Pecknold 1990), almost completely eliminated withdrawal symptoms. Also, this long discontinuation period provides the clinician adequate time to distinguish withdrawal symptomatology from relapse, as well as allowing patients to adapt to transient or even permanent symptoms that occur.

With discontinuation of effective pharmacotherapy of panic disorder, several outcomes are generally observed. Some patients discontinue medication without difficulty and fully maintain most, if not all, of their improvement. Some patients discontinuing effective benzodiazepine-type treatment develop transient withdrawal symptomatology. This is apparently highly dependent on the rate of tapering; following rapid tapering in one trial, 35% of patients developed significant withdrawal symptoms (Pecknold et al. 1988). However, with a slower tapering, recent evidence has suggested that the percentage of withdrawal symptoms is much smaller (Pecknold 1990).

The phenomenon of rebound, when symptoms are transiently worse than even prior to treatment, can occur. This level of symptomatology is highly distressing to patients and physicians, but generally peaks within the first week and resolves in the second or third week after discontinuation. Other patients relapse to their original level of symptomatology or partially relapse to a lower level of symptomatology. Evidence is limited and generally contradictory on the percentage of patients who relapse. Reported figures vary from 20%–30% (Zitrin et al. 1983) to 70%–80% (Sheehan 1986; Versiani et al. 1987), but the differences in these studies may be related to the definition of relapse used, which ranges from return of one or more panic attacks to full clinical relapse.

There are few formal data regarding the long-term outcome of patients discontinued from effective medication treatment of panic disorder. However, in the first phase of this study in 1974, Wittchen (1990) found that the disorder had remitted in 33% of the patients, whereas 40% of the patients had episodic courses and another 40% had chronic courses. On further follow-up 7 years later, only 20% were in a remitted state, 45% had episodic courses, and 60% had chronic courses. Wittchen's assessment of the data was that panic disorder is "at best persistent and at worst chronic and worsening" (Wittchen 1990). Katschnig et al. (1991) studied a cohort of patients followed up 4–6 years after acute treatment with alprazolam, imipramine, or placebo as part of the large Cross-National Collaborative Panic Study Phase II Trial. The general trend for these patients was improvement, with approximately one-third of the patients developing an asymptomatic state during this period, although almost 20% remained chronically ill.

Summary

At this point in time, I posit that there is no "one best medicine" for treatment of panic disorder but that each of the three major classes have advantages and disadvantages (see Table 5–2). The tricyclic antidepressants have been well studied, have some generic forms, and can be given once daily. One disadvantage is that at least 20%–30% of patients initially experience an activation, amphetamine-like syndrome that, if not well managed, can lead to discontinuation in as many as one-third to two-thirds of patients. Patients also rarely demonstrate significant efficacy in less than 6–12 weeks. The traditional anticholinergic side effects are frequent, as is orthostatic hypotension. The MAOIs share many of the advantages and disadvantages of the tricyclic antidepressants, including delayed onset, the activation syndrome, and weight gain, but also seem to produce more difficulty with orthostatic hypotension and insomnia. Perhaps the greatest drawback of the MAOIs is the special diet required, which is particularly frightening to many panic patients. The benzodiazepine-type medications are the only class with a rapid onset (1–2 weeks) and significant efficacy against background and anticipatory anxiety. In addition, they are well tolerated. Their principal difficulties include sedation, the necessity for multiple daily dosing (with shorter acting benzodi-

Table 5–2.   Advantages and disadvantages of various antipanic agents

Antipanic agent	Advantages	Disadvantages
Tricyclic antidepressants	Administered in single daily dose Provide prophylaxis against recurrent depression Are well studied Some available in generic form	Have delayed onset Cause activation syndrome Cause anticholinergic effects Cause orthostatic hypotension Can affect sexual performance Cause mania (bipolar patients)
Monoamine oxidase inhibitors	May serve as a better antiphobic Provide prophylaxis against recurrent depression	Require restricted diet Carry risk of hypertensive, hyperpyrexic reactions Have delayed onset Cause insomnia Cause orthostatic hypotension Cause weight gain Can affect sexual performance Cause mania (bipolar patients)
Benzodiazepines	Have rapid onset Are well tolerated Are effective against anticipatory anxiety Few are available in generic form	Carry risk of withdrawal symptoms Cause sedation Administered in multiple daily doses Can affect sexual performance

azepines), and their potential for development of withdrawal symptomatology on discontinuation.

There are few data that suggest that a particular patient might respond particularly well to one or another class of medications. However, recently Briggs and colleagues (A. C. Briggs, D. D. Stretch, S. Brandon, unpublished data, 1991) reported from the large Cross-National Collaborative Panic Study Phase II Trial that there may be some differences in the patient groups that respond to alprazolam and imipramine. They reported that the patient group with prominent respiratory symptoms of shortness of breath, choking, fear of dying, and more spontaneous panic attacks appeared to respond better to imipramine. Conversely, the group with more prominent cardiovascular symptoms of palpitations, dizziness, nausea, and more situational attacks appeared to respond better to alprazolam. This should be a fruitful area of future research.

Symptomatic predictors of a poor response have included high initial levels of symptomatology, obsessionalism, depression, and personality disorders (Ballenger et al. 1984; Lesser et al. 1988; C. L. Woodman, R. Noyes, Jr., J. C. Ballenger, G. Seivers, D. Mihalko, R. B. Lydiard, unpublished data, 1992). The individual clinician's response to an initial outcome should include examination of the dosage and length of the trial, as inadequate medication trials have been the primary factor associated with poor response. At that point, the clinician should logically ask whether a change of medication or the addition of behavior treatment is appropriate.

In summary, pharmacotherapy of panic disorder begins with an aggressive but careful dosage-finding strategy in order to obtain maximum initial response. In most patients, the goal should be to reach a nearly asymptomatic state or a return to "almost normal." Treatment and changes in treatment should always be responsive to the patient's social and economic situation as well as functional adjustment. Psychological management of patients, whether it involves formal behavior therapy or psychotherapy, needs to be sensitive, responsive, available, knowledgeable, and confident to effectively deal with these gratifying but at times difficult-to-treat patients.

The remaining unresolved issues in the pharmacological treatment of panic disorder for which there are simply insufficient data include 1) the matching of treatment to individual patients, 2) the optimal length of treatment, 3) relapse rates, and 4) treatment of patients resistant to initial pharmacotherapy. The optimal treatment or combination of treatments is also still unknown and often follows the individual clinician's ideas or training. An issue currently being researched is whether the ideal treatment of panic disorder is pharmacological or purely behavioral, involving primarily in vivo exposure or cognitive therapy.

Many clinicians and some recent research studies (Mavissakalian 1990b; Swinson 1990) point to the combination of pharmacotherapy and behavior treatment as the best treatment. Certainly, the accumulated evidence indicates that pharmacotherapy and behavioral exposure treatments are effective individually but are also additive in their effects (Mavissakalian 1990b). It is both logical and supported by considerable research that the most effective and probably efficient treatment of panic disorder involves a combination of pharmacotherapy and exposure-based treatments.

References

Amin MM, Ban TA, Pecknold JC, et al: Clomipramine (Anafranil) and behavior therapy in obsessive-compulsive and phobic disorders. J Int Med Res 5:33–37, 1977

Ballenger JC: A comparison of 2 mg and 6 mg/day in the treatment of panic disorder patients. Paper presented at the Panic Disorder and Biological Research Workshop, Washington, DC, April 15–16, 1986

Ballenger JC, Sheehan DV, Jacobson G: Antidepressant treatment of severe phobic anxiety. Paper presented at the annual meeting of the American Psychiatric Association, Toronto, Canada, May, 1977

Ballenger JC, Peterson GA, Laraia M, et al: A study of plasma catecholamines in agoraphobia and the relationship of serum tricyclic level to treatment response, in Biology of Agoraphobia. Edited by Ballenger JC. Washington, DC, American Psychiatric Press, 1984, pp 27–63

Ballenger JC, Howell EF, Laraia M, et al: Comparison of four medicines in panic disorder. Paper presented at the annual meeting of the American Psychiatric Association, Chicago, IL, May 14, 1987

Ballenger JC, Burrow GD, DuPont RLJ, et al: Alprazolam in panic disorder and agoraphobia: results from a multicenter trial, I: efficacy in short-term treatment. Arch Gen Psychiatry 45:413–422, 1988

Burrows GD: Long-term treatment of panic disorder. Paper presented at Panic and Anxiety: A Decade of Progress, Geneva, Switzerland, June 21, 1990

Charney DS, Woods SWS, Goodman WIC, et al: Drug treatment of panic disorder: the comparative efficacy of imipramine, alprazolam, and trazodone. J Clin Psychiatry 47:580–586, 1986

Charney DS, Woods SW: Benzodiazepine treatment of panic disorder: a comparison of alprazolam and lorazepam. J Clin Psychiatry 50:418–423, 1989

Cross-National Collaborative Panic Study, Second Phase Investigators: Drug treatment of panic disorder: comparative efficacy of alprazolam, imipramine, and placebo. Br J Psychiatry 160:191–202, 1992

Curtis GC, Massana J, Udina C, et al: Maintenance drug therapy of panic disorder. Paper presented at the annual meeting of the American Psychiatric Association, New York, May 12–17, 1990

Den Boer JA, Westenberg HGM, Kamerbeek WDJ, et al: Effect of serotonin uptake inhibitors in anxiety disorders: a double-blind comparison of clomipramine and fluvoxamine. Int Clin Psychopharmacol 2:21–31, 1987

Den Boer JA, Westenberg HGM: Effect of a serotonin and noradrenaline uptake inhibitor in panic disorder: a double-blind comparative study with fluvoxamine and maprotiline. Int Clin Psychopharmacol 3:59–74, 1988

Doctor RM: Major results of a large-scale pretreatment survey of agoraphobics, in Summary of Modern Treatment. Edited by Dupont R. New York, Brunner/Mazel, 1982, pp 215–230

Escobar JI, Landbloom RP: Treatment of phobic neurosis with clomipramine: a controlled clinical trial. Current Ther Research 20:680–685, 1976

Gorman J, Liebowitz MR, Fyer AJ, et al: An open trial of fluoxetine in the treatment of panic attacks. J Clin Psychopharmacol 7:329–332, 1987

Johnston DG, Troyer IE, Whitset SF: Clomipramine treatment of agoraphobic women: an eight-week controlled trial. Arch Gen Psychiatry 45:453–459, 1988

Kahn RS, Westenberg HGM, Verhoeven WMA, et al: Effect of a serotonin precursor and uptake inhibitor in anxiety disorders: a double-blind comparison of 5-hydroxy-tryptophan, clomipramine and placebo. Int Clin Psychopharmacol 2:33–45, 1987

Karabanow O: Double-blind controlled study in phobias and obsession. J Int Med Res 5(5):42–48, 1977

Katschnig H, Stolk J, Klerman GL, et al: Discontinuation experiences and long-term treatment follow-up of participants in a clinical drug trial for panic disorder, in Biological Psychiatry International Congress, Series 968, Vol 1. Edited by Racagni G, Brunello N, Fukuda T. New York, Elsevier, 1991, pp 657–660

Klein DF: Delineation of two drug-responsive anxiety syndromes. Psychopharmacologia 5:397–408, 1964

Klein DF: Psychopharmacologic treatment of panic disorder. Psychosomatics 25 (suppl 10):32–35, 1984

Klein DF, Fink M: Psychiatric reaction patterns to imipramine. Am J Psychiatry 119:432–438, 1962

Klerman GL, Coleman JH, Purpura RP: The design and conduct of the Upjohn Cross-National Panic Study. Psychopharmacol Bull 22:59–75, 1986

Lesser IM, Rubin RT, Pecknold JC, et al: Secondary depression in panic disorder and agoraphobia, I: frequency, severity, and response to treatment. Arch Gen Psychiatry 45:437–443, 1988

Lydiard RB: Successful utilization of maprotiline in a patient intolerant of tricyclics. J Clin Psychopharmacol 7:113–114, 1987

Lydiard RB, Ballenger JC: Antidepressants in panic disorder and agoraphobia. J Affect Disord 13:153–168, 1987

Lydiard RB, Morton A, Zealberg J, et al: A placebo-controlled, double-blind study of desipramine in panic disorder. Paper presented at the annual meeting of the New Clinical Drug Evaluation Unit (NCDEU), Washington, DC, May 1992a

Lydiard RB, Lesser IM, Ballenger JC, et al: A fixed-dose study of alprazolam 2 mg, alprazolam 6 mg, and placebo in panic disorder. J Clin Psychopharmacol 12(2):96–103, 1992b

Mavissakalian M: Relationship of dose/plasma concentrations on imipramine to the treatment of panic disorder with agoraphobia, in Clinical Aspects of Panic Disorder. Edited by Ballenger JC. New York, Wiley-Liss, 1990a, pp 211–218

Mavissakalian M: Differential efficacy between tricyclic antidepressant and behavior therapy of panic disorder, in Clinical Aspects of Panic Disorder. Edited by Ballenger JC. New York, Wiley-Liss, 1990b, pp 195–210

Mavissakalian M, Perel JM: Clinical experiments in maintenance and discontinuation of imipramine therapy in panic disorder with agoraphobia. Arch Gen Psychiatry 49:318–323, 1992

Mavissakalian M, Perel J, Michelson L: The relationship of plasma imipramine and 7-demethylimipramine to improvement in agoraphobia. J Clin Psychopharmacol 4:36–40, 1984

Muskin PR, Fyer AJ: Treatment of panic disorder. J Clin Psychopharmacol 1:81–90, 1981

Nagy LM, Krystal JH, Woods SW, et al: Clinical and medication outcome after short-term alprazolam and behavioral group treatment of panic disorder. Arch Gen Psychiatry 46:993–999, 1989

Noyes R, Garvey MJ, Cook BL, et al: Problems with tricyclic antidepressant use in patients with panic disorder or agoraphobia: results of a naturalistic follow-up study. J Clin Psychiatry 50(5):163–169, 1989

Pecknold JC: Discontinuation studies: short-term and long-term. Paper presented at the Panic Awareness for the Clinician Symposium, Carlsbad, CA, November 27–29, 1990

Pecknold JC, Swinson RP, Kirch K, et al: Alprazolam in panic disorder and agoraphobia: results from a multicenter trial, II: discontinuation effects. Arch Gen Psychiatry 45:429–436, 1988

Raskin A: Role of depression in the antipanic effects of antidepressant drugs, in Clinical Aspects of Panic Disorder. Edited by Ballenger JC. New York, Wiley-Liss, 1990, pp 169–180

Sheehan DV: Current views on the treatment of panic and phobic disorders. Drug Ther Hosp 7:74–93, 1982

Sheehan DV: Tricyclic antidepressants in the treatment of anxiety disorders. Paper presented at the annual meeting of the American Psychiatric Association, Washington, DC, May 10–16, 1986

Sheehan DV, Ballenger J, Jacobson G: Treatment of endogenous anxiety with phobic, hysterical, and hypochondriacal symptoms. Arch Gen Psychiatry 37:51–59, 1980

Sheehan DV, Davison J, Manschreck J, et al: Lack of efficacy of a new antidepressant (bupropion) in the treatment of panic disorder with phobias. J Clin Psychopharmacol 3:28–31, 1983

Spier SA, Tesar GE, Rosenbaum JF, et al: Treatment of panic disorder and agoraphobia with clonazepam. J Clin Psychiatry 47:238–242, 1986

Swinson RP: Nondrug therapies of panic disorder and agoraphobia. Paper presented at Panic Awareness for the Clinician Symposium, Carlsbad, CA, November 27–29, 1990

Tesar GE, Rosenbaum JF, Pollack MH, et al: Clonazepam versus alprazolam in the treatment of panic disorder: interim analysis of data from a prospective double-blind, placebo-controlled trial. J Clin Psychiatry 48 (Oct suppl):16–19, 1987

Versiani M, Costa e Silva JA, Klerman GL: Treatment of panic disorder with alprazolam, clomipramine, imipramine, tranylcypromine or placebo. Paper presented at the annual meeting of the American College of Neuropsychopharmacology. San Juan, Puerto Rico, December 7–11, 1987

Wittchen HU: Epidemiology of panic disorder: progress and unresolved issues. Paper presented at Panic and Anxiety: A Decade of Progress, Geneva, Switzerland, June 1990

Zitrin CM, Klein DF, Woermer MG, et al: Treatment of phobias, I: comparison of imipramine hydrochloride and placebo. Arch Gen Psychiatry 40:125–138, 1983

Chapter 6

The Long-Term Course
of Panic Disorder

Heinz Katschnig, M.D., and
Michaela Amering, M.D.

The natural history of panic disorder (i.e., the longitudinal course of the untreated condition) is unknown. Also unknown is whether or not the course of panic disorder is chronic or even chronically progressive. Is it episodic? How many patients recover spontaneously?

Lack of such knowledge is unfortunate, as having it would provide a yardstick against which to measure the efficacy of therapeutic activities. Such a measure (or measures) would be especially important in resolving the opposing claims by psychopharmacologists on the one hand that panic disorder is a chronic condition that requires long-term pharmacological treatment, and by behavior and cognitive therapists on the other hand, who tend to show—albeit only for small samples of patients so far—that relatively short interventions provide a long-term cure. Do these opposing views reflect selection of different types of patients with different severity and different natural histories? We will know only after we have elucidated the natural history of panic disorder.

There are several reasons for the deplorable lack of knowledge on the natural history of panic disorder. The general reason is that it is difficult to identify cases that have remained untreated over a long time period; in fact, this dilemma is valid for most medical conditions for which no data exist on the course prior to the availability of treatment. A more specific reason is that panic disorder was defined as a disease entity only in 1980 in DSM-III (American Psychiatric Association 1980), so that there has been little time for long-term observation of the disorder's development. No study is available for panic disorder comparable to that by Eugen

Bleuler (1972) on schizophrenia, in which he followed patients who had been diagnosed by his father (Bleuler 1911/1950) over their whole lifetime. Matussek et al.'s (1965) study on the course of endogenous depression prior to the introduction of treatment is another example of such a long-term study. Both studies will probably never be repeated, because they were carried out when no efficacious treatment was available for those disorders over most of the time covered.

The definition of panic disorder in DSM-III was followed by the propagation of pharmacological and behavior treatments. More and more patients are being treated now, and the course of their disorder is thus being altered by that treatment, making it difficult to determine the untreated, natural course of panic disorder. However, because the clinical condition had not been unknown before 1980 but had only been defined differently or subsumed under the term *anxiety neurosis,* studies from the pre–DSM-III era can be used to estimate panic disorder's natural history. Such data will be briefly reviewed here. In addition, after a brief review of some newer follow-up studies of DSM-III–defined clinical samples, results will be presented from a 2- to 6-year follow-up study of participants in a large, international, multicenter drug trial. Finally, an attempt will be made to construct a longitudinal model from published cross-sectional Epidemiologic Catchment Area data on the fate of persons who have experienced panic attacks.

Course of Panic Disorder Prior to the Widespread Use of Medication

Keller (1990) and Hirschfeld (1992), using an earlier summary paper by Marks and Lader (1973), commented on seven follow-up studies (Blair et al. 1957; Eitinger 1955; Ernst 1959; Greer and Crawley 1966; Harris 1938; Miles et al. 1951; Wheeler et al. 1950) carried out before the definition of panic disorder in DSM-III and long before the widespread use of pharmacological and behavior treatments of panic disorder. Among others, the terms *anxiety state, anxiety neurosis,* and *neurocirculatory asthenia* were used by these authors. The definitions of panic used in these seven studies were neither comparable among themselves nor comparable with studies using DSM criteria. However, these studies had rather long follow-up periods (up to 20 years in the Wheeler et al. study). The overall conclusion of these studies was that a rather large proportion of patients (41%–59%) continued to experience symptoms and that psychosocial outcome was usually better than symptomatic outcome.

Follow-Up Studies of DSM-III– or DSM-III-R–Defined Panic Disorder Patients

Since the introduction of DSM-III and the widespread use of standardized diagnostic interview techniques, results of panic disorder studies have become more comparable. However, very few such follow-up studies have been completed to date, and, except for one study (Katschnig et al. 1991; see below), the numbers of patients used were rather small and the follow-up durations short.

The two most well-designed and relevant studies were carried out by Noyes and colleagues. In the first study (Noyes et al. 1989), 107 patients who had panic disorder or agoraphobia with panic attacks and who had participated in a clinical drug trial with imipramine were reinterviewed on average 2.5 years after leaving the trial. More than 80% were found to be symptomatic at follow-up, but less than 50% reported panic attacks and less than 40% reported phobic avoidance during the 3 months before the interview. In the second study (Noyes et al. 1990), 89 panic disorder patients who had participated in a placebo-controlled clinical trial of alprazolam and diazepam received a structured interview 3 years after the trial. Forty-one percent of the patients were found well or markedly improved at follow-up.

Maier and Buller (1988) followed 77 panic disorder patients (as determined by DSM-III-R criteria) from a variety of treatment settings over 1 year and found that 2 out of 5 patients had a marked decrease in panic attacks and phobic avoidance. However, most patients had received pharmacotherapy during follow-up.

Other follow-up studies have included mainly or even exclusively agoraphobic patients who do not fulfill DSM-III criteria for panic disorder (Faravelli and Albanesi 1987; Mavissakalian and Michelson 1986; Nagy et al. 1989); one study also included patients with anxiety neurosis or phobia (Krieg et al. 1987). The results of these four studies simply are not comparable with the panic disorder studies above and are not considered here (for a full discussion see Hirschfeld 1992).

Follow-Up on Patients From the Cross-National Collaborative Panic Study

The Cross-National Collaborative Panic Study was a multicenter, double-blind, randomized drug trial carried out in 15 countries in Europe and North and Latin America. The original population in the study consisted of 1,647 panic disorder patients, diagnosed according to a modified version of DSM-III criteria. All subjects took part in either the Phase I drug trial (in which alprazolam and placebo were compared [see Ballenger et al. 1988]) or the Phase II drug trial (in which alprazolam, imipramine, and placebo were compared [Cross-National Collaborative Panic Study, Second Phase Investigators 1992]). Most subjects completed an 8-week trial protocol; in some centers the study was extended to 8 months. After 8 weeks, alprazolam and imipramine were found to be equally efficient and both were found to be superior to placebo.

Katschnig et al. (1991) reported on the largest ($N = 367$) and longest follow-up (2–6 years, median 4 years) investigation carried out so far, in which patients from the Cross-National Collaborative Panic Study were studied. Roughly one-quarter ($n = 423$) of the original sample from seven sites in North America and Europe were chosen to be reassessed 2–6 years after leaving the drug trial. A special follow-up interview was constructed, focusing on 1) comparisons of symptoms and disabilities between the poststudy year and the year before the interview (the "current year") and 2) current medication use. A total of 367 patients (86.8% of those to be followed) could be reinterviewed. The patterns of course could be analyzed for a subsample of 220 patients.

Only 24% of the 367 patients reported having experienced no panic attacks during the poststudy year. There was some improvement between the poststudy year and the current year, when the percentage of patients experiencing no panic attacks rose to 39%, leaving 61% who experienced at least occasional panic attacks.

Global phobic fear and avoidance were measured on an 11-point scale (0 = no phobic avoidance, 10 = maximum phobic avoidance). During the poststudy year, 39% of all patients reported no or only mild phobic avoidance (a score of 0–4), with a substantial increase to 60% during the current year. The same pattern could be found for work, family, and social disabilities, with, however, a much larger improvement for most disabilities (e.g., the proportion of patients with no or only mild work disability increased from 48% to 82% between the poststudy year and the current year).

Forty-five percent of all patients were not taking any psychotropic medication at the time of the follow-up interview. Twenty-three percent were taking benzodiazepines alone, 12% an antidepressant, and 9% both. Eleven percent were using other psychotropic drugs.

None of the above variables (symptoms, disabilities, or current medication use) showed differences in outcome in relationship to the type of medication received during the original drug trial. Buller and Amering (1991) showed for the same study population that patients who had panic disorder without agoraphobia did better than those with agoraphobia.

The patterns of the symptomatic course of panic disorder were analyzed for 220 patients (see Figure 6–1). Thirty-one percent of these patients had recovered and had stayed well until the follow-up interview, but a severe, chronic course was found in 19%. The remaining 50% showed intermediate patterns of course. There were no suicides reported. Three patients had developed malignant neoplasms and had subsequently died.

From these data a differentiated picture about the long-term course of panic disorder emerged. One in five panic disorder patients had a severe, chronic course, but nearly one in three patients did excellently 4 years following the clinical trial. However, 50% of all patients showed recurrent or mild chronic symptomatology. Although panic attacks still occurred in three of five patients, disabilities had largely disappeared.

It has to be kept in mind that these results were obtained from a naturalistic follow-up study of patients who had taken part in a clinical drug trial. Such patients clearly constitute a selected group: on the one hand, they were chosen for a drug trial because they had reached a certain degree of symptom severity; on the

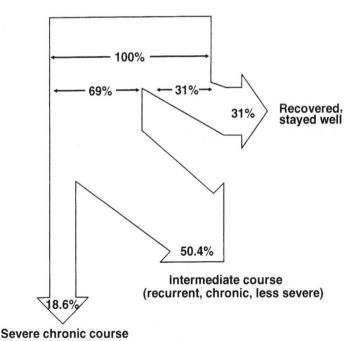

Figure 6–1. Cross-National Collaborative Panic Study follow-up data. Follow-up duration = median 4 years; *N* = 220 patients. *Source.* Based on data from Katschnig et al. 1991.

other hand, exclusion criteria of clinical drug trials would tend to prevent co-morbid patients from being included in the study population. This exclusion means that drug trial patients had a less severe disorder in this respect than many other patients.

Keeping these qualifications in mind, four explanations are possible for the relatively good outcome in a large subgroup of patients (Katschnig et al. 1991): 1) a favorable natural history of the disorder in a subgroup of patients (i.e., it is possible that different subtypes of panic disorder have different natural histories); 2) a statistical "regression to the mean" effect (due to the fact that patients selected for a clinical drug trial tend to be more severely ill); 3) the effect of unsystematic and uncontrolled treatments received during follow-up (treatment was not controlled in this naturalistic follow-up study); and finally, 4) a "sleeper" effect of unintended nonpharmacological factors operating during the original treatment study, especially "cognitive factors" working through self-monitoring (Nelson 1977) by means of a diary and in vivo exposure mechanisms (Telch et al. 1985), which patients might have inadvertently learned during the trial.

Fate of Persons Who Experience Panic Attacks

A hypothetical model of the fate of persons who have had at least one panic attack, based on results from the Epidemiologic Catchment Area (ECA) study (Klerman et al. 1991; Weissman 1988), is shown in Figure 6–2. About 10% of the general population experience at least one panic attack in a lifetime. One in six of these individuals (or 1.6% of the total population) goes on to develop panic disorder as defined in DSM-III; approximately one-third of those (0.5%) also fulfill criteria for agoraphobia, whereas two-thirds (1.1%) do not. It is interesting that a substantial minority of patients who experience panic attacks without fulfilling panic disorder criteria also develop agoraphobia (1.2%). Of the remaining persons, 4.8% (or roughly one-half of those experiencing any panic attacks) have isolated attacks without agoraphobia. Finally, one-third experience recurrent panic attacks without agoraphobia.

Such cross-sectional data can by no means represent the true development of the disorder, but they can give a hint of the size of the problem. These figures can be verified only by a true prospective study starting with patients experiencing their first panic attack.

Conclusion

It is difficult to imagine how to elucidate the true natural history of panic disorder. Better approximations than studying the naturalistic course of panic disorder in patients who have taken part in a clinical drug trial are conceivable. An approach worth exploring would be to include less severely ill patients. Another, rather costly, possibility would be to conduct a prospective study of cases identified in community surveys of the ECA type. A more feasible approach would be to conduct a follow-up study of cases identified in general practice, cases that would

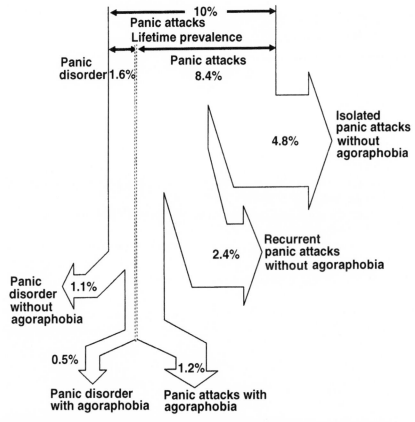

Figure 6–2. Hypothetical longitudinal model of the fate of persons experiencing panic attacks. *Source.* Derived from Epidemiologic Catchment Area study data reported by Klerman et al. 1991; Weissman 1988.

represent a broader spectrum of degrees of severity than highly selected drug study populations. This study would also include patients not fulfilling full criteria for panic disorder. On the other hand, follow-up studies should also be carried out on comorbid patients of the type most frequently seen in outpatient departments— panic patients who experience depression, suicidal ideation, and drug and alcohol abuse. These patients constitute a large group from a public health point of view, but they are excluded from clinical drug trials. All these studies should preferably be prospective, similar to the Harvard Anxiety Panic Disorder Research Project (HARP) study presently being carried out (Keller et al. 1990).

Thus, although the results of the available studies suggest that the long-term outcome of panic disorder is not as gloomy as usually thought, this picture might be corrected in one or the other direction by future research.

References

American Psychiatric Association: Diagnostic and Statistical Manual of Mental Disorders, 3rd Edition. Washington, DC, American Psychiatric Association, 1980

Ballenger JC, Burrows GD, DuPont RL, et al: Alprazolam in panic disorder and agoraphobia: results from a multicenter trial, I: efficacy in short-term treatment. Arch Gen Psychiatry 45:413–422, 1988

Blair R, Gilroy JM, Pilkington F: Some observations on outpatient psychotherapy: follow-up of 235 cases. BMJ 1:318–321, 1957

Bleuler E (1911): Dementia Praecox or the Group of Schizophrenias. Translated by Zinkin J. New York, International University Press, 1950

Bleuler M: Die schizophrenen Geistesstörungen im Lichte langjähriger Kranken- und Familiengeschichten. Stuttgart, Thieme, 1972

Buller R, Amering M: Follow-up in subtypes of panic disorder. Biol Psychiatry 29 (suppl 11):290S, 1991

Cross-National Collaborative Panic Study, Second Phase Investigators: Drug treatment of panic disorder: comparative efficacy of alprazolam, imipramine, and placebo. Br J Psychiatry 160:191–202, 1992

Eitinger L: Studies in neurosis. Acta Psychiatrica et Neurologica Scandinavica 30 (suppl 101):5–47, 1955

Ernst K: Die Propuose der Neurosen. Berlin, Springer-Verlag, 1959

Faravelli C, Albanesi G: Agoraphobia with panic attacks: one-year prospective follow-up. Compr Psychiatry 28:481–486, 1987

Greer S, Crawley RH: Some observations on the natural history of neurotic illness (Archdall Medical Monograph 3). Sydney, Australia, Australian Medical Publishing, 1966

Harris A: The prognosis of anxiety states. BMJ 2:649–654, 1938

Hirschfeld RMA: The clinical course of panic disorder and agoraphobia, in Handbook of Anxiety, Vol 5. Edited by Burrows GD, Roth M, Noyes RJ. New York, Elsevier, 1992, pp 105–119

Katschnig H, Stolk JM, Klerman GL, et al: Discontinuation and long-term follow-up of participants in a clinical drug trial for panic disorder. Biol Psychiatry 1:657–660, 1991

Keller M: The natural history of panic disorder and depression prior to the widespread use of medication. Paper presented at the annual meeting of the New Clinical Drug Evaluation Unit (NCDEU) Program, Key Biscayne, FL, May 20–June 1, 1990

Klerman GL, Weissman MM, Ouellette R, et al: Panic attacks in the community: social morbidity and health care utilization. JAMA 265:742–746, 1991

Krieg JC, Bronisch T, Wittchen HU, et al: Anxiety disorders: a long-term prospective and retrospective follow-up of former inpatients suffering from an anxiety neurosis or phobia. Acta Psychiatr Scand 76:36–47, 1987

Maier W, Buller R: One-year follow-up of panic disorder. European Archives of Psychiatry and Neurological Sciences 238:105–108, 1988

Marks IM, Lader M: Anxiety states (anxiety neurosis): a review. J Nerv Ment Dis 156:3–18, 1973

Matussek P, Halbach A, Troeger U: Endogene Depression. München-Berlin, Urban and Schwarzenberg, 1965

Mavissakalian M, Michelson L: Two-year follow-up of exposure and imipramine treatment of agoraphobia. Am J Psychiatry 143:1106–1112, 1986

Miles HHW, Barrabes EL, Finesinger JE: Evaluation of psychotherapy: with a follow-up study of 62 cases of anxiety neurosis. Psychosom Med 13:83–105, 1951

Nagy LM, Krystal JH, Woods SW, et al: Clinical and medical outcome after short-term alprazolam and behavioral group treatment in panic disorder. Arch Gen Psychiatry 46:993–999, 1989

Nelson RO: Methodological issues in assessment via self-monitoring, in Behavioral Assessment: New Directions in Clinical Psychology. Edited by Cone JD, Hawkins RP. New York, Brunner/Mazel, 1977, pp 217–240

Noyes R, Garvey MJ, Cook BL: Follow-up study of patients with panic disorder and agoraphobia with panic attacks treated with tricyclic antidepressants. J Affect Disord 16:249–257, 1989

Noyes R, Reich J, Christiansen J, et al: Outcome of panic disorder: relationship to diagnostic subtypes and comorbidity. Arch Gen Psychiatry 47:809–818, 1990

Telch MJ, Agras WS, Taylor CB: Combined pharmacological and behavioral treatment for agoraphobia. Behav Res Ther 23:325–335, 1985

Weissman MM: The epidemiology of panic disorder and agoraphobia, in American Psychiatric Press Review of Psychiatry, Vol 7. Edited by Frances AJ, Hales RE. Washington, DC, American Psychiatric Press, 1988, pp 54–66

Wheeler EO, White PD, Reed EW, et al: Neurocirculatory asthenia (anxiety neurosis, effort syndrome, neurasthenia): a twenty year follow-up study of one hundred and seventy-three patients. JAMA 142:878–889, 1950

Yonkers KA, Ellison JM, Shera DM, et al: Pharmacotherapy observed in a large prospective longitudinal study on anxiety disorders. Psychopharmacol Bull 28:131–137, 1992

Chapter 7

New and Experimental Pharmacological Treatments for Panic Disorder

Jack M. Gorman, M.D.

Existing pharmacological treatments for panic disorder are highly effective and safe. The standard medication treatments are the heterocyclic antidepressants (particularly imipramine), monoamine oxidase inhibitors (MAOIs), and alprazolam, a benzodiazepine. These agents have been reported to have success rates of 70%–90% in blocking panic attacks. However, they do not effect a permanent cure, in that after drug discontinuation many patients experience relapse, although this may not be evident for prolonged periods of time. The medications also have some drawbacks. Because of the side effects of imipramine, some patients do not easily tolerate it. MAOIs also provoke a number of unpleasant side effects so that they are not recommended as the drug of first choice. And although the side effects of benzodiazepines like alprazolam are few, their prolonged use may lead to physical dependency, a possibility that concerns some patients and clinicians.

Because of side effect considerations, it is important that new and more specific medications for the treatment of panic disorder be developed. Ultimately, a medication that would "cure" the illness would be desirable. In the absence of definitive cure, however, new antipanic medications are sought that would have fewer side effects, more rapid onset of action, and the capacity to be administered over long periods of time to patients who relapse frequently after medication discontinuation.

Drugs That Affect Serotonin Transmission

Of particular recent interest are drugs that selectively block presynaptic neuronal reuptake of serotonin (5-hydroxytryptamine [5-HT]). Three such agents are currently available: fluoxetine, sertraline, and paroxetine. Investigators in two uncontrolled studies (Gorman et al. 1987; Schneier et al. 1990) have documented that fluoxetine is capable of blocking panic attacks in patients with panic disorder. In a double-blind, placebo-controlled comparison of the experimental, selective 5-HT reuptake blocker fluvoxamine with the 5-HT$_2$ receptor antagonist ritanserin, Den Boer and Westenberg (1990) showed fluvoxamine to be superior to placebo in reducing panic attacks and avoidance behavior. Other 5-HT reuptake blockers are cericlamine and venlafaxine.

Many clinicians in the United States already prescribe fluoxetine and sertraline for panic patients, often as the drug of first choice. The 5-HT reuptake blockers have a favorable side effect profile compared with currently available antipanic drugs: they do not adversely affect blood pressure or other cardiovascular functions, do not induce weight gain, have no anticholinergic side effects, and do not produce physical dependency. However, some patients have a hypersensitivity reaction characterized by increased anxiety, agitation, and insomnia when fluoxetine treatment is initiated at a 20-mg/day dosage. Consequently, initiation of therapy at lower dosages is often recommended. It is clear that use of selective 5-HT reuptake blockers is a promising area of antipanic treatment that has already found a place in standard practice and that should be the subject of further controlled trials.

The success of fluoxetine, sertraline, and other selective 5-HT reuptake blockers challenges earlier hypotheses that panic attacks are caused by abnormalities in the noradrenergic transmission system. According to current data, fluoxetine and sertraline have no acute effects on noradrenergic reuptake or receptors. It is possible, however, that chronic use may alter the noradrenergic system. Nevertheless, the antipanic effect of fluoxetine and sertraline has led to work implicating the serotonergic system in the pathophysiology of panic (Sheehan et al. 1988). Interestingly, a nonselective 5-HT reuptake blocking drug, clomipramine, which is a heterocyclic compound similar in molecular structure to imipramine, appears to be effective in blocking panic (Gloger et al. 1981), possibly at lower dosages than are required with imipramine. The fact that lower dosages of clomipramine may be effective is significant because clomipramine is a more potent 5-HT reuptake blocker than imipramine, again implicating the serotonergic system.

The efficacy of the 5-HT reuptake blockers in treating panic prompts consideration of other classes of drugs that specifically affect the serotonergic system. Of interest here is that many such drugs that appear effective in relieving generalized anxiety disorder (GAD) do not seem to have an antipanic effect. The fact that drugs affecting different aspects of serotonergic neurotransmission have differential effects on panic and GAD suggests interesting neurobiological differences between GAD and panic disorder. For example, the specific 5-HT2 receptor antagonist ritanserin was not as good as fluvoxamine or better than placebo in treating panic (Den Boer and Westenberg 1990). The antipanic effects of specific 5-HT3 antagonists, such as granisetron and ondansetron, have not yet been reported.

Another very interesting class of drug that affects the serotonin system is the group of 5-HT1A partial agonists. One of these drugs, buspirone, is currently marketed in the United States for the treatment of GAD. Several well-controlled trials have shown that buspirone is equally as effective as benzodiazepines in the treatment of GAD (Rickels 1990). On the other hand, there are reports, substantiated by clinical practice, that buspirone does not block panic attacks (Sheehan et al. 1990). The authors of one uncontrolled study (Gastfriend and Rosenbaum 1989) did find, however, that buspirone offered an adjunctive effect when added to benzodiazepines in treating panic. Other drugs in the class of 5-HT1A agonists, each with a slightly different pharmacological profile than buspirone, that should be studied with respect to panic disorder include gepirone, ipsapirone, zalospirone, and metanopirone.

Monoamine Oxidase Inhibitors

As mentioned earlier, MAOIs are highly potent in blocking panic attacks, but their side effects limit their use mainly to patients who are refractory to other treatments. There is great interest, therefore, in developing MAOIs with fewer adverse effects. A class of reversible MAOIs may have this property. Anecdotal reports suggest that one such agent, moclobemide, may have antipanic properties. Other drugs in this class are brofaromine and zacopride. These drugs should be tested in panic patients as soon as possible.

Benzodiazepines

The success of alprazolam in treating panic disorder has reopened consideration of the role of benzodiazepines in panic. Previously, it was believed that benzodiazepines were effective only for GAD patients. The antipanic effects of alprazolam challenged this notion. At first, investigators suggested that alprazolam might have some unique pharmacological properties that distinguished it from other benzodiazepines, and that these properties could potentially explain the drug's antipanic effect. This possibility may indeed be the case, but more recently it has been shown that other high-potency benzodiazepines are effective in treating panic (Tesar 1990). Both controlled and uncontrolled trials have shown that lorazepam (Charney and Woods 1989; Schweizer et al. 1988) and clonazepam (Herman et al. 1987; Tesar et al. 1987) are effective antipanic medications. An investigational triazolobenzodiazepine, adinazolam, which is similar in structure to alprazolam, has been shown to be effective in blocking panic in a double-blind comparison with alprazolam (Pyke and Greenberg 1989).

Benzodiazepines have few side effects and are medically safe. Contrary to popular belief, tolerance (or tachyphylaxis) to benzodiazepines is rare. For patients who need to stay on medications for prolonged periods of time because they relapse after drug discontinuation, an argument can be made that benzodiazepines are the most reliable and medically safe agents for long-term therapy. The main drawback to benzodiazepine treatment of panic is that many patients experience a withdrawal syndrome when the medication is discontinued. Withdrawal symptoms can be moderated, but not entirely eliminated, by gradual tapering of the drug. Also, the sedative side effects of benzodiazepines, although usually mild and transient, can be bothersome in treating panic.

Consequently, there is interest in a group of medications called *benzodiazepine partial agonists* that may not have sedative side effects or the same potential for physical dependency as traditional benzodiazepines. These drugs typically potentiate the central nervous system action of the inhibitory neurotransmitter gamma-aminobutyric acid (GABA) by interacting with the benzodiazepine-GABA receptor complex. Some have partial benzodiazepine inverse agonist properties, as are seen with compounds of the beta-carboline class. Suriclone is one such benzodiazepine partial agonist that de Jonghe et al. (1989) compared with lorazepam and placebo in the treatment of a mixed group of patients with GAD and panic disorder. The antipanic effects of suriclone were modest, and more studies are indicated. There have also been preliminary reports of antipanic effects of another benzodiazepine partial agonist, abecarnil, in treating panic ("Promising therapy for anxiety, panic" 1991). Other drugs in this class include bretazenil, CGS-20625, divaplon, and ZK-91296.

Other Classes of Drugs

For theoretical reasons, there has always been interest in the possible effects of antihypertensive drugs in treating panic disorder. Many theorists believe that panic attacks arise because of instability or hyperactivity in the autonomic nervous system, and that antihypertensive drugs generally act either centrally or peripherally to decrease autonomic activity. For the most part, however, antihypertensive drugs have not proven useful in treating panic. Propranolol, a beta-adrenergic receptor–blocking drug, is active both centrally and peripherally. Interestingly, it has not been found useful for treating panic disorder (Munjack et al. 1989). As mentioned earlier, there is evidence that hyperactivity of the noradrenergic system may at least partially cause panic. Clonidine, an alpha2-adrenergic receptor agonist, decreases central noradrenergic tone and does block panic attacks. However, unlike other effective antipanic drugs, patients appear to become tolerant to the effects of clonidine after relatively short periods of time, and panic attacks reoccur. One antihypertensive drug that may be effective in panic disorder is the calcium channel–blocking drug verapamil. In a small but controlled trial, verapamil demonstrated modest antipanic effects (Klein and Uhde 1988). Finally, there is anecdotal evidence that the antihypertensive drug acetazolamide may be effective in blocking panic. This is of theoretical interest because acetazolamide blocks the enzyme crucial to the conversion of carbon dioxide to bicarbonate, and therefore has potentially important effects on respiratory physiology. Some investigators believe that abnormalities in respiratory control are central to the pathogenesis of panic disorder.

It is now clear that stressful life events and cognitive factors play a role in the development of panic disorder. Nevertheless, the sudden and unexpected nature of panic attacks is reminiscent of a seizure, leading investigators to explore the possibility that anticonvulsant medications may be used for panic disorder. In one controlled study, Uhde et al. (1988) found that carbamazepine did not have antipanic effects. There is limited evidence that the GABA agonist valproate may have antipanic efficacy (Roy-Byrne et al. 1989), but this requires further study.

Several other medications deserve mention. Lithium is not useful as the sole agent in treating panic, but may be useful in potentiating the effects of antidepressants when prescribed for panic disorder (Camara 1990). The antidepressant trazodone, which has some 5-HT reuptake blocking effect, was shown in one study to block panic attacks (Mavissakalian et al. 1987), but in another study was found ineffective (Charney et al. 1986). Trazodone generally has not found a place in clinical practice for treating panic disorder. The new antidepressant bupropion appears devoid of antipanic effect (Sheehan et al. 1983). Electroconvulsive therapy is not useful in treating panic. Finally, the antipsychotic medications were originally, and incorrectly, called *major tranquilizers*. This misnomer has occasionally led to their being prescribed for panic disorder. Not only are antipsychotic medications ineffective in treating panic, they may make the panic patient worse.

Summary

In summary, a variety of medications are now being tested for antipanic effect. Some of them, like paroxetine, adinazolam, abecarnil, and gepirone, are investigational whereas others, like fluoxetine, acetazolamide, and valproate, are drugs that are currently marketed for other illnesses but are believed to have utility in blocking panic. These research efforts promise to improve the already excellent success rates in pharmacological blockade of panic.

References

Camara EG: Lithium potentiation of antidepressant treatment in panic disorder. J Clin Psychopharmacol 10:225–227, 1990

Charney DS, Woods SW, Goodman WK, et al: Drug treatment of panic disorder: the comparative efficacy of imipramine, alprazolam, and trazodone. J Clin Psychiatry 47:580–586, 1986

Charney DS, Woods SW: Benzodiazepine treatment of panic disorder: a comparison of alprazolam and lorazepam. J Clin Psychiatry 50:418–423, 1989

Den Boer JA, Westenberg HGM: Serotonin function in panic disorder: a double blind placebo controlled study with fluvoxamine and ritanserin. Psychopharmacology 102:85–94, 1990

de Jonghe F, Swinkels J, Tuynman-Qua H, et al: A comparative study of suriclone, lorazepam, and placebo in anxiety disorder. Pharmacopsychiatry 22:266–271, 1989

Gastfriend DR, Rosenbaum JF: Adjunctive buspirone in benzodiazepine treatment of four patients with panic disorder. Am J Psychiatry 146:914–916, 1989

Gloger S, Grunhaus L, Birmacher B, et al: Treatment of spontaneous panic attacks with clomipramine. Am J Psychiatry 138:1215–1217, 1981

Gorman JM, Liebowitz MR, Fyer AJ, et al: An open trial of fluoxetine in the treatment of panic attacks. J Clin Psychopharmacol 7:258–260, 1987

Herman JB, Brotman AW, Rosenbaum JF: Rebound anxiety in panic disorder patients treated with shorter-acting benzodiazepines. J Clin Psychiatry 48 (suppl):22–26, 1987

Klein E, Uhde TW: Controlled study of verapamil for treatment of panic disorder. Am J Psychiatry 145:431–434, 1988

Mavissakalian M, Perel J, Bowler K, et al: Trazodone in the treatment of panic disorder and agoraphobia with panic attacks. Am J Psychiatry 144:785–787, 1987

Munjack DJ, Crocker B, Cabe D, et al: Alprazolam, propranolol, and placebo in the treatment of panic disorder and agoraphobia with panic attacks. J Clin Psychopharmacol 9:22–27, 1989

Promising therapy for anxiety, panic. Clinical Psychiatry News 19(9):2, 27, 1991

Pyke RE, Greenberg S: Double-blind comparison of alprazolam and adinazolam for panic and phobic disorders. J Clin Psychopharmacol 9:15–21, 1989

Rickels K: Buspirone in clinical practice. J Clin Psychiatry 51 (suppl 9):51–54, 1990

Roy-Byrne PP, Ward NG, Donnelly PJ: Valproate in anxiety and withdrawal syndromes. J Clin Psychiatry 50 (suppl):44–48, 1989

Schneier FR, Liebowitz MR, Davies SO, et al: Fluoxetine in panic disorder. J Clin Psychopharmacol 10(2):119–121, 1990

Schweizer E, Fox I, Case G, et al: Lorazepam versus alprazolam in the treatment of panic disorder. Psychopharmacol Bull 24:224–227, 1988

Sheehan DV, Davidson J, Manschreck T, et al: Lack of efficacy of a new antidepressant (bupropion) in the treatment of panic disorder with phobias. J Clin Psychopharmacol 3:28–31, 1983

Sheehan DV, Zak JP, Miller JA, et al: Panic disorder: the potential role of serotonin reuptake inhibitors. J Clin Psychiatry 49 (suppl 8):30–36, 1988

Sheehan DV, Raj AB, Sheehan KH, et al: Is buspirone effective for panic disorder? J Clin Psychiatry 10:3–11, 1990

Tesar GE: High-potency benzodiazepines for short-term management of panic disorder: the U.S. experience. J Clin Psychiatry 51 (suppl 5):4–10, 1990

Tesar GE, Rosenbaum JF, Pollack MH, et al: Clonazepam versus alprazolam in the treatment of panic disorder: interim analysis of data from a prospective, double-blind, placebo-controlled trial. J Clin Psychiatry 48 (suppl):16–19, 1987

Uhde TW, Stein MB, Post RM: Lack of efficacy of carbamazepine in the treatment of panic disorder. Am J Psychiatry 145:1104–1109, 1988

Chapter 8

Mechanism of Action of Drugs Used in the Pharmacotherapy of Panic Disorder

George R. Heninger, M.D.

Over the past several years, the increased attention given to the anxiety disorders has resulted in the delineation and clarification of many clinical aspects of panic disorder, including the description of its clinical subtypes and its response to pharmacological and behavior treatments (Ballenger 1990a). A great deal of research has been conducted in laboratory animals, control subjects, and patients with panic disorder to clarify the possible neurobiological mechanisms that produce anxiety and panic attacks and the mechanisms involved in the therapeutic action of drugs. An overview of this current research indicates that anxiety symptoms and panic attacks can be generated by the administration of a number of quite different pharmacological, physiological, and environmental stimuli, and that different pharmacological agents are effective in treating patients with panic disorder (Ballenger 1990b). When these data are considered together, their diversity implies that multiple neurobiological mechanisms are involved.

Recent research has demonstrated the importance of several of the brain neurotransmitter systems in the genesis and modulation of anxiety, including the gamma-aminobutyric acid–benzodiazepine (GABA-BZ; Tallman and Gallager 1985), the norepinephrine (NE; Redmond and Huang 1979), the serotonergic (5-hydroxytryptamine [5-HT]; Pecknold 1990), the purinergic (Uhde 1990), and several peptide systems (Bradwejn et al. 1991). Davis (1992) showed that the neurocircuits involved in these neurotransmitter systems are complex, they are connected to each other in both a serial and parallel fashion, and drug effects in one of the systems may interact with other systems to increase or decrease anxiety.

91

A wide range of medical conditions produce symptoms of anxiety, including cardiovascular, respiratory, metabolic, immunological, and neurological disorders. External factors such as diet and drugs have also been known to produce syndromes similar and in many cases identical to those observed in patients diagnosed with idiopathic panic disorder. The large number of medical diagnostic labels for anxiety and anxiety disorders reflects the heterogeneity and nonspecificity of the anxiety symptoms; this diversity may be related to the complexity and interconnectedness of the neurobiological systems regulating anxiety.

The pharmacological treatments for panic disorder have direct or indirect effects on many neurotransmitter systems, including those mentioned above. The neurobiological mechanisms known to be involved in the regulation of these systems are very complex; due to space limitations, only a brief description of the neurotransmitter systems affected by drugs used to treat panic disorder can be given.

The Gamma-Aminobutyric Acid–Benzodiazepine System

Up to 30% of the neurons in the brain use the GABA-BZ transmitter system, which primarily involves the smaller interneurons. The widespread use, broad efficacy, and rapid onset of benzodiazepines in the treatment of anxiety and panic disorder demonstrate the importance of the GABA-BZ system (Tallman and Gallager 1985). It is of considerable importance that, in both humans and laboratory animals, benzodiazepine agonists have been demonstrated to be anxiolytic, whereas the inverse agonists are anxiogenic (Braestrup 1982).

The GABA-BZ receptor complex can be altered in two directions by different drugs. Those drugs that increase chloride flux are called *agonists,* and those that produce a net decrease in chloride flux are called *inverse agonists. Antagonists* are in the middle, producing no change in chloride flux, but they do block the effects of both the agonists and the inverse agonists. It has been clearly shown in many animals studies (e.g., Braestrup 1982; Ninan et al. 1982) that the agonists are anxiolytic and that the inverse agonists are anxiogenic.

Some data indicate that panic disorder patients may have an abnormality in the GABA-BZ system because they appear to be subsensitive to some of the agonist effects of benzodiazepines, and because antagonists that have been shown to produce no effects in control subjects appear to be mildly anxiogenic in patients with panic disorder (Darragh et al. 1983; Woods et al. 1990). This insensitivity suggests that there may be a shift in the GABA-BZ receptor complex to an inverse agonist configuration or that panic disorder patients may have an endogenous benzodiazepine-like compound that is blocked by antagonists, thus producing anxiety. Chronic stress can shift the GABA-BZ complex to a more inverse agonist–type configuration so that animals that have failed to cope with repeated shocks are more vulnerable to seizures (Davis 1992). The ability of stress to shift the GABA-BZ complex to this type of configuration may be what is seen when environmental stresses affect the functioning of this system in patients with panic disorder or other stress-related clinical conditions, such as posttraumatic stress disorder (PTSD) or depression.

The important role of the GABA-BZ system in panic disorder can be demonstrated by administering different benzodiazepines to reverse the anxiety and panic symptoms produced in panic disorder patients and control subjects by numerous anxiogenic and panicogenic drugs or stimuli. In all instances, the administration of a benzodiazepine to either control subjects or patients blocked the anxiogenic effect of these procedures (Charney and Heninger 1985).

The major liability to using benzodiazepines to treat anxiety and panic disorder is the development of side effects, such as sedation, and the long-term development of tolerance, dependence, and withdrawal liability (Gallager et al. 1988). Recent research with laboratory animals (Tallman and Gallager 1985) has demonstrated that benzodiazepines have multiple anxiolytic, sedative-hypnotic, anticonvulsive, and muscle relaxant properties. There is new evidence that these specific behavioral effects of benzodiazepines may be produced by stimulation of different benzodiazepine receptor subtypes. Because the molecular biology of the benzodiazepine receptor complex has many different subunits, which can result in a large number of different receptor subtypes, current research suggests that drugs may be developed that are specific to one behavioral effect without producing another (e.g., producing an anxiolytic effect without the sedative-hypnotic, anticonvulsive, or muscle relaxant effects). It is possible that with the proper development of drugs that react with specific receptor subtypes, treatment can be more accurately directed at specific symptoms without the liabilities of the sedative and addictive properties of these compounds.

The Norepinephrine System

There is a great deal of evidence, primarily from studies with laboratory animals, that the NE system is involved in the symptomatic expression of anxiety. The NE system is one of the primary systems involved in the flight-or-fight reaction, and agonists of the epinephrine and NE system that primarily act outside the brain can produce anxiety and panic attacks (Pohl et al. 1990). Drugs that block the alpha2-receptors also produce anxiety and panic attacks (Charney et al. 1984). The alpha2-adrenergic receptor system is located on cell bodies and terminals of NE neurons; when stimulated, it reduces the rate of cell firing and the amount of norepinephrine released (Cedarbaum and Aghajanian 1977). When the alpha2-receptors are blocked, there is increased cell firing and increased norepinephrine release. Drugs that are effective in the long-term treatment of panic disorder, such as imipramine and monoamine oxidase inhibitors (MAOIs), have been found to reduce alpha2-adrenergic receptor sensitivity in both laboratory animals and patients with panic disorder.

The most prominent cell group in the brain containing norepinephrine is the locus coeruleus (LC), whose axons project widely to most brain areas, where they make contact with a large variety of other neurons in the cerebral cortex, hippocampus, other limbic system structures, the thalamus, and the midbrain. The firing rate and norepinephrine release of these neurons is regulated by a variety of other receptors in addition to presynaptic alpha2-receptors. Inhibitory inputs to the LC include serotonin, opiate receptors, and GABA-BZ receptors. There are also numerous excitatory inputs to the LC, including acetylcholine, substance P, corticotropin-releasing factor (CRF), and other peptides and excitatory amino acids. A number of stimuli have been shown to increase the firing rate of the LC, including hypoglycemia, noxious and non-noxious sensory stimuli, autonomic effects (e.g., distension of the stomach, bladder, or colon), hypoglycemia, reduced blood pressure or blood volume, hypercapnia (increased CO_2), thermoregulatory change, and stress or threat from the environment (Redmond and Huang 1979).

Thus LC function is one of the important regulators and modulators of input from the NE system to other brain areas that could increase or decrease anxiety. When recordings are made from the LC in laboratory animals placed in fearful situations, (e.g., a cat exposed to a dog), there is a fourfold increase in the firing rate of the LC neurons (Abercrombie and Jacobs 1987). Mild stimulation of this system in monkeys produces behaviors that appear to be related to anxiety, such as eye scanning, grasping and clutching, and head and body turning. When lesions are produced in the LC of monkeys, they demonstrate a loss of emotional aspects of fear, such as a slow retreat from threats; there is also increased approach and eye contact with higher ranking monkeys and humans, which is normally an anxiogenic response (Redmond et al. 1976). The LC system has also been shown to be sensitive to chronic stress as animals exposed to inescapable shock are more sensitive to drugs that increase LC firing (Weiss and Uhde 1990).

The pharmacology of the LC system has been used to study the role of the NE system in panic disorder. The drug yohimbine increases blood pressure and the production of 3-methoxy-4-hydroxyphenylglycol (MHPG), a metabolite of NE in plasma. By blocking the alpha$_2$-adrenergic receptor with yohimbine, an increase in LC firing in animals can be demonstrated (Cedarbaum and Aghajanian 1977). Charney et al. (1984) showed that, when panic disorder patients are given yohimbine, a subgroup of them experience a panic attack. The patients having a panic attack show an increased level of MHPG in the plasma as well as increased ratings of anxiety, increased blood pressure, and release of the stress hormone cortisol. In contrast, stimulation with the alpha$_2$-agonist clonidine produces decreases in blood pressure and MHPG. Charney and Heninger (1986) demonstrated that, when panic disorder patients are given clonidine, there is blunting of the sedation response to clonidine and a greater fall in blood pressure and plasma MHPG. A consistent finding across all studies has been a blunted growth hormone response to the clonidine. Taken together, these data suggest that there is a possible abnormality in the regulation of the alpha$_2$-adrenergic system in panic disorder. The increased responsiveness to yohimbine may be specific to patients with panic disorder because it is not seen in other psychiatric diagnostic groups (Charney et al. 1990). The anxiety ratings and changes in MHPG in the panic disorder patients (who have a panic attack following yohimbine) are increased in comparison with patients with generalized anxiety disorder, depression, obsessive-compulsive disorder, or schizophrenia.

Cerebral blood flow has been monitored following yohimbine administration using single photon emission computed tomography (SPECT) in an attempt to more directly evaluate the sensitivity of the alpha$_2$-adrenergic system in the brains of patients with panic disorder. In their study using SPECT, Woods et al. (1988a) measured blood flow following yohimbine, and compared changes in the panic disorder patients with those in control subjects. Their findings demonstrated that yohimbine produced an approximately 10% decrease in cerebral blood flow in the panic disorder patients, whereas yohimbine produced no change in the control subjects. This outcome is consistent with those in a number of studies using laboratory animals where stimulation of the LC produced a decrease in cerebral blood flow. Thus the data suggest that panic disorder patients are abnormally sensitive to the effects of yohimbine, which increases output from the NE systems.

Southwick et al. (1993) studied patients with PTSD following yohimbine administration. Yohimbine produced panic attacks in 70% and flashbacks in 40% of the PTSD patients. The patients with the yohimbine-induced panic attacks had a greater yohimbine-induced increase in plasma MHPG, blood pressure, and heart rate than control subjects given yohimbine. In addition, yohimbine induced significant increases in PTSD symptoms as well as intrusive traumatic thoughts, emotional numbing, and grief. Thus, in another disorder where panic disorder is a frequent comorbid condition, the importance of the NE system in producing paniclike symptoms can be demonstrated.

Evidence for increased NE system function in high anxiety or paniclike states has not been seen in all studies, however. When panic disorder patients were given caffeine, which produces panic attacks, Uhde (1990) found no consistent change in MHPG. Similarly, when patients were given carbon dioxide or lactate, which produce panic attacks, there was again no change in the plasma level or MHPG (Carr et al. 1986; Woods et al. 1988b). It is possible that the panic attacks following administration of carbon dioxide and lactate were too transient to produce enough brain MHPG that would be observable in plasma. However, anxiety symptoms following caffeine consumption last for some hours, yet MHPG changes were still not seen. Thus MHPG may not be a sensitive indicator of the status of the brain NE system in all instances.

Drugs that affect the NE system, such as the NE uptake inhibitors (e.g., imipramine) and MAOIs, have been shown to be efficacious in the treatment of panic disorder. Because imipramine has both NE and 5-HT uptake inhibitory properties, it has not been possible to separate out clearly which of these two actions is more responsible for the antipanic effect. When Charney et al. (1986) studied patients over time, comparing their clinical response to imipramine with their response to alprazolam, the authors found that alprazolam acted within 1 or 2 days, whereas imipramine took much longer (4–5 weeks) to reach the equivalent clinical efficacy of alprazolam. Thus patients get a much more rapid relief of their anxiety and panic disorder symptoms following treatment with alprazolam or similar benzodiazepines. The NE uptake inhibitors, such as imipramine, take a longer period of time to work, although the NE uptake inhibitors and MAOIs do not have the tolerance and withdrawal liabilities of the benzodiazepines.

The Serotonergic System

The specific 5-HT uptake inhibitors, including fluvoxamine and fluoxetine, have been shown to be effective in treating panic disorder (Pecknold 1990). There is considerable evidence that the 5-HT system modulates anxiety in laboratory animals; a number of interactions between the 5-HT and noradrenergic system are known. (The anxiolytic effects of drugs that act on the 5-HT$_{1A}$ receptor system are described in detail in Chapter 7 of this volume.) Charney et al. (1990) found that the 5-HT agonists fenfluramine and m-chlorophenylpiperazine (MCPP) produced panic attacks in some susceptible individuals, but the precursors for 5-

HT—tryptophan and 5-hydroxytryptophan—did not produce panic attacks. This finding suggested a possible postsynaptic 5-HT supersensitivity related to panic disorder. The long-term administration of 5-HT uptake inhibitors or MAOI drugs could correct this putative supersensitive mechanism.

In a recent study by Goddard et al. (1990) in which yohimbine was given to patients before and after fluvoxamine treatment, it was found that fluvoxamine blunted the anxiogenic effects of yohimbine. In a control group treated with placebo, yohimbine was just as anxiogenic after placebo treatment as it was before. Fluvoxamine treatment, however, did not block the cortisol or the MHPG response to yohimbine, suggesting that the anxiolytic effects of fluvoxamine may involve actions on neuron systems outside the LC system. The 5-HT uptake inhibitors could be working at terminal sites such as the cortex, whereas the effects of benzodiazepines and drugs such as imipramine are much broader, involving both cortical and subcortical areas.

The results of another recent study by Cassano et al. (1988) have suggested that chlorimipramine is more effective in reducing panic attacks than treatment with imipramine. Because chlorimipramine has more 5-HT uptake properties than imipramine, this may be additional evidence that the 5-HT uptake inhibitors are more efficacious in treating panic disorder than those with NE uptake inhibitor properties. Currently, there is reliable evidence that the 5-HT uptake inhibitors are a viable and important treatment for panic disorder.

Neuropeptide Systems

The role of neuropeptide systems in panic disorder is being increasingly investigated, but treatment effects on these systems have not been studied. Cholecystokinin (CCK) is a small peptide located in many brain areas that appears relevant to anxiety. When CCK is administered to panic disorder patients, it produces panic attacks. In a study by Bradwejn et al. (1991; see Table 8–1), CCK was found to have a dose-related effect on panic symptoms in control subjects; at 25 µg, CCK produced panic in 17% of control subjects, 91% of panic disorder patients, and 92% of panic disorder patients with agoraphobia. At dosages of 0.6 µg/kg, pentagastrin, a slightly larger peptide, produced panic attacks in 100% of panic disorder patients but only 25% of control subjects. Thus CCK appears to be one of the more active stimulants for panic. Treatments to alter the responsiveness of the CCK receptor system are just now being started.

There is a blunted adrenocorticotropic hormone (ACTH) response to CRF infusion in patients with panic disorder (Gold et al. 1990). Blunting of ACTH would suggest that there is an increase in brain CRF in panic disorder. In laboratory animals CRF has been shown to be clearly anxiogenic. Specific antagonists to CRF have not yet been developed for human use, but some have been used in animals and have been shown to be anxiolytic (Sutton et al. 1982). Certainly as time progresses and research improves the understanding of these peptide systems, new treatments to reduce panic attacks in panic disorder patients will become increasingly available.

Neuroanatomical Aspects of Anxiety

There is considerable evidence from work in laboratory animals that the central nucleus of the amygdala is an important final common pathway involved in producing many of the behavioral and autonomic effects of anxiety (Davis 1992). There are many inputs to this brain nucleus from a variety of sensory systems, including the hippocampus, cerebral cortex, and limbic system. When this nucleus is stimulated, many of the autonomic and behavioral effects are similar to those observed in "anxious" animals. Abnormalities in panic disorder patients have been shown in the temporal lobe near the amygdala, and it has been shown through metabolic imaging studies that control subjects who become anxious show activation of the temporal lobe close to the amygdala (Reiman 1990). (The question of whether this is an artifact related to teeth clenching is currently being

Table 8–1. Panic-inducing effects of cholecystokinin (CCK)-like peptides

Subject group	Percentage of incidence of induced panic (number of subjects)			
	CCK (9 µg)	CCK (25 µg)	CCK (50 µg)	Pentagastrin (0.6 µg/kg)
Control subjects	11 (1/9)	17 (2/12)	47 (7/15)	25 (1/4)
Panic disorder patients		91 (10/11)		100 (5/5)
Panic disorder patients with agoraphobia		92 (11/12)		

Source. Adapted from Bradwejn et al. 1990.

investigated.) It has been well known for a considerable period of time that temporal lobe epilepsy has a major anxiety component. All of this taken together suggests that the neural pathways involving the amygdala and nearby areas could be critically important in the genesis of anxiety and panic attacks. Current research is focusing on drugs that modulate neural transmission in this area in order to more clearly understand the possible mechanisms involved that could serve as the basis for new treatments for panic disorder.

Summary

As has been briefly reviewed above, many pharmacological agents are anxiogenic, and thus any neurobiological theory of the pathogenesis of panic disorder must take into account the variety of possible neurobiological factors involved. A possible integrated model involving GABA-BZ system modulation of the NE and 5-HT systems, including peptide neural transmitter input to hippocampus and amygdala function, could be proposed. Such a model could account for the anxiogenic effects of the pharmacological stimuli and the anxiolytic effects of the treatments for panic disorder. The critical feature of such a model would be the multiple pathways involved in the pathogenesis of anxiety and panic disorder. Parts of this model can be tested through animal studies, which would allow the development of new drugs for the treatment of anxiety disorders and panic disorder. The most promising developments are in the molecular biology of receptor subunit cloning and the construction of a variety of receptor subtypes in the relevant neurotransmitter systems. This direction offers high promise for a much more rapid and specific development of drugs that would treat the symptoms of anxiety without producing unwanted side effects or the negative effects of tolerance and withdrawal.

The benzodiazepines are the most efficacious treatments for anxiety and panic disorder. However, the physical dependence and withdrawal stemming from long-term treatment with these drugs are a major liability. The recent reports of marked symptom reduction and long-term efficacy of behavior treatments need to be integrated into this model. It will be important to conduct neurobiological studies in patients treated by behavioral means to assess whether behavior treatment blocks the anxiogenic effects of panic-producing substances such as yohimbine, carbon dioxide, and lactate. If the behavior treatment is able to produce this type of blockade, we would have an important clue as to how the behavior treatment may be working. The long-term efficacy in terms of symptom reduction and overall behavioral and personal functioning needs continuous evaluation for both the pharmacological and behavior treatments. This type of evaluation will lead to a clearer understanding of the mechanisms involved, which could then generate the development of better treatments.

Because the pharmacological treatments are thought to mostly block symptom expression at a secondary level, future research should increasingly investigate the more fundamental molecular biological abnormalities involved. Onset of panic disorder occurs early in life (in the teens and early 20s), and there is a marked drop-off in the number of panic disorder patients after age 40. Thus the prevalence of panic disorder is markedly decreased after age 45. The role of stress- and age-related factors relevant to the development and maintenance of panic disorder through the young adult years needs to be much more carefully researched and understood. Only through the delineation of the mechanisms responsible for the onset of panic disorder in these young people can eventual preventive treatments be developed. It is through an improved understanding of the pathogenesis of panic disorder from the molecular level up through the biochemical, physiological, and symptomatic levels that more effective and preventive treatments will become available.

References

Abercrombie ED, Jacobs BL: Single-unit response of noradrenergic neurons in the locus coeruleus of freely moving cats, I: acutely presented stressful and nonstressful stimuli. J Neurosci 7:2837–2843, 1987

Ballenger JC (ed): Clinical Aspects of Panic Disorder: Frontiers of Clinical Neuroscience. Edited by Ballenger JC. New York, Alan R Liss, 1990a

Ballenger JC (ed): Neurobiology of Panic Disorder: Frontiers of Clinical Neuroscience. New York, Alan R Liss, 1990b

Bradwejn J, Koszycki D, Shriqui C: Enhanced sensitivity to cholecystokinin tetrapeptide in panic disorder: clinical and behavioral findings. Arch Gen Psychiatry 48:603–610, 1991

Braestrup C: Neurotransmitters and CNS disease. Lancet 1:1030–1034, 1982

Carr DB, Sheehan DV, Surman OS, et al: Neuroendocrine correlates of lactate-induced anxiety and their response to chronic alprazolam therapy. Am J Psychiatry 143:483–494, 1986

Cassano GB, Petraca A, Perugi G, et al: Clomipramine for panic disorder: the first 10 weeks of a long-term comparison with imipramine. J Affect Disord 14:123–127, 1988

Cedarbaum JM, Aghajanian GK: Catecholamine receptors on locus coeruleus: pharmacologic characterization. Eur J Pharmacol 44:375–385, 1977

Charney DS, Heninger GR: Noradrenergic function and the mechanism of action of anti-anxiety treatment, I: the effect of long-term alprazolam treatment. Arch Gen Psychiatry 42:458–462, 1985

Charney DS, Heninger GR: Abnormal regulation of noradrenergic function in panic disorders: effects of clonidine in healthy subjects and patients with agoraphobia and panic disorder. Arch Gen Psychiatry 43:1042–1054, 1986

Charney DS, Heninger GR, Brier A: Noradrenergic function in panic anxiety: effects of yohimbine in healthy subjects and patients with agoraphobia and panic disorder. Arch Gen Psychiatry 41:751–763, 1984

Charney DS, Woods SW, Goodman WK, et al: Drug treatment of panic disorder: the comparative efficacy of imipramine, alprazolam and trazodone. J Clin Psychiatry 47:580–586, 1986

Charney DS, Woods SW, Goodman W, et al: Serotonin function in anxiety, II: effects of the serotonin agonist, MCPP, in panic disorder patients, and healthy subjects. Psychopharmacology (Berl) 92:14–23, 1987

Charney DS, Woods SW, Krystal JH, et al: Neurobiological mechanisms of human anxiety, in The Biological Basis of Psychiatric Treatment, Vol 3. Edited by Pohl R, Gershon S. Basel, Switzerland, Karger, 1990, pp 242–283

Darragh A, Lambe R, Kenny M, et al: Tolerance of healthy volunteers to intravenous administration of the benzodiazepine antagonist Ro 15-1788. Eur J Clin Pharmacol 24:569–570, 1983

Davis M: The role of the amygdala in conditioned fear, in The Amygdala: Neurobiological Aspects of Emotion, Memory, and Mental Dysfunction. Edited by Aggleton JP. New York, Wiley-Liss, 1992, pp 255–306

Gallager DW, Heninger, C, Wilson MA: Chronic benzodiazepine agonist exposure and its consequences of GABA-benzodiazepine interactions, in Allosteric Modulation of Amino Acid Receptors: Therapeutic Implications. Edited by Barnard EA, Costa E. New York, Raven, 1988, pp 91–108

Goddard A, Charney D, Heninger GR, et al: Effects of the 5HT reuptake inhibitor fluvoxamine on anxiety induced by yohimbine (#487.1). Society for Neuroscience Abstracts 16:1177, 1990

Gold PW, Pigott T, Kling M, et al: Hypothalamic-pituitary-adrenal axis in panic disorder, in Neurobiology of Panic Disorder: Frontiers of Clinical Neuroscience. Edited by Ballenger JC. New York, Alan R Liss, 1990, pp 313–320

Ninan PT, Insel TR, Cohen RM, et al: Benzodiazepine receptor–mediated experimental "anxiety" in primates. Science 218:1332–1334, 1982

Pecknold JC: Serotonin abnormalities in panic disorder, in Neurobiology of Panic Disorder: Frontiers of Clinical Neuroscience. Edited by Ballenger JC. New York, Alan R Liss, 1990, pp 121–142

Pohl R, Yeragani V, Balon R, et al: Isoproterenol-induced panic: a beta-adrenergic model of panic anxiety, in Neurobiology of Panic Disorder: Frontiers of Clinical Neuroscience. Edited by Ballenger JC. New York, Alan R Liss, 1990

Redmond DE, Huang YH: New evidence for a locus coeruleus–norepinephrine connection with anxiety. Life Sci 25:2149–2162, 1979

Redmond DE, Huang YG, Snyder DR, et al: Behavioral changes following lesions of the locus coeruleus in macaca arctoides. Neuroscience Abstracts 1:472, 1976

Reiman EM: PET, panic disorder, and normal anticipatory anxiety, in Neurobiology of Panic Disorder: Frontiers of Clinical Neuroscience. Edited by Ballenger JC. New York, Alan R Liss, 1990, pp 245–270

Southwick SM, Krystal JH, Morgan CA, et al: Abnormal noradrenergic function in posttraumatic stress disorder. Arch Gen Psychiatry 50:266–274, 1993

Sutton RE, Koob GF, LeMoal M, et al: Corticotropin releasing factor produces behavioral activation in rats. Nature 297:331–333, 1982

Tallman JF, Gallager DW: The GABA-ergic system: a locus of benzodiazepine action. Annu Rev Neurosci 8:21–44, 1985

Uhde TW: Caffeine provocation in panic: a focus on biological mechanisms, in Neurobiology of Panic Disorder: Frontiers of Clinical Neuroscience. Edited by Ballenger JC. New York, Alan R Liss, 1990, pp 219–244

Weiss SB, Uhde TW: Animal models of anxiety, in Neurobiology of Panic Disorder: Frontiers of Clinical Neuroscience. Edited by Ballenger JC. New York, Alan R Liss, 1990, pp 3–30

Woods SW, Koster K, Krystal J, et al: Yohimbine alters regional cerebral blood flow in panic disorder. Lancet 2:678, 1988a

Woods SW, Charney DS, Goodman WK, et al: Carbon dioxide-induced anxiety: behavioral, physiologic and biochemical effects of 5% CO_2 in panic disorder patients and 5 and 7.5% CO_2 in healthy subjects. Arch Gen Psychiatry 45:43–52, 1988b

Woods SW, Charney DS, Silver JM, et al: Behavioral, biochemical and cardiovascular responses to the benzodiazepine receptor antagonist flumazenil in panic disorder. Psychiatry Res 36:115–127, 1990

Psychological Treatments of Panic Disorder

Effectiveness of Behavior Treatment for Panic Disorder With and Without Agoraphobia

David H. Barlow, Ph.D.

Treating Agoraphobia

Establishing the Effectiveness of Exposure-Based Treatment

As late as the 1960s, there were no proven effective psychological treatments for agoraphobia or panic. In fact, early behavior therapists, reflecting the tenor of the times, were reluctant to ask agoraphobic patients to expose themselves to any fear-provoking situations that might cause anything more than minimal anxiety in case the patients might be harmed. Although evidence had begun to accumulate that systematic desensitization was effective with simple phobic patients, in studies confined to agoraphobic patients this technique had not proven more effective than traditional psychotherapy; furthermore, overall improvements were small with both approaches (Barlow 1988; Emmelkamp 1982; Gelder and Marks 1966; Marks 1971).

In the mid-1960s, Agras et al. (1968) experimented with encouraging agoraphobic patients to expose themselves to real-life frightening situations. Since that time, investigators around the world have clearly demonstrated that exposure in vivo is the central ingredient in the behavior treatment of agoraphobia, and that this process is substantially more effective than any number of credible alternative psychotherapeutic procedures (Emmelkamp 1982; Marks 1987; Mathews et al. 1981; Mavissakalian and Barlow 1981; O'Brien and Barlow 1984). In the few studies in which in vivo exposure was not shown to be advantageous, either exposure in vivo was not the prime therapeutic modality (Klein et al. 1983) or treatment comparisons were confounded because patients were systematically encouraged to practice in vivo exposure in their home environment between sessions in all comparison groups (Mathews et al. 1976). In subsequent experiments, where this confounding factor was controlled for, results of systematic in vivo exposure became readily apparent (Greist et al. 1980; Leitenberg et al. 1970; Telch et al. 1985). The effectiveness of exposure-based procedures is also indirectly supported by the well-documented observation that agoraphobic patients do not improve over time without treatment. This phenomenon was first demonstrated by Agras et al. (1972), who followed a group of agoraphobic patients for 5 years before exposure-based treatment was widely available. No improvement was observed in the absence of treatment.

Demonstrating effectiveness of a psychotherapeutic procedure in controlled outcome studies is not the same as estimating the extent of that effectiveness with individual patients (i.e., the *clinical significance* of the treatment). Estimates of this measure of effectiveness in the behavior treatment of agoraphobia have been available for some time. They have indicated that the effects of exposure-based treatments are relatively consistent over a number of different studies conducted by clinicians in various parts of the world. The best estimates of outcome, when subjects who dropped out were excluded, have indicated that 60%–75% of agoraphobic patients completing treatment showed some clinical benefit (Barlow 1988; Clum 1989; Jansson and Öst 1982; Michelson and Marchione 1991). In an early review, Jansson and Öst (1982) summarized the clinical effectiveness based on 24 separate studies of exposure procedures (see Table 9–1). Subsequent meta-analyses by Trull et al. (1988) and Jacobson et al. (1988), in which the effects of exposure-based modalities were examined, arrived at similar conclusions. As with all treatments, attrition—averaging approximately 15% across a large number of studies—also subtracted from estimates of clinical effectiveness when all

Table 9–1. Outcome as global clinical ratings of exposure treatments for agoraphobia based on 24 studies at follow-up of at least 5 months (range 5 months to 5 years)

Improved (%)		Dropouts (%)	
Median	Range	Median	Range
70	58–83	12	0–35

Source. Reprinted from Jansson L, Öst LG: "Behavioral Treatments for Agoraphobia: An Evaluative Review." *Clinical Psychology Review* 2:311–336, 1982. Used with permission.

patients who began treatment were considered.

During the late 1970s and 1980s, after the effectiveness of exposure treatment had been established, a large number of studies were conducted on the optimal manner of administering exposure-based treatments. The major issues included the intensity of the treatment, the importance of the presence of a therapist, the addition of anxiety-reducing procedures such as relaxation and distraction, and other variables (see Barlow 1988 for a review). Generally, findings indicated that gradual, self-paced exposure seemed to have some advantages over more intensive exposure of a long duration in that attrition rates were reduced, excessive dependence on the therapist did not occur, and improvement continued after the end of treatment. In addition, and perhaps most importantly, intensive in vivo exposure was associated with a higher relapse rate than less intensive treatments (Hafner 1976; Jansson and Öst 1982), although there may be some qualifications to this conclusion (Chambless 1990; see also below). Several studies also suggested that minimal therapist involvement seemed sufficient to effect clinical improvement, unless patients were severely impaired, in which case more intensive therapeutic assistance was necessary (Ghosh and Marks 1987; Holden et al. 1983).

Follow-up studies of agoraphobic patients undergoing exposure-based treatment have revealed that clinically significant effects are maintained or even enhanced over long periods, particularly when treatment was more gradual and self-paced. A number of studies indicated that gains were maintained for periods of 4 years or more (Emmelkamp and Kuipers 1979; Jansson and Öst 1982; McPherson et al. 1980; Munby and Johnston 1980). Other follow-up studies confirmed this result (Burns et al. 1986; Cohen et al. 1984; Jansson et al. 1986). Jansson et al. (1986) added a formal program of maintenance exercises and noticed that an increasing percentage of patients participating in this program improved to a clinically significant degree at 7- and 15-month follow-up compared with those not receiving it. The authors concluded that a maintenance program of self-exposure to feared situations over at least 6 months following initial treatment would ensure continued improvement or preservation of treatment gains.

Improving Exposure-Based Treatments

Despite the gratifying results noted above, investigators have recognized the limitations of exposure-based procedures. Attrition rates have already been mentioned, although these can be ameliorated to some extent by careful introduction of the treatment and less intense, self-paced, exposure-based methods. Reported success rates of 60%–75% reflect the fact that 25%–40% of agoraphobic patients who complete treatment fail to benefit to any significant degree. A substantial percentage of the remaining 60%–75% may not reach clinically meaningful levels of functioning. For example, Marks (1971) reported that only 3 of 65 patients (4.6%) were completely symptom-free at 4-year follow-up. Mcpherson et al. (1980) reported that among patients who showed some improvement following behavior treatment, only 18% rated themselves as being completely free of symptoms. Typically, residual symptomatology in the forms of anticipatory anxiety, avoidance, and panic attacks was not uncommon (Michelson and Marchione 1991). In summary, exposure treatments are effective interventions for panic disorder with agoraphobia and the results are maintained over time, but many people do not benefit and many of those who do benefit are left with residual symptoms.

During the 1980s, several investigators experimented with additions to or substantial modifications of typical exposure-based procedures with the goal of enhancing effectiveness. Three of those innovations are briefly reviewed here.

One of the most dramatic innovations occurred in Germany where Fiegenbaum (1988) developed a 3- to 6-day intensive therapy program of almost continuous exposure involving travel by overnight train across Europe. During the trip considerable time was scheduled in crowded squares, on the tops of cathedral towers, and on cable cars riding to some of the highest mountains in Germany. In Fiegenbaum's hands, this dramatic treatment resulted in substantial improvement in 96% of his patients, with 76% reported as completely symptom-free at 5-year follow-up. This outcome is significantly better than a standard, graded-exposure approach, and the treatment used does not seem to be associated with a greater number of patients who drop out or refuse treatment. However, Fiegenbaum's results would have to be replicated in other centers as it seems unlikely that patients in other settings would readily accept this particular treatment approach.

The second, more extensively studied variation of the exposure format is one that includes the patient's spouse or partner in treatment. This type of treatment is part of a growing trend of incorporating the interpersonal system of the patient into treatment and is used with a number of disorders, such as alcoholism (McCrady 1985) and depression (Beach et al. 1990). In one study, Barlow et al. (1984) found that a group of agoraphobic patients treated with their spouses contained a significantly greater number of treatment responders at posttreatment (86%) than a group treated without their spouses (43%) (see Table 9–2). In a follow-up study of these patients, Cerny et al. (1987) found that the spouse group evidenced an increasingly more positive response than the nonspouse group at 1- and 2-year follow-ups, thus augmenting the between-group differences originally observed at posttreatment (see Table 9–3 and Figure 9–1). The fact that patients treated in the spouse-assisted format continued to improve across the follow-up period is consistent with the findings of several other studies in which patients treated with their spouses or significant others showed enhanced long-term functioning (Hand et al. 1974; Jannoun et al. 1980; Mathews et al. 1977; Munby and Johnston 1980).

In another well-controlled study pertaining to the inclusion of spouses in the treatment of panic disorder patients with agoraphobia, Arnow et al. (1985) evaluated whether the provision of an additional treatment component composed of a communications skills training package would significantly enhance treatment gains derived from a standard spouse-assisted, exposure protocol. At both posttreatment and 8-month follow-up, the authors found that patients treated in a communications training module showed a significantly greater response than a comparison group treated without the module. Based on the above-discussed results, further investigation into how incorporating patients' interpersonal systems into their treatment facilitates that treatment is warranted.

In the third innovation of exposure-based treatment, Michelson et al. (1989) compared a group of patients who had a cognitive therapy component added to their treatment with a group receiving graded exposure plus relaxation and another group receiving graded exposure only. At 3-month follow-up, the percentage of patients meeting a high end-state criterion was 87.5% in the group receiving a cognitive component, compared with only 47% in the group receiving relaxation combined with exposure, and 65% in the group receiving exposure alone. The results of many other studies have also suggested that enhanced benefit is gained by adding a cognitive component to exposure-based treatments (Barlow 1988); the method used in the Michelson et al. (1989) study provides a transition to newer cognitive-behavior approaches that target panic directly.

Treating Panic

Despite the above-discussed innovations, the results from exposure-based treatments remain less than satisfactory. As was already noted, improvement rates

Table 9–2. Treatment responders and nonresponders in spouse and nonspouse groups

	Responders	Nonresponders
Spouse	12	2
Nonspouse	6	8

Source. Reprinted from Barlow DH, O'Brien GT, Last CG: "Couples Treatment of Agoraphobia." *Behavior Therapy* 15:41–58, 1984. Used with permission.

from most studies indicated that the majority of patients (approximately 80%) are not cured and that a substantial minority (approximately 35%) fail to receive any substantial benefit whatsoever. When a spouse is systematically included in the treatment, the rates of clinical improvement seem to increase from approximately 65% to 90% (Arnow et al. 1985; Barlow et al. 1984; Mathews et al. 1977) and attrition is reduced, dropping to a rate of approximately 5% (Barlow 1988); however, the cure rate is still low.

Development of Panic Control Treatment

During the 1980s, psychologically oriented clinicians increasingly realized that exposure-based treatments concentrated on agoraphobic avoidance but ignored what had come to be considered the central feature of panic disorder with agoraphobia—panic attacks (Barlow 1988). Within this same time period, we (Barlow and Craske 1989) developed a cognitive-behavior protocol designed to target panic attacks directly. At the heart of this treatment program, referred to as *panic control treatment* (PCT), is systematic, structured exposure to feared internal sensations. While developing this approach, we devised a variety of ways to elicit feared internal sensations in the office, including sensations of depersonalization

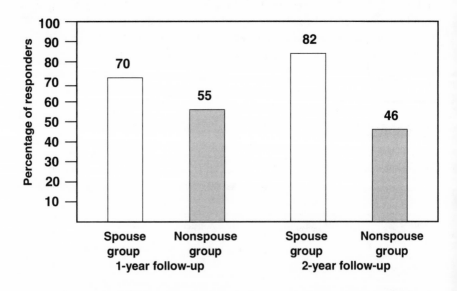

Figure 9–1. Percentage of participants in spouse and nonspouse treatment groups classified as responders at 1- and 2-year follow-up.

Table 9–3. Average client scores at posttreatment and 1- and 2-year follow-up for spouse and nonspouse groups: phobia measures

| | Spouse group | | | | | | Nonspouse group | | | | | |
| | Posttreatment | | 1-year follow-up | | 2-year follow-up | | Posttreatment | | 1-year follow-up | | 2-year follow-up | |
Variable name	Mean	N	Mean	N	Mean	N	Mean	N	Mean	N	Mean	N
Clinical rating	3.56 (1.60)	27	3.30 (1.35)	23	2.85 (1.56)	17	3.89 (1.72)	14	4.81 (1.86)	14	4.37 (1.56)	14
Agoraphobia subscale	17.33 (8.62)	27	13.78 (6.54)	18	11.88 (8.51)	17	20.17 (8.28)	12	21.79 (11.68)	12	20.80 (14.13)	5
Phobia self-rating	3.50 (1.10)	24	2.81 (1.51)	18	2.53 (1.63)	17	3.50 (1.73)	12	4.04 (2.55)	12	2.80 (1.10)	5

Note. Standard deviations appear in parentheses.
Source. Adapted from Cerny JA, Barlow DH, Craske M, et al.: "Couples Treatment of Agoraphobia: A Two-Year Follow-Up." *Behavior Therapy* 18:401–415, 1987. Used with permission.

and derealization. To this basic strategy we added a strong cognitive therapy component as well as a breathing retraining module.[1]

In this section I discuss studies that used PCT in treating panic disorder patients. To aid in examining the specificity of the PCT approach, all the studies I review are ones that targeted panic disorder patients who did not have substantial agoraphobic avoidance.

In open clinical trials, preliminary results from our protocol (Barlow et al. 1984) suggested significant improvement on all measures. More importantly, these treatment gains were maintained and even strengthened during an average follow-up period of 1 year. Gitlin et al. (1985) treated 11 patients with a similar approach and found 10 free of panic at postassessment as well as 5 months later. More recently, the same group of investigators (Shear et al. 1991) reported that 83% of 23 patients with panic disorder were panic-free after treatment.

In the first large-scale, controlled study of this approach (Barlow et al. 1989), three different treatment conditions—progressive muscle relaxation (PMR), PCT, and a combination of PMR and PCT (COMB)—were compared with a waiting-list condition (WLC). The PMR group was taught relaxation skills and then instructed to apply these skills during anxiety-provoking situations or when panic was imminent. Although PMR did not reduce panic attacks among individuals completing the treatment as effectively as did the other active treatment conditions, 60% of the PMR group achieved a panic-free status by the end of the 15-week program, compared with 87% of the patients receiving PCT either alone or in combination with PMR. In contrast, approximately 36% of the waiting-list control group was panic-free. When dropouts were included in the analysis and assumed to be continuing to panic, the significantly higher attrition rate in the PMR condition (33%) lowered the proportion of the PMR group who were panic-free to 40%, which was not significantly different from the 33% in the waiting-list control group, especially compared with 79% in the PCT group, and 74% in the COMB group. PCT, either alone or in combination with PMR, was significantly better than PMR or waiting list in this analysis.

In a related study, Klosko et al. (1990) compared the efficacy of PCT with that of alprazolam, placebo, and a waiting-list control condition in 57 patients with panic disorder with no more than mild agoraphobic avoidance. Alprazolam was

---

[1] At the same time, David Clark and his colleagues at Oxford were developing a similar treatment, placing somewhat more emphasis on the cognitive component. This chapter reviews results from our approach, whereas Dr. Clark's chapter (Chapter 10 of this volume) reviews a series of studies employing his protocol, but it is fair to say that Dr. Clark and I consider these treatment protocols to be quite similar cognitive-behavior approaches.

administered according to the guidelines used in the Upjohn-sponsored Cross-National Collaborative Panic Study (Ballenger et al. 1988). At posttreatment, once again, 87% of PCT patients were panic-free, compared with 50% for alprazolam patients, 36% for placebo patients, and 33% for the waiting-list control group. Differences between the PCT and alprazolam groups were not significant, although only the PCT group was significantly different from both the placebo and the waiting-list control groups on panic-free status.

In a more recent controlled study, Telch et al. (1993) used PCT to treat 34 panic disorder patients with agoraphobia. This group was compared with 33 patients in a delayed-treatment control group. The results indicated that 85.3% of the originally treated group were panic-free at posttest and that 83.3% were still panic-free at 6-month follow-up. Very little change was noted on this measure in the delayed-treatment control group at posttest.

Perhaps more importantly, Telch et al. (1993) calculated a measure of high end-state functioning, referred to as *composite recovery*. This conservative index indicates the proportion of subjects who achieved functioning within the normal range not only on measures of panic attacks but also on measures of anxiety and avoidance. On this index, 63.6% of the panic disorder patients were in the normal range of functioning after treatment compared with 9.1% of the delayed-treatment control group.

Clinicians have attempted to use these procedures in settings other than where they originated, such as in pharmacologically oriented clinics. For example, in the Department of Psychiatry at Columbia University and the New York State Psychiatric Institute, clinicians reported that 74% of 19 patients who completed treatment with PCT were panic-free and 90% were moderately or significantly improved (Welkowitz et al. 1991).

Another method of ascertaining therapeutic effectiveness of PCT is to examine the number of panic disorder patients responding with a panic attack to biological challenge procedures both before and after treatment. Shear et al. (1991) examined six patients who had panicked during sodium lactate infusion prior to treatment with the Cornell version of PCT (Barlow et al. 1984). After treatment, only one of these patients reported having a panic attack and four out of six were free of panic based on the Acute Panic Inventory (Gorman et al. 1983).

At the Center for Stress and Anxiety Disorders in Albany, Brown et al. (1990) examined 42 patients' responses to inhalation of 5.5% CO_2. Prior to PCT, 57.1% of 42 panic disorder patients with agoraphobia met criteria for a panic attack during inhalation of CO_2, following the "liberal" criteria commonly used in these studies to determine the presence of panic of moderate intensity. After treatment, the percentage of patients panicking dropped to 28.6%. Using more conservative criteria that required the reporting of a severe panic attack, the figures were 35.7% pretreatment and 11.9% posttreatment (see Figure 9–2).

Follow-Up of Patients Treated With Panic Control Treatment

Craske et al. (1991) published data on a 2-year follow-up of patients treated in the Barlow et al. (1989) study (see Figure 9–3). At the 2-year follow-up, when patients who had dropped out during the active treatment phase (and who were presumed to be continuing to panic) were included in the analyses, 81% of the PCT subjects were panic-free compared with 43% of the COMB subjects and 36% of the PMR subjects. For the majority of the remaining variables (e.g., general anxiety, depression), patients evidenced maintenance of treatment gains or continued improvement. Craske et al. (1991) speculated that a dilution effect or perhaps a detrimental effect of relaxation procedures accounted for the somewhat lower success of the combination treatment in comparison with PCT alone at 2-year follow-up. It is also important to note that, although over 80% of the patients treated with PCT were panic-free after 2 years, only 50% of these patients met criteria for high end-state functioning at that period. A closer analysis indicated that, although the majority of the subjects were panic-free, some continued to evidence mild agoraphobic avoidance. Craske et al. concluded that this feature may need to be targeted

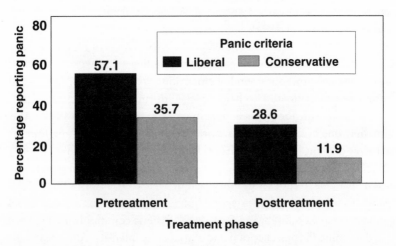

Figure 9–2.   Percentage of subjects ($N = 42$) reporting panic in response to CO_2 inhalation.

separately in treatment, as elimination of panic may not ensure the amelioration of all agoraphobic avoidance. These findings also suggested that reliance on panic-free status as the central measure of treatment outcome, even in those patients with little or no agoraphobic avoidance, may be an overly optimistic indicator of treatment success.

In one other study reporting a follow-up, Coté et al. (1990) compared the efficacy of therapist-directed PCT with a minimal therapist contact variation of PCT in 21 panic disorder patients with agoraphobic avoidance. At posttreatment, over 82% of the patients in both conditions were panic-free and 90% of the patients were panic-free at 6-month follow-up.

Summary and Conclusions

Although substantial evidence has been amassed in a relatively short period of time on the effectiveness of behavior treatments for panic disorder, many ques-

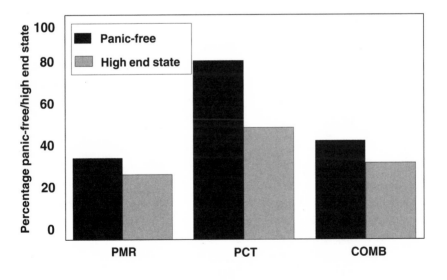

Figure 9–3. Panic-free and end-state status at 24-month follow-up. PMR = progressive muscle relaxation. PCT = panic control treatment. COMB = PMR plus PCT.
Source. Based on data from Craske et al. 1991.

tions remain unanswered and much work lies ahead. PCT and closely related approaches seem quite effective for panic attacks and associated anxiety; however, there is evidence that panic attack reduction in isolation is a rather narrow target in many cases of panic disorder with or without agoraphobia, and that more comprehensive approaches may be required to bring the maximum number of people into the normal range of functioning.

Currently an investigation is under way in the Center for Stress and Anxiety Disorders in Albany, as well as in several other centers, on the utility of combining PCT or closely related treatments with optimally delivered, exposure-based procedures. It is possible that this combination may provide a significant advantage for the majority of people who have panic disorder with agoraphobia, but particularly for those who have agoraphobic avoidance. This possibility derives from the fact that panic intensity and frequency and the extent of avoidance have been found to be weakly correlated at best (Craske et al. 1988), and that successful completion of PCT may result in partial, but not complete, reduction in agoraphobic avoidance. On the other hand, successful reduction of agoraphobic avoidance through exposure-based procedures may result in partial, but not complete, reduction of panic attacks.

In addition, the strategy of actively incorporating the interpersonal system of the patient into treatment has not yet been attempted with PCT, although results from combining this element with exposure-based treatments look very promising. Based on clinical experience, there is every reason to believe that incorporating the interpersonal system into PCT may provide additional advantages.

Somewhat beyond the scope of this chapter is the coming stage of research in which combinations of psychosocial and pharmacological treatments for panic disorder with and without agoraphobia will be considered. Recently we (D. H. Barlow, M. K. Shear, J. M. Gorman, and S. W. Woods) began a large-scale collaborative study sponsored by the National Institute of Mental Health in conjunction with the psychiatry departments of Cornell, Columbia, and Yale Universities to examine the relative effectiveness of PCT and imipramine treatments separately and in combination. This large study will allow sufficient statistical power to detect beneficial interaction effects. Other studies will examine these two approaches introduced in various sequences.

Finally, PCT and related treatments have not been widely disseminated or evaluated outside the specialty anxiety clinics. This is a potential disadvantage when compared with more widely available pharmacological treatments. In an attempt to facilitate this dissemination, user-friendly workbooks presenting PCT for self-directed treatment under minimal clinical supervision are now available (Barlow and Craske 1989) and initial results are encouraging. For example, as noted above, Coté et al. (1990) reported that home-based treatment delivered in this way was as effective as office-based treatment for patients with panic disorder without significant agoraphobic avoidance. Similar reports have appeared concerning patients with more substantial agoraphobic avoidance (McNamee et al. 1989). Nevertheless, at present these treatments for panic attacks remain, for the most part, unavailable to the public at large.

References

Agras WS, Leitenberg H, Barlow DH: Social reinforcement in the modification of agoraphobia. Arch Gen Psychiatry 19:423–427, 1968

Agras WS, Chapin HN, Oliveau DC: The natural history of phobia. Arch Gen Psychiatry 26:315–317, 1972

Arnow BA, Taylor CB, Agras WS, et al: Enhancing agoraphobia treatment outcome by changing couple communication patterns. Behavior Therapy 16:452–467, 1985

Ballenger JC, Burrows G, DuPont R, et al: Alprazolam in panic disorder and agoraphobia: results from a multicenter trial, I: efficacy in short-term treatment. Arch Gen Psychiatry 45:413–422, 1988

Barlow DH: Anxiety and Its Disorders: The Nature and Treatment of Anxiety and Panic. New York, Guilford, 1988

Barlow DH, Craske MG: Mastery of Your Anxiety and Panic. Albany, NY, Graywind Publications, 1989

Barlow DH, O'Brien GT, Last CG: Couples treatment of agoraphobia. Behavior Therapy 15:41–58, 1984

Barlow DH, Craske M, Cerny J, et al: Behavioral treatment of panic disorder. Behavior Therapy 20:261–282, 1989

Beach SRH, Sandeen EE, O'Leary KD: Depression in Marriage: A Model for Etiology and Treatment. New York, Guilford, 1990

Brown TA, Rapee RM, Antony MM, et al: Patterns of responding to hyperventilation and carbon dioxide inhalation following behavioral treatment of panic disorder. Paper presented at the annual meeting of the Association for Advancement of Behavior Therapy, San Francisco, CA, November 1990

Burns LE, Thorpe GL, Cavallaro LA: Agoraphobia eight years after behavioral treatment: a follow-up study with interview, self-report, and behavioral data. Behavior Therapy 17:580–591, 1986

Cerny JA, Barlow DH, Craske M, et al: Couples treatment of agoraphobia: a two-year follow-up. Behavior Therapy 18:401–415, 1987

Chambless DL: Spacing of exposure sessions in treatment of agoraphobia and simple phobia. Behavior Therapy 21:217–229, 1990

Clum GA: Psychological interventions versus drugs in the treatment of panic. Behavior Therapy 20:429–457, 1989

Cohen SD, Monteio W, Marks IM: Two-year follow-up of agoraphobics after exposure and imipramine. Br J Psychiatry 144:276–281, 1984

Coté G, Gauthier JG, Laberge B, et al: Clinic-based versus home-based treatment with minimal therapist contact for panic disorder. Paper presented at the meeting of the Association for Advancement of Behavior Therapy, San Francisco, CA, November 1990

Craske MG, Rapee RM, Barlow DH: The significance of panic expectancy for individual patterns of avoidance. Behavior Therapy 19:577–592, 1988

Craske MG, Brown TA, Barlow DH: Behavioral treatment of panic: a two-year follow-up. Behavior Therapy 22:289–304, 1991

Emmelkamp PMG: Phobic and Obsessive-Compulsive Disorders: Theory, Research, and Practice. New York, Plenum, 1982

Emmelkamp PMG, Kuipers ACM: Agoraphobia: a follow-up study four years after treatment. Br J Psychiatry 128:86–89, 1979

Fiegenbaum W: Long-term efficacy of ungraded versus graded massed exposure in agoraphobics, in Panic and Phobias, 2: Treatments and Variables Affecting Course and Outcome. Edited by Hand I, Wittchen HU. New York, Springer-Verlag, 1988, pp 83–88

Gelder MG, Marks IM: Severe agoraphobia: a controlled prospective trial of behavior therapy. Br J Psychiatry 112:309–319, 1966

Ghosh A, Marks IM: Self-treatment of agoraphobia by exposure. Behavior Therapy 18:3–16, 1987

Gitlin B, Martin J, Shear MK, et al: Behavior therapy for panic disorder. J Nerv Ment Dis 173:742–743, 1985

Gorman JM, Levy GF, Liebowitz MR, et al: Effect of acute β-adrenergic blockade on lactate-induced panic. Arch Gen Psychiatry 40:1079–1082, 1983

Greist JH, Marks IM, Berlin F, et al: Avoidance versus confrontation of fear. Behavior Therapy 11:1–14, 1980

Hafner RJ: Fresh symptom emergence after intensive behavior therapy. Br J Psychiatry 129:378–383, 1976

Hand I, Lamontagne Y, Marks IM: Group exposure (flooding) in vivo for agoraphobics. Br J Psychiatry 124:588–602, 1974

Holden AE, O'Brien GT, Barlow DH, et al: Self-help manual for agoraphobia: a preliminary report of effectiveness. Behavior Therapy 14:545–556, 1983

Jacobson NS, Wilson L, Tupper C: The clinical significance of treatment gains resulting from exposure-based interventions for agoraphobia: a reanalysis of outcome data. Behavior Therapy 19:539–554, 1988

Jannoun L, Munby M, Catalan J, et al: A home-based treatment program for agoraphobia: replication and controlled evaluation. Behavior Therapy 11:294–305, 1980

Jansson L, Öst LG: Behavioral treatments for agoraphobia: an evaluative review. Clinical Psychology Review 2:311–336, 1982

Jansson L, Jerremalm A, Öst LG: Follow-up of agoraphobic patients treated with exposure in vivo or applied relaxation. Br J Psychiatry 149:486–490, 1986

Klein DF, Zitrin CM, Woerner MG, et al: Behavior therapy and supportive psychotherapy: are there any specific ingredients? Arch Gen Psychiatry 40:139–153, 1983

Klosko JS, Barlow DH, Tassinari RB, et al: A comparison of alprazolam and behavior therapy in the treatment of panic disorder. J Consult Clin Psychol 58:77–84, 1990

Leitenberg H, Agras WS, Edwards JA, et al: Practice as a psychotherapeutic variable: an experimental analysis within single cases. J Psychiatr Res 7:215–225, 1970

Marks IM: Phobic disorders four years after treatment: a prospective follow-up. Br J Psychiatry 118:683–686, 1971

Marks I: Fears, phobias and rituals. New York, Oxford University Press, 1987

Mathews AM, Johnston DW, Lancashire M, et al: Imaginal flooding and exposure to real phobic situations: treatment outcome with agoraphobic patients. Br J Psychiatry 129:362–371, 1976

Mathews AM, Teasdale J, Munby M, et al: A home-based treatment program for agoraphobia. Behavior Therapy 8:915–924, 1977

Mathews AM, Gelder MG, Johnston DW: Agoraphobia: Nature and Treatment. New York, Guilford, 1981

Mavissakalian M, Barlow DH (eds): Phobia: Psychological and Pharmacological Treatment. New York, Guilford, 1981

McCrady BS: Alcoholism, in Clinical Handbook of Psychological Disorders: A Step-by-Step Treatment Manual. Edited by Barlow DH. New York, Guilford, 1985, pp 245–298

McNamee G, O'Sullivan G, Lelliott P, et al: Telephone-guided treatment for housebound agoraphobics with panic disorder: exposure versus relaxation. Behavior Therapy 20:490–497, 1989

McPherson FM, Brougham L, McLaren S: Maintenance of improvement in agoraphobic patients treated by behavioral methods—four year follow-up. Behav Res Ther 18:150–152, 1980

Michelson LK, Marchione K: Behavioral, cognitive, and pharmacological treatments of panic disorder with agoraphobia: critique and synthesis. J Consult Clin Psychol 59:100–114, 1991

Michelson LK, Marchione K, Greenwald M: Cognitive-behavioral treatments of panic disorder with agoraphobia: a comparative outcome investigation. Paper presented at the symposium, Emerging Issues in Assessment and Treatment of Anxiety Disorders, at the meeting of the Association for Advancement of Behavior Therapy, Washington, DC, November 1989

Munby J, Johnston DW: Agoraphobia: the long-term follow-up of behavioral treatment. Br J Psychiatry 137:418–427, 1980

O'Brien GT, Barlow DH: Agoraphobia, in Behavioral Treatment of Anxiety Disorders. Edited by Turner SM. New York, Plenum, 1984, pp 143–185

Shear MK, Ball G, Fitzpatrick M, et al: Cognitive-behavioral therapy for panic: an open study. J Nerv Ment Dis 179:467–471, 1991

Telch MJ, Agras WS, Taylor CB, et al: Combined pharmacological and behavioral treatment for agoraphobia. Behav Res Ther 23:325–335, 1985

Telch MJ, Lucas JA, Schmidt NB, et al: Group cognitive-behavioral treatment of panic disorder. Behav Res Ther 31:279–287, 1993

Trull TJ, Nietzel MT, Main A: The use of meta-analysis to assess the clinical significance of behavior therapy for agoraphobia. Behavior Therapy 19:527–538, 1988

Welkowitz LA, Papp LA, Cloitre M, et al: Cognitive-behavior therapy for panic disorder delivered by psychopharmacologically oriented clinicians. J Nerv Ment Dis 179:472–476, 1991

Chapter 10

Cognitive Therapy for Panic Disorder

David M. Clark, D.Phil.

C ognitive therapy is a recently developed, brief psychological treatment for panic. It is based on the cognitive theory (Beck et al. 1985; Clark 1986; Margraf et al. 1986; Salkovskis 1988) of panic disorder, which proposes that individuals who experience panic attacks do so because they have an enduring tendency to misinterpret benign bodily sensations as indications of impending physical or mental catastrophe (e.g., palpitations indicate an impending heart attack). This cognitive abnormality is said to lead to a positive feedback loop in which misinterpretations of bodily sensations produce increases in anxiety, which in turn strengthen the sensations, thus producing a vicious circle that culminates in a panic attack.

Empirical support for the cognitive theory comes from studies that have demonstrated that 1) panic disorder patients are more likely to misinterpret bodily sensations than other anxious patients or nonpsychiatric control subjects (Chambless and Gracely 1989; Clark et al. 1988; Foa 1988); 2) activating these negative interpretations produces panic attacks in panic disorder patients (Clark et al. 1988); and 3) cognitive procedures that prevent panic disorder patients from misinterpreting the sensations induced by pharmacological challenge tests, such as those using CO_2 and lactate, block panic attacks induced in the laboratory (Clark et al. 1991; Sanderson et al. 1990).

If the cognitive theory of panic is correct, it should be possible to treat naturally occurring panic attacks by helping patients identify and change their misinterpretations of bodily sensations. Several cognitive-behavior treatment packages that attempt to achieve these goals have been devised, the most prominent of which are probably cognitive therapy (CT) as developed by Clark,

Salkovskis, and Beck (Clark 1989; Salkovskis and Clark 1991) and panic control treatment (PCT) as devised by Barlow and colleagues (Barlow and Cerny 1988; Barlow and Craske 1989). Both treatments aim at changing patients' appraisals of the bodily sensations that trigger panic. There is considerable overlap in the procedures used to achieve this aim; however, there is also a difference of emphasis. PCT is a broad-based treatment that includes a wide range of cognitive, behavior, and coping techniques, including extensive interoceptive exposure and relaxation training. CT, on the other hand, focuses more exclusively on directly changing misinterpretations of bodily sensations, has rather less interoceptive exposure, and does not include relaxation training. In this chapter I cover evaluations of the CT package.

Controlled Trials of Cognitive Therapy

Early indications that CT might be an effective treatment for panic were provided by five case series (Clark et al. 1985; Kopp et al. 1986; Michelson et al. 1990; Salkovskis et al. 1986; Sokol et al. 1989) reported by groups in England, the United States, and Hungary. In each series, consecutively referred panic disorder patients showed substantial reductions in panic frequency. Investigators in two of the studies (Clark et al. 1985; Sokol et al. 1989) also reported on long-term follow-up (1–2 years), finding that the gains made in treatment were maintained at follow-up. These initial encouraging results have been confirmed in five recent controlled trials, which are reviewed below. Two further controlled trials, one in the Netherlands and one in the United States, are still in progress.

Beck et al. 1992

The aim of this trial was to investigate the role of nonspecific therapy factors. Thirty-three patients meeting DSM-III (American Psychiatric Association 1980) criteria for panic disorder or agoraphobia with panic attacks were randomly allocated to either 12 weeks of CT or 8 weeks of brief supportive therapy. When assessed after 4 and 8 weeks, the patients given CT had improved significantly more than those given supportive therapy, according to self- and clinician ratings of panic frequency and the Beck Anxiety Inventory (Beck et al. 1988). At 8 weeks, 71% of CT patients were panic-free as opposed to 25% of brief supportive therapy patients. At the end of the cognitive treatment (12 weeks), 94% of CT patients were panic-free, and at 1-year follow-up, 87% were panic-free.

Clark et al. 1990

The main aim of this trial was to compare CT with alternative, empirically validated psychological and pharmacological treatments for panic disorder. Each alternative treatment was chosen because it previously had been shown to be more effective than placebo treatment. The psychological treatment was Öst's applied relaxation treatment (Clark 1989; Öst 1987), which involves training in a highly specialized and portable relaxation technique in conjunction with graded exposure to feared situations. It was chosen because, in a recent controlled trial, Öst (1988) found that applied relaxation was significantly more effective than traditional relaxation training plus exposure. The pharmacological treatment was imipramine, chosen because it repeatedly has been shown to be more effective than placebo medication (Fyer and Sandberg 1988) and is as effective as alprazolam—the leading alternative pharmacological treatment.

Sixty-four patients meeting DSM-III-R (American Psychiatric Association 1987) criteria for panic disorder were randomly assigned to either CT, applied relaxation, imipramine (up to 325 mg/day [mean dosage = 233 mg/day], verified by blood plasma levels), or a waiting-list control condition. Patients receiving CT or applied relaxation had up to 12 sessions in the first 3 months and up to 3 booster sessions in the next 3 months. Patients receiving imipramine had a similar number of sessions, reached the maximum dosage after an average of 7.5 weeks, and were then maintained at that dosage until 6 months, after which medication was gradually withdrawn. Patient and independent assessor ratings were taken prior to treatment and after 3, 6, and 15 months.

Comparisons between treatment groups and waiting-list control subjects at the 3-month point indicated that all three treatments were effective in reducing panic (see Figure 10–1) and generalized anxiety. Comparisons among the three treatment groups indicated that CT was significantly more effective than applied relaxation or imipramine, both initially (at 3 months) and in the long term (at 15 months), but did not differ from imipramine at 6 months. This pattern is illustrated in Figure 10–2.

It has often been suggested that CT may be particularly effective at producing sustained therapeutic change. Analysis of the long-term outcome data from this study provided some support for this suggestion. Patients treated with imipramine were significantly ($P < .05$) more likely to relapse and require further treatment than patients treated with CT (40% versus 5%). The percentages of patients who were panic-free at 15 months after receiving no additional treatment for panic during follow-up were 80% in the CT group, 47% in the applied relaxation group, and 50% in the imipramine group.

The cognitive theory of panic predicts that long-term outcome will depend on the extent to which misinterpretations of bodily sensations have changed during the course of treatment (Clark 1986). In particular, patients who continue to misinterpret bodily sensations at the end of treatment should have a worse clinical outcome during the follow-up period than patients who have ceased to do so. Analysis of the long-term (15-month) outcome data from this study provided some support for this hypothesis. Measures of misinterpretation of bodily sensations taken at the end of treatment were significant predictors of subsequent symptomatology.

Michelson and Marchione 1989

This study's aim was to investigate whether CT enhanced the effects of exposure in treatment of agoraphobia with panic. Seventy-two patients meeting DSM-III criteria for agoraphobia with panic were randomly allocated to CT plus graded exposure, relaxation training plus graded exposure, or graded exposure alone. Patients had up to 16 sessions in small groups. Patient and independent assessor ratings were completed at pre-, mid-, and posttreatment and at 3-month follow-up.

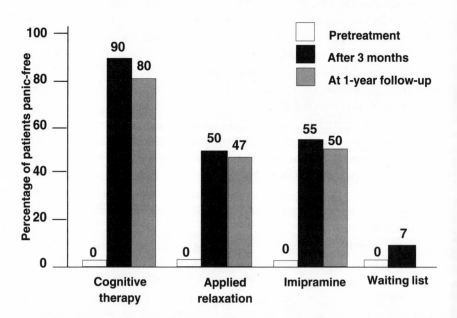

Figure 10–1. Percentage of patients panic-free and receiving no extra treatment. *Source.* Clark DM, Gelder MG, Salkovskis PM, et al.: "Cognitive Therapy for Panic: Comparative Efficacy." Paper presented at the annual meeting of the American Psychiatric Association, New York, May 15, 1990.

The results showed that all three treatments were associated with significant reductions in panic, anxiety, and phobic avoidance. However, where there were significant between-group differences, these consistently favored CT plus graded exposure. All patients in this condition successfully completed a one-mile behavioral avoidance test at the end of treatment and at follow-up. A significantly greater proportion of patients treated with CT plus exposure (79%) were panic-free than of those treated with exposure alone (39%). Patients treated with relaxation training plus exposure were midway between the two treatments, with 62% of patients being panic-free. CT patients also scored higher than patients in the other two treatment groups on a composite measure of improvement that took into account changes in phobic anxiety as well as panic.

Öst 1991

The aim of this study was to compare CT with applied relaxation. Thirty-six patients meeting DSM-III-R criteria for panic disorder were randomly allocated to

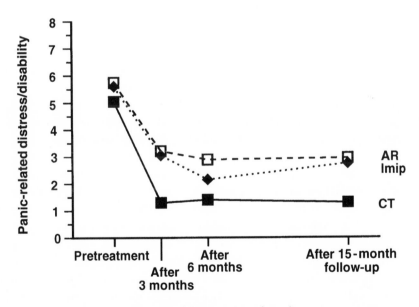

Figure 10–2. Panic-related distress/disability in patients from three treatment groups. AR = applied relaxation treatment. Imip = imipramine treatment. CT = cognitive therapy. *Source.* Clark DM, Gelder MG, Salkovskis PM, et al.: "Cognitive Therapy for Panic: Comparative Efficacy." Paper presented at the annual meeting of the American Psychiatric Association, New York, May 15, 1990.

either CT or applied relaxation. The cognitive treatment was similar to that used by Beck et al. (1992) and Clark et al. (1990). Applied relaxation was identical to that described by Öst (1987), and slightly different from that used by Clark et al. (1990). Assessments were conducted at pre- and posttreatment and at 1-year follow-up. At this time, complete data are available only for the pre- and posttreatment assessments.

Pre- to posttreatment comparisons indicated that CT and applied relaxation were both associated with substantial improvements on ratings of panic frequency, panic-related distress/disability, the Beck Anxiety Inventory (Beck et al. 1988), the Hamilton Anxiety Scale (Hamilton 1959), and the Beck Depression Inventory (Beck et al. 1978). There were no significant differences between the treatments. By the end of treatment, 74% of CT patients and 65% of applied relaxation patients were panic-free.

One-year follow-up data are currently available for 26 out of 36 patients. These data indicate that the gains made in treatment were maintained at follow-up. Eighty percent of these 26 CT patients were panic-free and had received no additional treatment at the 1-year follow-up.

Margraf and Schneider 1991

The aim of this study was to investigate the active ingredients in CT. Treatment usually involves a complex mixture of cognitive and behavior procedures. The cognitive procedures include identifying and challenging patients' evidence of their misinterpretations, substituting more realistic interpretations, and restructuring images. The behavior procedures include inducing feared sensations (by hyperventilation, exercise, and attentional focus) and exposing the patient to feared situations.

To determine whether the cognitive and behavior procedures are separately effective, patients meeting DSM-III-R criteria for panic disorder who were not taking any psychotropic medication were allocated to 10 weeks of either pure cognitive treatment, pure behavior treatment, combined cognitive-behavior treatment, or a waiting-list control condition. Preliminary results based on 16–22 patients per group are shown in Figure 10–3. Comparisons with the waiting-list control group indicated that all three active treatments were effective in reducing panic frequency, agoraphobic avoidance, and anxiety (as assessed by the Hamilton Anxiety Scale [Hamilton 1959]). There were no significant differences among the three active treatments. Cognitive theory predicts that the main mechanism of change in psychological treatments will be change in misinterpretations of bodily sensations. Consistent with this prediction, Margraf and Schneider found that change in panic-related cognitions was positively correlated with clinical improvements, whereas change in self-exposure was not.

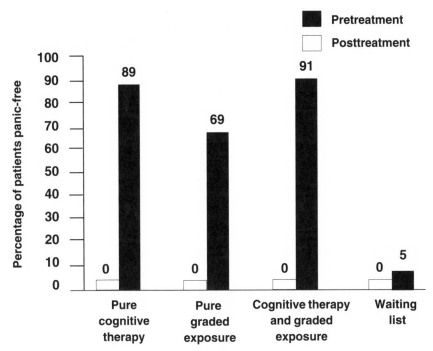

Figure 10–3. Percentages of patients in three treatment groups and a waiting-list control group who were panic-free. *Source.* Margraf J, Schneider S: "Outcome and Active Ingredients of Cognitive-Behavioral Treatments for Panic Disorder." Paper presented at the annual meeting of the Association for the Advancement of Behavior Therapy, New York, November 26, 1991.

General Considerations

The results described above are remarkably consistent. In trials conducted in five different centers and four countries (England, Germany, Sweden, and the United States), between 74% and 95% of patients became panic-free after 3 months of CT; these gains were maintained at follow-ups lasting up to 1 year (see Table 10–1). The studies varied in the proportion of patients who had agoraphobia. In Öst's (1991) study, most patients had panic disorder with no agoraphobic avoidance. In Clark et al.'s (1990) and Margraf and Schneider's (1991) studies, the majority of patients suffered from panic disorder with mild or moderate agoraphobic avoidance, and in Michelson and Marchione's (1989) study, all patients had agoraphobia with panic. It therefore appears that CT is effective across the full spectrum of panic disorder with or without agoraphobia.

Table 10–1. Controlled trials of cognitive therapy in panic disorder

Study	Patients	Treatments	Percentage (number) of panic-free patients	
			Posttreatment	At follow-up
Beck et al. 1992	DSM-III panic disorder (82%) and agoraphobia with panic attacks (18%)	1. CT 2. ST	94 (16/17) 25 (4/16)[a]	87(13/15)[b] —
Clark et al. 1990	DSM-III-R panic disorder (19% no avoidance) (48% mild avoidance) (33% moderate avoidance)	1. CT 2. AR 3. IMIP 4. WL	90 (18/20) 50 (10/20) 55 (11/20) 7 (1/16)	80 (16/20)[b,c] 47 (9/19)[b,c] 50 (10/20)[b,c] —
Michelson and Marchione 1989	DSM-III agoraphobia with panic	1. CT + GE 2. RT + GE 3. GE	79 (19/24)[d] 63 (15/24)[d] 38 (9/24)[d]	— — —
Öst 1991	DSM-III-R panic disorder (78% no avoidance) (22% mild avoidance)	1. CT 2. AR	74 (14/19) 65 (11/17)	80 (12/15)[b,c] 82 (9/11)[b,c]
Margraf and Schneider 1991	DSM-III-R panic disorder (22% no avoidance) (78% mild or moderate avoidance)	1. Pure CT 2. Pure GE 3. Combined 4. WL	89 (16/18)[d] 69 (11/16)[d] 91 (20/22)[d] 5 (1/20)	— —
Total across all studies for cognitive therapy			85 (87/102)	82 (41/50)

Note. CT = cognitive therapy. ST = supportive therapy. AR = applied relaxation. IMIP = imipramine. GE = graded exposure. WL = waiting list. RT = relaxation training. [a] At 8 weeks, which is the end of supportive therapy. At this time 71% of CT patients were panic-free. [b] 1-year follow-up. [c] Percentage of patients panic-free at follow-up and who received no additional treatment during the follow-up period. [d] 4-week follow-up.

In any trial of treatments for panic, a proportion of patients will be taking psychotropic medication prior to entry into the trial. There are two ways of dealing with this problem. The first is to withdraw all such medications. The second is to accept only patients who have been on a stable dosage for several months without showing any further improvement and then require them not to increase their medication during the trial. Both strategies were used in the above studies, and CT appears to have achieved essentially similar results whichever strategy was employed. In the trials by Michelson and Marchione (1989) and by Margraf and Schneider (1991), all psychotropic medications were withdrawn prior to the start of the trial. In the trials by Beck et al. (1992), Clark et al. (1990), and Öst (1991), patients had been on a stable dosage for several months without showing improvement and were asked not to increase their medication during the trial. In fact, in all three of these latter trials, patients treated with CT showed significant reductions in psychotropic medication, presumably as a consequence of increased confidence in their ability to control panic.

Conclusions

1. CT is an effective treatment for panic disorder, with between 74% and 95% of patients becoming panic-free after 3 months of treatment.
2. Effectiveness of the treatment is not entirely due to nonspecific factors, as CT has been shown to be more effective than supportive therapy (Beck et al. 1992) or a version of applied relaxation training that was judged equally credible (Clark et al. 1990). The effectiveness of treatment is also not entirely attributed to exposure to feared situations, as this was common to all treatments in Clark et al.'s (1990) trial and Michelson and Marchione's (1989) trial. In both trials, CT was superior to the alternative treatments.
3. The gains obtained with CT were largely maintained at 1- and 2-year follow-ups.
4. Both the immediate (3 months) and the longer term (15 months) responses to CT compared favorably with responses to imipramine and applied relaxation. CT was associated with a significantly lower relapse rate than imipramine.
5. Component analyses suggested that both the cognitive and the behavior procedures in CT packages are effective and operate through cognitive change.
6. There is preliminary evidence that sustained improvement after the end of treatment depends on cognitive change occurring during the course of treatment.

Questions for Future Research

Two questions that need to be addressed by future research are briefly discussed below.

Treatment of Nonresponders

In the studies reviewed above, between 5% and 26% of patients failed to become panic-free during a 3-month course of CT. Although it is possible that a number of these patients might become panic-free with additional cognitive treatment, some are likely to continue to experience residual panic symptoms. Further investigation of possible treatments for these individuals would be most helpful. Some of these patients may benefit from combined cognitive and pharmacological treatment; this question could be addressed by a large-scale trial that includes a combined treatment condition.

Development of a Briefer Form of Cognitive Therapy

Ninety percent of patients treated in Clark et al.'s (1990) study became panic-free when given up to 12 sessions of CT. However, analysis of the session-by-session data revealed that these patients achieved their panic-free status after an average of only 5.5 treatment sessions. This suggests that it should be possible to develop a briefer form of cognitive treatment. In Oxford, we (D. Clark, P. Salkovskis, A. Hachmann) are currently experimenting with a version of CT that uses a self-help manual and requires only four sessions with the therapist. If this treatment is as effective as the full version of CT, it will be possible to offer the treatment at a much lower cost and to many more individuals.

References

American Psychiatric Association: Diagnostic and Statistical Manual of Mental Disorders, 3rd Edition. Washington, DC, American Psychiatric Association, 1980

American Psychiatric Association: Diagnostic and Statistical Manual of Mental Disorders, 3rd Edition, Revised. Washington, DC, American Psychiatric Association, 1987

Barlow DH, Cerny JA: Psychological Treatment of Panic. New York, Guilford, 1988

Barlow DH, Craske MG: Mastery of Your Anxiety and Panic. Albany, NY, Graywind Publications, 1989

Beck AT, Ward CH, Mendelson M, et al: An inventory for measuring depression. Arch Gen Psychiatry 4:561–571, 1961

Beck AT, Epstein N, Brown G, et al: An inventory for measuring clinical anxiety: psychometric properties. J Consult Clin Psychol 56:893–897, 1988

Beck AT, Emery G, Greenberg RL: Anxiety Disorders and Phobias. New York, Basic Books, 1985

Beck AT, Sokol L, Clark DA, et al: Focused cognitive therapy of panic disorder: a crossover design and one-year follow-up. Am J Psychiatry 147:778–783, 1992

Chambless DL, Gracely EJ: Fear of fear and the anxiety disorders. Cognitive Therapy and Research 13:9–20, 1989

Clark DM: A cognitive approach to panic. Behav Res Ther 24:461–470, 1986

Clark DM: Anxiety states: panic and generalized anxiety, in Cognitive Behavior Therapy for Psychiatric Problems: A Practical Guide. Edited by Hawton K, Salkovskis P, Kirk J, et al. Oxford, England, Oxford University Press, 1989

Clark DM, Salkovskis PM, Chalkley AJ: Respiratory control as a treatment for panic attacks. J Behav Ther Exp Psychiatry 16:23–30, 1985

Clark DM, Salkovskis PM, Gelder MG, et al: Tests of a cognitive theory of panic, in Panic and Phobias 2: Treatments and Variables Affecting Course and Outcome. Edited by Hand I, Wittchen HU. New York, Springer-Verlag, 1988

Clark DM, Gelder MG, Salkovskis PM, et al: Cognitive therapy for panic: comparative efficacy. Paper presented at the annual meeting of the American Psychiatric Association, New York, May 15, 1990

Clark DM, Gelder MG, Salkovskis PM, et al: Cognitive mediation of lactate-induced panic. Paper presented at the annual meeting of the American Psychiatric Association, New Orleans, May 14, 1991

Foa EB: What cognitions differentiate panic disorder from other anxiety disorders?, in Panic and Phobias 2: Treatments and Variables Affecting Course and Outcome. Edited by Hand I, Wittchen HU. New York, Springer-Verlag, 1988

Fyer AJ, Sandberg DP: Pharmacological treatment of panic disorder, in American Psychiatric Press Review of Psychiatry, Vol 7. Edited by Frances AJ, Hales RE. Washington, DC, American Psychiatric Press, 1988

Hamilton M: The assessment of anxiety states by rating. Br J Med Psychol 32:50–55, 1959

Kopp M, Milhaly K, Vadasz P: Agoraphobics ex panikneurotikus betegek legzesi kontroll keyelese. Ideggyogyaszati Szemle 39:185–196, 1986

Margraf J, Schneider S: Outcome and active ingredients of cognitive-behavioral treatments for panic disorder. Paper presented at annual meeting of the Association for Advancement of Behavior Therapy. New York, November 26, 1991

Margraf J, Ehlers A, Roth WT: Biological models of panic disorder and agoraphobia: a review. Behav Res Ther 24:553–567, 1986

Michelson L, Marchione K: Cognitive, behavioral, and physiologically based treatments of agoraphobia: a comparative outcome study. Paper presented at the annual meeting of the Association for Advancement of Behavior Therapy, Washington, DC, November 1989

Michelson L, Marchione K, Greenwald M, et al: Panic disorder: cognitive-behavioral treatment. Behav Res Ther 28:141–153, 1990

Öst LG: Applied relaxation: description of a coping technique and review of controlled studies. Behav Res Ther 25:397–410, 1987

Öst LG: Applied relaxation versus progressive relaxation in the treatment of panic disorder. Behav Res Ther 26:13–22, 1988

Öst LG: Cognitive therapy versus applied relaxation in the treatment of panic disorder. Paper presented at the European Association of Behavior Therapy meeting, Oslo, Norway, September 1991

Salkovskis PM: Phenomenology, assessment and the cognitive model of panic, in Panic: Psychological Perspectives. Edited by Rachman S, Maser J. New Jersey, NJ, Lawrence Erlbaum, 1988

Salkovskis PM, Clark DM: Cognitive therapy for panic disorder. Journal of Cognitive Psychotherapy 5:215–226, 1991

Salkovskis PM, Jones DRO, Clark DM: Respiratory control in the treatment of panic attacks: replication and extension with concurrent measurement of behavior and pCO_2. Br J Psychiatry 148:526–532, 1986

Sanderson WC, Rapee RM, Barlow DH: The influence of an illusion of control on panic attacks induced via inhalation of 5.5% carbon dioxide enriched air. Arch Gen Psychiatry 46:157–162, 1990

Sokol L, Beck AT, Greenberg RL, et al: Cognitive therapy of panic disorder: a non-pharmacological alternative. J Nerv Ment Dis 177:711–716, 1989

Chapter 11

Psychological Treatment of Panic: Mechanisms

S. Rachman, Ph.D.

Most of the recent progress in the psychological treatment of panic disorder has been accomplished by clinical researchers who have approached the subject from a cognitive point of view and whose methods of treatment have been derived directly from cognitive theory (see Rachman and Maser 1988). Accordingly, in this analysis I emphasize cognitive theory and therapy; however, it is first necessary to place this new theory in its historical context.

Noncognitive Theories for Explaining the Mechanisms of Panic

The introduction of innovative psychological methods for reducing fear and anxiety can be traced to Wolpe's (1958) research. We now possess five techniques for reducing fear: desensitization, therapeutic modeling, in vivo exposure, flooding, and cognitive therapy (CT). However, despite many energetic efforts, we still do not have a wholly satisfactory explanation for the therapeutic effects of these techniques (Barlow 1988; Rachman 1991), and it is unclear whether one or several mechanisms are involved.

Previous explanations that have survived include Wolpe's (1958) original theory of *reciprocal inhibition,* which gives a plausible explanation of desensitization but cannot easily accommodate the effects of flooding or CT. Reciprocal inhibition has proven surprisingly difficult to test in a thoroughly rigorous manner despite the clarity of Wolpe's exposition. The *habituation model,* introduced by Lader and Wing (1966) and elaborated by Lader and Mathews (1968), has the great merit of simplicity and is based on the widely observed phenomenon of habituation, but has difficulty accounting for rapid and sudden changes in fear and for fears that decline in the absence of exposures. Moreover, in the continuing absence of an independent measure of habituation, the model cannot be proven false (D. M. Clark, personal communication, June 1988; Rachman 1991). The related theory of *extinction* encounters the same difficulties as the habituation theory. Marks (1987) suggested that therapeutic changes are attributable to re-peated exposures to the fear-provoking stimulus; such exposure is indeed a pow-erful reducer of fears and panic (Margraf and Schneider 1991). This is, however, a procedural description, not an explanation, and has difficulty accounting for those instances in which fear persists despite many repetitions of exposure. Furthermore, it is incapable of explaining the reductions of fear that occur without exposures (de Silva and Rachman 1981). In the Margraf and Schneider (1991) study, for example, patients who received pure CT without exposures experienced large reductions in panic; no less than 86% of them were panic-free at the end of 15 sessions. Cognitive theory, with its deduced therapy, is the latest recruit in the attempt to explain panic; until recently it was used mainly in the treatment of depression.

Cognitive Deductions and Explanations for Panic

The leading proponents of a cognitive approach to the treatment of panic are Barlow (1988), who emphasizes the internal as well as the external cues for panic, Beck (1988), and Clark (1986, 1988). According to Clark, "panic attacks result from the catastrophic misinterpretation of certain bodily sensations" (1986, p. 462). From this hypothesis, the following can be deduced:

1. A reduction in catastrophic cognitions should reduce the episodes of panic.
1a. The elimination of the catastrophic cognitions should lead to the cessation of panic.
2. The substitution of noncatastrophic interpretations of these bodily sensations should reduce episodes of panic.
3. However, there is another, less obvious deduction, namely, that a reduction in the relevant bodily sensations should reduce the opportunities for catastrophic misinterpretations and, hence, should be followed by a decline in the episodes of panic.

4. Reduction or elimination of the catastrophic cognitions should be followed by a generalized reduction in fear and panic episodes.
5. The enduring reduction of these cognitions should be accompanied by a lasting reduction in the occurrence and intensity of panic episodes.
5a. A return of these cognitions or a restoration of their high believability will be followed by a return of fear and a recurrence of panic episodes.

Most panic disorder patients endorse or describe more than one catastrophic cognition and several bodily "symptoms"; in fact, the DSM-III-R (American Psychiatric Association 1987) criteria for panic disorder require the endorsement of at least three such bodily sensations. Leaving aside for the moment the complexities of deciding which of the several cognitions and bodily sensations are critical, we can turn to the evidence pertaining to these deductions.

1. There is evidence that after successful treatment of panic disorder, patients do report significantly fewer negative cognitions than they did prior to treatment (Clark et al. 1991; Margraf and Schneider 1991).
2. There is also some indirect evidence to support the second deduction. An encouragingly high percentage of patients are free of panic attacks at the conclusion of treatment (see Table 11–1). In the most recent controlled studies, between 71% and 90% of patients who received CT were panic-free at the end of treatment. However, we do not have specific information about the nature and number of the remaining cognitions, if any, of the panic-free patients.
3. So far there is no quantitative evidence that pertains directly to the third deduction (i.e., the extent to which successfully treated patients make fresh but benign interpretations of their bodily sensations). Clinical reports suggest that this change does take place.
4. In two studies in which successful treatment of panic disorder was reported (Clark et al. 1991; Margraf and Schneider 1991), patients reported fewer bodily sensations than they did prior to treatment.

The evidence pertaining to deductions 1 and 1a is positive; the evidence for deductions 2–4 is also positive, but limited in quantity, and is derived from a clinical experiment on claustrophobic patients (Booth and Rachman 1992; see below).

There are indications that the improvements achieved in reducing panic remain stable, and that there is a positive correlation between reduction of the negative cognitions during treatment and the maintenance of improvements (see Clark et al. 1991; Margraf and Schneider 1991). However, it is possible that cognitions predict the stability of change even though they are not the vehicle of

Table 11–1. Controlled studies of cognitive therapy versus other treatment modalities

Study	Treatment groups	Mean panic frequency	Other measures included	Results	% Panic-free (posttreatment)	Follow-up (duration)
Clark et al. 1991	WL, CT, RT, IM (n = 16 each; all with exposure)	±3	HAS BAS Sensations Avoidance	All treatment groups benefited; CT most effective. RT and IM comparable. Scores on anxiety scales declined.	CT = 90 IM = 55 RT = 50 WL = 7	3- and 12-month follow-up, minimal change. Misinterpretation of bodily sensations predicts improvement from posttreatment to 1-year follow-up.
Margraf and Schneider 1991	CT, GE, CT + GE, WL (n = 20 each)	1–3/ week	HAS BDI Avoidance SCL BSQ CS	All treatment groups benefited, with few between-group differences. Treatment success correlated with therapist variables; pretreatment cognitions, bodily sensations, and fear; and exposure.	CT = 86 (93)[a] GE = 62 (77)[a] CT + GE = 67 (80)[a] WL = 7	
Beck et al., in press	CT (n = 17), ST (n = 16) (half on medication)	5.2/ week	BDI BAS	CT patients significantly improved on all panic measures and on BDI and BAS. No significant improvements in ST group, except on BDI (exposure in CT group?).	CT = 71 ST = 25	At 1-year follow-up, gains stable for 13/15.

Study	Treatment conditions		Assessment scales	Results	Outcome	Follow-up
Barlow et al. 1989	CT, AZ, PL, WL (n = 15 each)	Severity = 5 on ADIS	HAS BDI	CT included exposure to internal/external cues. CT more effective than PL but same as AZ on panic frequency and severity. Intensity of cognitive symptoms declined in CT, AZ, and PL groups. On disorder severity, no difference between CT, AZ, and PL at posttreatment.	CT = 86 AZ = 50 PL = 36	2-week follow-up.
Barlow et al. 1989	RT, WL, GE + CT, GE + CT + RT (practice exercises common) (n = 10–16 each)	1.5/ week	HAS BDI Monitoring CS	Equal reductions in severity in all 3 treatment groups. Scores on anxiety and depression scales declined in all 3 groups, as did scores on CS.	GE + CT + RT = 87 GE + CT = 85 RT = 60 WL = 36	No changes in 6-month follow-up period.
Öst, in press	CT, AR	4/week	HAS BAS BDI	Large, equal reductions in panic frequency across groups.	CT = 75 AR = 65	At 1-year follow-up, patients showed steady or further improvement.

Note. **Treatment conditions:** CT = cognitive therapy; RT = relaxation training; IM = imipramine; WL = waiting list; GE = graded exposure; ST = supportive therapy; AZ = alprazolam; PL = placebo; AR = applied relaxation. **Assessment scales:** HAS = Hamilton Anxiety Scale; BAS = Beck Anxiety Scale; HRSD = Hamilton Rating Scale for Depression; BDI = Beck Depression Inventory; SCL = Symptom Checklist; BSQ = Bodily Symptoms Questionnaire; CS = Chambless Cognitions Scale; ADIS = Anxiety Disorder Interview Schedule.
[a]Number in parentheses indicates percentage of patients panic-free at 4-week follow-up.

change. Furthermore, Margraf and Schneider found other predictors of stability (e.g., in the patient-therapist relationship). All of these results certainly are consistent with the cognitive approach to therapy.

It is worth noting that, even after successful therapy, a number of patients have continued to report some negative cognitions (e.g., Margraf and Schneider 1991); presumably these are noncritical cognitions, or, if they are critical, they are no longer strongly believed. Patients have also continued to report bodily sensations, and these remaining sensations too must be noncritical or now interpreted in a benign manner. From this, one can deduce that some cognitions are critical (the so-called *key cognitions;* see below) and that some bodily sensations may be critical also. In testing the major therapeutic deductions, it will be necessary to identify the critical cognitions and bodily sensations in advance.

Altered Cognitions: Cause, Consequence, or Correlate?

The decline in cognitions and bodily sensations observed after successful treatment is, of course, open to more than a single interpretation. These declines may produce the reduction of panic attacks. It is also possible that these declines are a consequence of the reduced episodes of panic and not the cause. It is further possible that the declines in cognitions may be correlates of the reduction in the panic episodes (some critics have suggested that the cognitions and their decline may be mere epiphenomena [e.g., Seligman 1988; Wolpe and Rowan 1989]).

One reason for giving serious consideration to these alternative explanations arises from the fact that, in Margraf and Schneider's (1991) study, the patients who received pure exposure treatment without cognitive manipulations showed improvements as large as the patients receiving pure CT. Moreover, cognitions declined to the same extent in both groups. In a similar vein, Booth and Rachman (1992) found that the fears and negative cognitions of claustrophobic patients showed large declines, regardless of whether the patients received exposure treatment or pure cognitive treatment (see Figure 11–1). It appears that negative cognitions can decline after a direct attack or an indirect attack.

Accounting for the Effects of Noncognitive Treatments on Cognitions

A satisfactory cognitive explanation needs to account for the declining cognitions that occur after an indirect treatment, such as exposure. The most obvious possibility is that, with each exposure, the patient acquires fresh, disconfirmatory evidence (e.g., experienced no heart attack, did not lose control). The accumulation of this personal, direct, disconfirmatory evidence weakens the catastrophic cognitions. However, one is nevertheless left to ponder why the direct assault on cognitions is not more effective than the indirect, incidental effects of exposure, as seen in the studies by Margraf and Schneider (1991) and Öst (in press). However, the results of the Clark et al. (1991) study (in which all patients were asked to carry out regular homework exposure exercises) were consistent with the idea that the effects of indirect attacks on the negative cognitions were significantly weaker than those achieved by a direct cognitive assault.

There is an even more difficult problem: how to account for the therapeutic effects of drugs such as imipramine, and the fact that, in the Clark et al. (1991) study, negative cognitions showed a small but significant decline after such drug treatment. Skeptics may argue that it was the provision of weekly exposure exercises that produced the therapeutic improvements in the CT group and in the

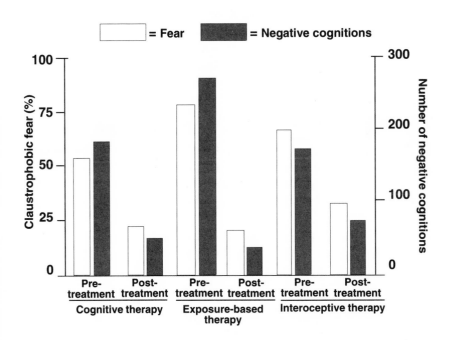

Figure 11–1.   Decline in claustrophobic fear and in negative cognitions after three interventions.   *Source.* Data from Booth and Rachman 1992.

imipramine group, and they can point to the powerful effects achieved by exposure treatment in the Margraf and Schneider (1991) study. However, the interpretation of the results of imipramine treatment and CT in terms of exposure fails to
explain why in the Clark et al. (1991) study the applied relaxation group, and
indeed the imipramine group, both of which had weekly self-exposure exercises,
did significantly less well than did the patients who received CT plus the exposure
exercises. It also fails to explain the absence of a relationship between the amount
of exposure and the extent of improvement (Margraf and Schneider 1991).

A cognitive explanation of the improvements in the imipramine group can be
based on the putative effects of the drug on bodily sensations. Perhaps, it can be
argued, there were fewer opportunities to make catastrophic cognitions because
the bodily sensations were muted by the drug (there is an overall decline in bodily
sensations after imipramine treatment) (Clark et al. 1991). This explanation is
plausible, but imipramine can increase heart rate, one of the bodily sensations that
is said to be implicated in many cases of panic disorder (e.g., "I fear that I will have
a heart attack and die."), and hence imipramine may provide *more* opportunities
for certain catastrophic cognitions. Perhaps the patients attributed the bodily
sensations to the drug, and "knowing" their origin, found them less alarming. To
clarify the psychological action of imipramine, studies of the drug's effects on
bodily sensations and how they are interpreted will need to be undertaken. To rule
out the effects of exposure, steps will need to be taken to prevent any change in
self-exposure during the analysis of cognitive changes.

Accounting for Reductions in Other Symptomatology

Cognitive explanations, no less than those based on ideas of habituation or extinction, need to account for the breadth of the therapeutic changes reported in the
relevant studies (Booth and Rachman 1992; Clark et al. 1991; Margraf and Schneider 1991). In all of these studies, successfully treated groups also showed reductions in depression and in general anxiety. The decline in anxiety raises few
problems, but it is not immediately clear why exposure treatment or CT should
reduce other problems. It seems unlikely that the reduction of panic, important
although it undoubtedly is, can account for the broad reduction of depression.

Conditions for Change

No satisfactory evaluation of the effects of CT can ignore the context from which
the cognitive theory emerged and the evidence pertaining to the validity of the
cognitive explanation for the nature and the causes of panic disorder (see Clark
1988; Rachman 1991; Rachman and Maser 1988; Seligman 1988; Teasdale 1988;

for present purposes, only a brief account is provided here). Clark and his colleagues showed that people who experienced panic attacks made a greater number of more intensely negative interpretations of bodily sensations than did other people. There are meaningful links between cognitions and bodily sensations (Marks et al. 1991; Rachman and Levitt 1988). For example, varying the instructions given to panic disorder patients prior to their undergoing the lactate challenge test affects the probability that a panic episode will occur; as another example, panic episodes can be induced by cognitive or other psychological manipulations (Rachman 1991).

Cognitive theory has been criticized for being nonexclusive, unrelated to traditional cognitive psychology (e.g., Seligman 1988), incomplete (Rachman 1991), unable to account for important phenomena (Klein and Klein 1989), and indistinguishable from conditioning theory (Wolpe and Rowan 1989). These complex theoretical matters will be sorted out in time, but to return to the therapeutic mechanisms of CT, we need to ascertain whether the reduction or elimination of key cognitions is the critical element in this form of therapy. We already know that the direct modification of cognitions can be *sufficient* for treatment success (see Table 11–1), but we also know that direct modification is not *necessary* for such success (e.g., exposure alone can be as effective as CT; imipramine and other medications can produce therapeutic improvements).

As mentioned earlier, the possibility that cognitions can be modified indirectly, as in exposure exercises, or perhaps even by imipramine, remains open. Failure to demonstrate that such indirect action is capable of reducing negative cognitions will limit the generality of the cognitive theory. So too will a failure to demonstrate that the reduction or elimination of panic occurs only if the negative cognitions are changed, whether by direct or indirect means. In essence, we need to find out whether the reduction or removal of the catastrophic cognitions is a necessary condition for the decline or elimination of panic attacks. It must be determined whether panic attacks can be reduced or eliminated despite the persistence of negative cognitions. We also need to know whether the reduction or removal of these cognitions can be accomplished by indirect means, and if so, how this is achieved.

Complexities

The above analytical tasks appear to be straightforward, but unfortunately there are several obstacles.

Defining Key Cognitions

As mentioned earlier, one is obliged to consider the probable existence of *key cognitions* (i.e., critical cognitions that are responsible for the panic attacks and whose removal is necessary for elimination of the attacks). During treatment, patients may express not one but several cognitions and endorse several cognitions from standard lists, such as that constructed by Chambless (1988). Also, during the course of treatment, other often idiosyncratic cognitions emerge. It is unlikely that all of these cognitions are equally critical, and we know that even after successful treatment some patients continue to endorse a diminished number of negative cognitions. Given that treatment is successful, these remaining cognitions cannot be regarded as critical. How, then, can we determine in advance, as we will need to do, which cognitions are critical and which are not?

The key cognitions may serve special functions. They may serve to drive fear and probably stitch together different types of fearful cognitions. There are various ways in which one can define and measure key cognitions, none of them simple or straightforward. One begins with the content, frequency, and intensity of the cognition. Unfortunately, it is not possible to depend entirely on the patient's description and rating of these cognitions because it cannot be assumed that the patient's information is always reliable and consistent (e.g., Nisbett and Wilson 1977). Therapist ratings also depend largely on the information provided by the patient. Another approach to the matter is to construct a scale for determining the degree of distortion contained in a cognition and the amount of functional impairment associated with it. Perhaps one of the most promising ways of measuring a cognition is to connect its content to the occurrence of avoidance behavior or other observable consequences. Methods for determining the connections between different fears already exist (e.g., Rachman 1991), and these, with some tailoring, can be adapted to the fearful cognitions that play a part in panic.

Understanding the Effects of Clusters of Cognitions

There is another layer of complexity because combinations or clusters of cognitions are more influential than single cognitions (Marks et al. 1991; Rachman et al. 1987). The probability of panic is greater when a patient has two or more threatening cognitions.

Understanding the Sequence of Events

Another obstacle arises from the need for control over the timing of events. If the reductions in negative cognitions are no more than correlates of panic reduction, or if the cognitive changes follow rather than precede the reduction of panic, we need to study the sequence of events with care. Reductions in fear are easier to observe and record, but they can occur slowly—over weeks, rather than minutes. In cases of panic, the measures typically range over days or weeks (e.g., the number of panic attacks recorded per week or even per month). Thus if the patient records a decline in panic attacks, say from four per week to one per week, when exactly did this change take place?

Cognitive changes can be even more difficult to track. It is true that in treatment major changes can occur suddenly (e.g., Öst 1989; Rachman and Whittal 1989), and it is therefore possible to time the change in these instances. In many clinical or experimental occurrences, however, the cognitive shifts are slow to develop, changing over weeks rather than minutes (e.g., the CT group in the Booth and Rachman 1992 study). To make matters worse, the changes in fear and in fearful cognitions can and undoubtedly often do occur even when the affected person is separated from and out of contact with the fear-provoking stimulus (Rachman 1991). It is not possible to determine precisely when the change occurred, assuming, of course, that there is a complete change in the first place. So we are left with the awkward task of timing the sequence of changes in the cognitions and in the episodes of panic, knowing that these changes may take place over an extended period and that the determination of a precise point of change will in many instances be impossible.

In the midst of these complexities and obstacles, it is worth drawing attention to the fact that useful progress has been made in developing methods to tackle these critical questions. For example, Salkovskis et al. (1991) were able to show in a preliminary study that cognitive treatment that is focused on specific cognitions produces larger and quicker changes than therapy that is more broadly aimed. In addition, we have early indications from the claustrophobia experiment (Booth and Rachman 1992) that the *believability* of the cognitions plays a major part in therapy. A single, strongly believed cognition may be more important than four or five cognitions with low believability (Shafran et al. 1993). Furthermore, the believability of the cognitions appears to have a clear influence on the return of fear. This same experiment produced preliminary evidence of the centrality of certain cognitions; when the presumably key cognition of "feeling trapped" was reduced, most of the other cognitions collapsed and fear declined sharply.

Determining How Many Processes Are Involved

The fact that there are several procedures that dependably reduce fear inevitably gives rise to considerations about whether these changes can be accounted for by a single process, or whether the therapeutic end is achieved by several different processes (see Barlow 1988; Rachman 1991). The finding that exposure and cognitive treatments were equally effective in the Margraf and Schneider (1991) study, despite clear procedural differences, raises the possibility that at least two processes are involved. If so, it is reasonable to expect that a combination of the two processes should produce an additive effect that is greater than that produced by either process acting alone. It is a curiosity of many of these forms of treatment that additive effects are not always demonstrable (e.g., Rachman et al. 1979), and, in the case of panic, the results from Margraf and Schneider's combined procedure produced no evidence of an additive effect. However, because there was virtually no room for demonstrating an additive effect, as the CT and the exposure therapy acting alone each produced results that were close to the ceiling, it is not reasonable at present to rule out the possibility of additive effects. In the absence of such evidence, it is simpler and more parsimonious to propose that a single process is responsible for the large and stable improvements in panic disorder that are being reported.

Having considered the cognitive explanation and the habituation theory, we turn to a different approach, exemplified by the work of Lang (1970, 1985) on the nature of fear. In brief, Lang argued that fear consists of at least three kinds of components—verbal, behavioral, and psychophysiological—and that these three are loosely coupled. In these terms, the two main psychological treatments for panic, CT and exposure, are aimed at different components of the fear structure: CT is directed at the verbal component and exposure treatment is aimed at the behavioral component. Direct modification of any one of the three components often leads to a modification in one or the other of the remaining components, albeit at a different pace. So, for example, if the therapist reduces the patient's false interpretation of his or her bodily sensation (e.g., interpreting a racing heart as the sign of a heart attack), then this misinterpretation generally is followed by a reduction in avoidance behavior. Similarly, a reduction in avoidance produced by repeated exposure exercises generally is followed or accompanied by a reduction in negative and false interpretations of bodily sensations. What Lang has called the *fear structure* can be changed by engineering a modification in one of the components of that structure. It is worth mentioning that the fear structure can be changed without evoking the fear response, even though that is often the most effective way of proceeding (de Silva and Rachman 1981). It is likely that cognitive processes can reduce all three components of fear—all three of which are components of panic.

The possibility that a single process is responsible for the therapeutic effects of two different psychological procedures remains plausible, but the possibility that a single process is responsible for the effects of a psychological and a pharmacological procedure is less plausible. There is no obvious connection between CT and the administration of imipramine. One procedure changes brain chemistry and the other rearranges cognitions. They involve different levels of action, consist of different operations, and follow different time courses. Nevertheless, the effects sometimes are comparable in breadth and speed (e.g., Clark et al. 1991), even if not in overall magnitude. The only noteworthy connection is the finding that, after taking imipramine, patients reported small but significant decreases in negative cognitions (Clark et al. 1991). The unexpected fact that negative cognitions decline during pharmacological treatment emphasizes again that these negative cognitions are amenable to change by several means, not only by direct modification. As noted above, in a recent clinical experiment Booth and Rachman (1992) found that the negative cognitions of claustrophobic patients declined significantly—and equally—after exclusively cognitive or exclusively exposure treatment.

Ideally, a cognitive explanation of CT should be broad enough to explain the cognitive changes that follow other forms of therapy, notably exposure and pharmacology. These broad and unexpected reductions in negative cognitions need not lead to the conclusion that negative cognitions are too insubstantial and ephemeral to provide any useful clues to mechanisms. There is a limit beyond which we need not go because there are methods, such as applied relaxation or interoceptive retraining, that produce only moderate changes in panic, or, for that matter, in claustrophobia, and are not accompanied or followed by such large reductions in negative cognitions (Figure 11–1). There is a connection between decreased negative cognitions and therapeutic progress. Moreover, the persistence of negative cognitions at the end of treatment is a partial predictor of poor long-term outcome (Clark et al. 1991; Margraf and Schneider 1991) and of the return of fear (Shafran et al. 1993).

To settle the question of whether cognitions are mere correlates, or even consequences of panic, it will be necessary to show that the reductions in panic are conditional on the decline of negative cognitions. So far, we have only a small amount of tantalizing evidence on this point. In a series of case studies, Salkovskis et al. (1991) showed that reductions in panic seemingly were dependent on the direct reduction of negative cognitions. Replication of this work on a larger scale is desirable. Evidence that therapeutic progress is conditional on the reduction of negative cognitions, even when methods other than CT are used, would be especially convincing. Indirect evidence includes the finding that reductions in claustrophobia were incomplete in those subjects who endorsed an excessive number of negative cognitions (Rachman and Levitt 1988), suggesting that these cognitions may impede the reduction of fear. However, if it can be shown that panic is reduced despite the persistence of key negative cognitions, then the cognitive explanation must be dismissed or severely qualified.

Incidentally, a full explanation of the mechanisms of treatment must find a place for the failures of a waiting-list control condition (Clark et al. 1991), brief supportive therapy (Beck et al., in press), and the relative failure of applied relaxation (Clark et al. 1991). What is the missing ingredient? Is it exposure or cognitive modification? In one sense, the difficulty in explaining the effects of therapy arises from an excess of success, for there are at least two methods that produce significant reductions in panic (exposure or CT), and another two that produce at least moderate reductions in panic (imipramine or applied relaxation).

Conclusions

The cognitive explanation for the results of CT is the best supported at present. Indeed, there is currently no plausible alternative explanation for the effects of CT.

Therapeutic reductions in the frequency and intensity of panic are associated with reductions in negative cognitions. The magnitude of the therapeutic improvements is impressive. In addition, there is a growing amount of indirect evidence for CT, mainly in the form of support for the underlying theory of panic causation. CT is legitimately deduced from the theory, and the theory itself is gaining some support. This intellectual cohesiveness is an added source of strength.

It remains to be shown that the reduction of panic is conditional on the reduction of critical negative cognitions. The temporal relations between cognitive change and panic reductions need close investigation, and a variety of other questions need to be answered. On a broader scale, we need to determine the extent to which the cognitive explanation can account for the therapeutic effects of exposure treatment and pharmacological treatment. As a first step we need to investigate the cognitive changes that accompany these other treatments. While aiming for a parsimonious explanation of the effects of therapy, we should leave open the possibility that a single explanation may prove unattainable.

References

American Psychiatric Association: Diagnostic and Statistical Manual of Mental Disorders, 3rd Edition, Revised. Washington, DC, American Psychiatric Association, 1987

Barlow D: Anxiety and Its Disorders. New York, Guilford, 1988

Barlow D, Craske M, Cerny J, et al: Behavioral treatment of panic disorder. Behavior Therapy 20:261–282, 1989

Beck A: Cognitive approaches to panic disorder, in Panic: Psychological Perspectives. Edited by Rachman S, Maser J. Hillsdale, NJ, Lawrence Erlbaum, 1988, pp 91–110

Beck A, Ward CH, Mendelson M, et al: An inventory for measuring depression. Arch Gen Psychiatry 4:561–571, 1961

Beck A, Sokol L, Clark DA, et al: Focused cognitive therapy of panic disorder (in press)

Booth R, Rachman S: The reduction of claustrophobia. Behav Res Ther 30:207–221, 1992

Chambless DL: Cognitive mechanisms in panic disorder, in Panic: Psychological Perspectives. Edited by Rachman S, Maser J. Hillsdale, NJ, Lawrence Erlbaum, 1988, pp 205–218

Clark DM: A cognitive approach to panic. Behav Res Ther 24:461–470, 1986

Clark DM: A cognitive model of panic attacks, in Panic: Psychological Perspectives. Edited by Rachman S, Maser J. Hillsdale, NJ, Lawrence Erlbaum, 1988, pp 71–90

Clark DM, Salkovskis P, Hackmann A, et al: A comparison of cognitive therapy, applied relaxation, and imipramine in the treatment of panic disorder. Paper presented at the annual meeting of the American Association for the Advancement of Behavior Therapy, New York, November 1991

de Silva P, Rachman S: Is exposure a necessary condition for fear-reduction? Behav Res Ther 19:227–232, 1981

Hamilton M: The assessment of anxiety states by rating. Br J Med Psychol 32:50–55, 1959

Hamilton M: A rating scale for depression. J Neurol Neurosurg Psychiatry 23:56–62, 1960

Klein D, Klein H: The nosology of anxiety disorders: a critical review of hypothesis testing about spontaneous panic, in Psychopharmacology of Anxiety. Edited by Tyrer P. Oxford, UK, Oxford University Press, 1989, pp 163–195

Lader M, Mathews A: A physiological model of phobia anxiety and desensitization. Behav Res Ther 6:411–418, 1968

Lader M, Wing L: Physiological Measures, Sedative Drugs and Morbid Anxiety. London, Oxford University Press, 1966

Lang P: Stimulus control, response control and desensitization of fear, in Learning Approaches to Therapeutic Behavior Change. Edited by Levis D. Chicago, IL, Aldine Press, 1970, pp 64–82

Lang P: The cognitive psychophysiology of emotion: fear and anxiety, in Anxiety and the Anxiety Disorders. Edited by Tuma A, Maser J. Hillsdale, NJ, Lawrence Erlbaum, 1985, pp 219–230

Margraf J, Schneider S: Outcome and active ingredients of cognitive-behavioral treatments for panic disorder. Paper presented at the annual meeting of the American Association for the Advancement of Behavior Therapy, New York, November 1991

Marks I: Fears, Phobias, and Rituals. Oxford, UK, Oxford University Press, 1987

Marks M, Basoglu M, Alkubaisy T, et al: Are anxiety symptoms and catastrophic cognitions directly related? Journal of Anxiety Disorders 5:247–254, 1991

Nisbett R, Wilson T: Telling more than we can know: verbal reports on mental processes. Psychol Rev 84:231–259, 1977

Öst L: One-session treatment for specific phobias. Behav Res Ther 27:1–8, 1989

Öst L: Applied relaxation, exposure in vivo, and cognitive methods in the treatment of panic disorder. Behav Res Ther (in press)

Rachman S: Fear and Courage, 2nd Edition. New York, WH Freeman, 1991

Rachman S, Levitt K: Panic, fear reduction and habituation. Behav Res Ther 26:199–206, 1988

Rachman S, Maser J (eds): Panic: Psychological Perspectives. Hillsdale, NJ, Lawrence Erlbaum, 1988

Rachman S, Whittal M: Fast, slow and sudden reductions in fear. Behav Res Ther 27:613–620, 1989

Rachman S, Cobb J, Grey S, et al: The behavioral treatment of obsessional-compulsive disorders, with and without clomipramine. Behav Res Ther 17:467–472, 1979

Rachman S, Levitt K, Lopatka C: Panic: the links between cognitions and bodily symptoms. Behav Res Ther 25:411–424, 1987

Salkovskis P, Clark D, Hackmann A: Treatment of panic attacks using cognitive therapy without exposure or breathing retraining. Behav Res Ther 29:161–166, 1991

Seligman MEP: Competing theories of panic, in Panic: Psychological Perspectives. Edited by Rachman S, Maser J. Hillsdale, NJ, Lawrence Erlbaum, 1988, pp 321–330

Shafran R, Booth R, Rachman S: The reduction of claustrophobia: cognitive analyses. Behav Res Ther 31:75–85, 1993

Teasdale T: Cognitive models and treatments for panic: a critical evaluation, in Panic: Psychological Perspectives. Edited by Rachman S, Maser J. Hillsdale, NJ, Lawrence Erlbaum, 1988, pp 189–220

Wolpe J: Psychotherapy by Reciprocal Inhibition. Stanford, CA, Stanford University Press, 1958

Wolpe J, Rowan V: Panic disorder: a product of classical conditioning. Behav Res Ther 27:583–585, 1989

Chapter 12

A Review of Psychosocial Treatments for Panic Disorder

Dianne L. Chambless, Ph.D., and Martha M. Gillis, M.A.

Given the emotional, economic, and social costs of panic disorder (e.g., Markowitz et al. 1989), promoting the identification and availability of effective treatments should be a priority on our national mental health agenda. Although it is heartening to observe the important advances in pharmacological treatment, it is also vital that we consider psychological alternatives to pharmacotherapy. The seeming ease of prescribing medication can be deceptive. In the long run, if clinicians rely solely on pharmacological approaches, they must face problems such as the side effects of both short-term and chronic use of medication, relapse after withdrawal, and patients' noncompliance with medication regimens. Furthermore, we must consider that approximately 10% of the panic disorder population abuses alcohol (Bibb and Chambless 1986), which may interact dangerously with medication. Because the majority of those with panic disorder are women in the childbearing years, the possible effects of medication on the developing fetus and nursing infant must give us pause.

In this chapter we argue that there are abundant empirical data documenting the efficacy of psychological treatments. There is little systematic evidence concerning the availability of the effective psychological treatments, but it appears that relatively few people with panic disorder receive appropriate treatment (Taylor et al. 1989). This state of affairs seems to result, at least in part, from ill-informed referral practices of the health care professionals whom patients who experience panic first contact and the lack of mental health professionals aware of and trained

Preparation of this manuscript was supported by NIMH Grant 5 R01-MH44190-03.

149

in specific and effective treatment approaches. Public ignorance about panic disorder and financial constraints are other important factors.

Although many American practitioners are psychodynamic in orientation (e.g., Norcross and Prochaska 1982), there is almost no research on the efficacy of psychoanalytical approaches for panic disorder. The authors of Chapters 9–11 discuss the cognitive and behavior treatment of panic; our review provides a broader overview, focusing on the effectiveness of cognitive and behavior treatments. Current research seems to be focused on the panic attacks that are the defining feature of panic disorder. This is a welcome and long overdue development. One should recall, however, that the majority of those who seek treatment for panic disorder have developed phobic anxiety and avoidance, ranging from subtle deficits in functioning to incapacitating agoraphobia. Thus we begin by reviewing the findings on treatment of phobic avoidance in panic disorder patients with agoraphobia. Subsequently, we review the literature on treatment aimed at reducing panic attacks, and survey the evidence of those treatments' effects on the high level of general anxiety commonly found in this population and on the cognitive aspects of panic anxiety.

Efficacy of Psychological Treatments for Phobic Avoidance

Exposure-Based Treatments

After a comprehensive review of 24 empirical studies of behavior treatment for agoraphobia, Jansson and Öst (1982) concluded that both imaginal flooding and in vivo exposure (exposure in real life to phobic situations) consistently yielded significant improvement for agoraphobic patients, whereas systematic desensitization did not. Other studies have indicated that cognitive modification approaches, such as self-instructional training or rational emotive therapy, are less effective than exposure therapy (e.g., Emmelkamp et al. 1978, 1986).

Because in vivo exposure has generally been found to have more powerful effects than imaginal flooding, it has become the standard behavior treatment for agoraphobia. Exposure therapy is effective whether carried out with the therapist or by the patient alone with direction and structure provided by the therapist. In follow-up studies of clinical status 1–9 years after treatment, patients treated with exposure therapy have, by and large, maintained their gains on self-report, behavioral, and physiological measures (Emmelkamp and Kuipers 1979; Jansson et al.

1986; Munby and Johnston 1980). Moreover, with a maintenance program of written instructions for self-directed exposure and occasional telephone contact with the therapist, patients have continued to improve significantly (Jansson et al. 1986). Such studies tell us that statistically significant changes reliably occur, but how clinically important are these changes?

Trull et al. (1988) conducted a meta-analysis of 22 published studies of various behavior treatments in which the same outcome measure (the Fear Questionnaire—Agoraphobia Subscale [Marks and Matthews 1979]) was used. To form a comparison group, these authors collected data on this measure from a randomly selected community sample of people who had never received treatment for a phobia. Across all studies, the 454 agoraphobic patients scored two standard deviations (SDs) above the community norms before treatment, whereas their scores fell to within 0.5 SDs of the community group after treatment and at follow-up. Expressed in percentile scores, patients began treatment at the 97th percentile for community norms and finished at the 68th percentile (66th at follow-up). Similar effects were obtained on depression scores on the Beck Depression Inventory (Beck and Steer 1987). Patients who had received in vivo exposure, especially in the form of self-directed exposure, fared better than those whose treatment was not exposure based. Thus, after an average of 13 hours of treatment, agoraphobic patients were clinically improved on self-reported depression and avoidance behavior. These group averages, however, hide considerable within-sample variability in treatment response. How well did the individual patient do?

Using a 50% reduction in agoraphobic fear and avoidance as their criterion of improvement, Jansson and Öst (1982) found that 58%–83% (median 70%) of agoraphobic patients who completed treatment with in vivo exposure benefited markedly from treatment. An average of 12% dropped out. Jacobson et al. (1988) used a statistically based criterion for improvement—the Reliable Change Index. (A patient who has improved approximately 2 standard errors of the pre- to posttreatment difference scores is considered to have reliably changed.) These authors reanalyzed the raw data from 11 published studies of exposure-based treatments for agoraphobia (imaginal and in vivo). Considering a variety of measures, most but not all of which were measures of phobia, Jacobson et al. found that 58% of the patients had improved reliably at posttest (60% at follow-up). Using their criterion for clinically significant change (reliable change plus the patient's having moved within the normal range on the measure in question), 27% of the patients were recovered at posttest and 34% at follow-up. Patients showed most improvement on the main phobias they had targeted for treatment, with 90% reliably changing on this measure. Broader measures of phobia showed lower rates (38.5%) of reliable change.

Increasing the Effectiveness of Exposure-Based Treatment

The results of exposure-based treatment are, on the one hand, very heartening. Although agoraphobia had previously proven refractory to a variety of treatments, the majority of patients now show meaningful change with exposure therapy. On the other hand, 30%–40% fail to benefit from exposure therapy, and 65% stop short of recovery. In addition, many patients continue to seek pharmacological or psychological treatments after short-term treatment with exposure therapy, thereby telling us that they think their treatment was insufficient or the results were unstable (Munby and Johnston 1980). Accordingly, researchers' attention has turned to how to improve the effects of exposure-based treatments, frequently by adding additional components to a treatment package.

Investigators have examined the additive effects of medication, spousal involvement, relaxation training, and cognitive strategies in combination with exposure-based treatment.

▮ **Adding medications.** Although the results are somewhat variable (e.g., Marks et al. 1983), on the whole, patients who received imipramine plus exposure therapy improved more on avoidance behavior than did those who took a placebo (Mavissakalian and Michelson 1986a; Telch et al. 1985; Zitrin et al. 1980). The effects seemed to occur at a daily dosage of greater than 150 mg (Mavissakalian and Michelson 1986a), a level that is often difficult for agoraphobic patients to reach because they are very sensitive to the side effects of tricyclics. Mavissakalian and Michelson (1986a) reported that, of those who did reach this therapeutic level, 75% were functioning well on phobic measures at posttest, versus about 30% of those on placebo or daily dosage levels of less than 125 mg. However, subsequent to drug withdrawal, the beneficial effects of imipramine are largely lost, probably due to the higher relapse rate of the imipramine-treated subjects (Mavissakalian and Michelson 1986b).

Study results on the effects of benzodiazepines are even less promising. Neither acute doses of benzodiazepines plus exposure therapy (e.g., Hafner and Marks 1976) nor daily low doses of benzodiazepines plus exposure therapy (Gray 1991) have proved more effective than placebo plus exposure therapy. At the dosage level advocated for reduction of panic attacks (e.g., 4–6 mg/day), the high potency benzodiazepine alprazolam actually reduced the benefits of exposure therapy during the follow-up period (Marks et al. 1991). In contrast to those who received placebo plus exposure therapy, those who received alprazolam plus exposure therapy had a high relapse rate after drug withdrawal. We may conclude that, unless patients remain on medication indefinitely, tricyclics have only short-term benefit for patients receiving exposure treatment where avoidance behavior is concerned, and benzodiazepines have none at all.

▮ **Adding other psychological components.** What of attempts to augment the effects of exposure therapy through the addition of other psychological treatments? In four studies (Michelson et al. 1988, 1989; Öst et al. 1984, 1989) the incremental effects of relaxation training to exposure therapy were examined, with patients being taught relaxation techniques to apply in phobic situations. In all studies the combined treatment was no more effective than exposure therapy alone. Similarly disappointing results emerged from six studies (Emmelkamp and Mersch 1982; Emmelkamp et al. 1986; Michelson et al. 1988, 1989; Öst et al. 1989; Williams and Rappoport 1983) in which 6–16 sessions of various cognitive modification techniques (paradoxical intention, self-statement training, rational emotive therapy, and Beck's and Emery's cognitive therapy [CT]) were paired with exposure therapy.

Related to, but somewhat different from, the studies on cognitive modification are those on respiratory control. In this treatment, agoraphobic patients who recognize hyperventilation-induced symptoms to be similar to those of their panic attacks are trained to reattribute anxiety symptoms to hyperventilation, and are taught slow, diaphragmatic breathing to counteract such symptoms. In two controlled studies (Bonn et al. 1984; de Ruiter et al. 1989), breathing retraining did not add significantly to the effects of exposure therapy on avoidance behavior at posttest. Indeed, de Ruiter et al. (1989) found exposure therapy alone to be more effective, perhaps because the group receiving exposure therapy plus breathing retraining had only half as much exposure treatment. However, at 6-month follow-up, Bonn et al. (1984) found their breathing retraining plus exposure therapy group to fare significantly better than the exposure therapy–alone subjects on a number of variables, including phobic anxiety and avoidance. Hence, de Ruiter et al.'s follow-up data will be of great interest when they are available.

In a final set of studies, the usefulness of addressing the agoraphobic's interpersonal system in combination with exposure treatment has been examined. Kleiner et al. (1987) treated agoraphobic women with exposure therapy or exposure therapy plus training in interpersonal problem solving; the combination treatment was no more effective at posttest or follow-up. Other investigators have included the agoraphobic patient's spouse in educational and treatment interventions, with the spouse assisting the agoraphobic patient in carrying out exposure homework assignments. The results have been mixed, perhaps due to differences in levels of spousal involvement. Whereas Barlow et al. (1984; see also Cerny et al. 1987) found that including spouses in all 12 treatment sessions led to superior treatment results at posttest and follow-up, Cobb et al. (1984) discerned no additional benefit from including spouses in their brief intervention.

In the preceding studies, spouses were involved in treatment, but marital therapy per se was not conducted. Arnow et al. (1985) first treated agoraphobic patients with exposure therapy and then assigned patients and their spouses to either couples communication and problem-solving training or couples relaxation training (the latter intended as a placebo). Couples in the communication group were more positive in their communication patterns after the training, and the phobic partners in the communication group showed significantly superior responses on self-report and behavioral measures of phobic avoidance at posttest and at 8-month follow-up. It is important to note that, on the whole, these couples were not maritally distressed. Rather, learning to communicate more effectively about the patient's phobia appeared to have significantly enhanced treatment response. Such data suggest that helping agoraphobic patients' families support efforts by the patients to change may improve the benefits derived from exposure therapy. Also congruent with this conclusion are the data gathered by Munby and Johnston (1980), who found that, at long-term follow-up, agoraphobic patients whose spouses were included in treatment were less likely to have sought additional treatment than were patients who were treated individually. It is important to replicate Arnow et al.'s (1985) marital therapy study, and it is surprising that this has not been done yet.

Summary of Treatment for Phobic Avoidance

The preceding review informs us that in vivo exposure and its variants (e.g., applied relaxation) are the most demonstrably effective treatments for avoidance behavior in panic disorder patients with agoraphobia. Approximately 60% of patients make very substantial changes with treatment and 34% recover. These results are well maintained or increased at follow-up. Our concern needs to be focused on that 40% of patients who do not benefit markedly and on increasing the number in the recovered category. In general, the addition of time-limited pharmacotherapy or other psychological interventions has not added to the long-term effectiveness of exposure therapy, but attention to the agoraphobic patient's interpersonal system seems to be bearing fruit. Additional National Institute of Mental Health–supported studies in this area are being conducted by David Barlow and his group at the State University of New York at Albany and collaboratively by Gail Steketee and Dianne Chambless at Boston University and American University, respectively.

Generalized Anxiety, Panic, and Fear of Fear

Avoidance behavior is only one aspect of panic disorder. Other important symptoms include generalized anxiety, panic attacks, and the patient's fear of anxiety, variously called *anxiety sensitivity* or *fear of fear*. Published empirical reviews of the effectiveness of psychosocial treatments for these symptoms are largely lacking (for an exception, see Clum's 1989 review comparing behavioral and pharmacological interventions for panic attacks), especially where the newer, and quite powerful, treatments are considered. Accordingly, for this chapter, the literature on behavior and cognitive-behavior treatments has been summarized by converting treatment findings into effect sizes. We include only studies in which the diagnosis of all subjects was agoraphobia or panic disorder without agoraphobia; furthermore, of necessity, our sample of studies is restricted to those for which the authors provided means and standard deviations for the measures across treatments.

Two types of effect sizes were calculated using Smith and Glass's delta (1977). Because most studies compared the effects of one treatment with another, rather than contrasting the results of a treatment group to a waiting-list control or placebo, crude pretest-posttest and pretest–follow-up effects were first computed with the following formula:

$$(M_{pretest} - M_{posttest}) / SD_{pretest}$$

Where meaningful groups of studies with similar treatments could be formed, average effect sizes weighted for sample size were calculated. These are presented in Tables 12–2 through 12–7 and Table 12–9. Second, we calculated controlled effect sizes for those studies with waiting-list or placebo controls (see Tables 12–8 and 12–10). The number of subjects reported to be panic-free is noted when authors provided these data, and dropout data are presented in weighted average

Table 12–1. Dropout rates for psychosocial treatment of agoraphobia and panic disorder

Treatment method	Weighted average (%)	Range (%)
Exposure in vivo (may include coping skills)	16	3–25
Relaxation (usually applied)	12	5–33
Cognitive therapy (may include interoceptive exposure)	8	0–24

Table 12–2. In vivo exposure with agoraphobia: pretest to posttest effects

Study	No. of sessions	Anxiety	No. of panic attacks	Fear of fear	% Panic-free
Craske et al. 1989	11	1.46	0.33	0.89	57
de Ruiter et al. 1989	8	0.33	0.00	0.83	—
Marks et al. 1991	6	8.00	3.90	—	43
Michelson et al. 1988	12	0.99	—	—	50
Öst et al. 1989	12	—	—	0.93	—
Telch et al. 1985	6	—	0.53	—	—
Weighted average[a]		1.08	0.29	0.89	54

[a]Outlier (Marks et al. 1991) excluded.

form (see Table 12–1). When multiple measures of a construct were used, effect sizes within each study were averaged. To facilitate comparisons across treatments, average effect sizes are depicted graphically in Figures 12–1 through 12–5.[1]

Exposure-Based Treatment

As shown by the data in Table 12–1, our review of more recent studies of exposure therapy found that the treatment continues to be well tolerated by patients, with an average dropout rate of 16%. The effects of six studies (Craske et al. 1989; de Ruiter et al. 1989; Marks et al. 1991; Michelson et al. 1988; Öst et al. 1989; Telch et al. 1985) using in vivo exposure therapy alone (plus pill placebo in two cases) are depicted in Table 12–2. Because the effect sizes for the Marks et al. (1991) study

---

[1] To provide some convention for the evaluation of effect sizes, Cohen (1988) suggests that researchers consider 0.2, 0.5, and 0.8 to be small, medium, and large effect sizes, respectively. However, note that the importance of an effect size does not correspond completely with its absolute size. For example, the effect size for the benefits of zidovudine (AZT) for survival in people with acquired immunodeficiency syndrome is small (Rosenthal 1990), but, given the consequences of the untreated condition, of great practical significance.

were widely discrepant from the remainder, these have not been included in the weighted averages. Patients who received an average of 10 sessions of exposure treatment showed large changes on generalized anxiety and fear of fear, but the effects on the number of panic attacks per week were small. It should be noted, however, that, because these patients participated in studies where agoraphobia was the defining symptom for treatment entry, most samples did not have high rates of weekly panic episodes before treatment (the only exception was the Marks et al. sample, which had extremely severe symptoms). Hence, restriction of range may limit our ability to assess exposure therapy's effectiveness for this variable. Table 12–3 contains the follow-up effect sizes indicating that exposure therapy's effects are well maintained or even somewhat increased after an average period of 6 months. An average of 54% of the patients were panic-free at posttest and 63% at follow-up.

Applied Relaxation

Seven study samples (Barlow et al. 1989; Clark et al. 1991; Marks et al. 1991; Michelson et al. 1988; Öst 1988; Öst and Westling 1991; Öst et al. 1989) of the effects of relaxation training were located. In all cases except the Marks et al. (1991) study, the treatment was applied relaxation training wherein, via imaginal or in vivo exposure, patients were taught to apply their relaxation skills when

Table 12–3. In vivo exposure with agoraphobia: pretest to follow-up effects

Study	Follow-up length (months)	Effect sizes Anxiety	No. of panic attacks	Fear of fear	% Panic-free
Craske et al. 1989	6	1.50	0.54	1.18	67
Marks et al. 1991	9	11.70	6.00	—	77
Michelson et al. 1988	3	1.15	—	—	43
Öst et al. 1989	12	—	—	1.13	—
Telch et al. 1985	4.5	—	0.22	—	—
Weighted average[a]		1.34	0.40	1.16	63

[a]Outlier (Marks et al. 1991) excluded.

anxious. In other research, Öst (1988) showed that applied relaxation is superior to progressive muscle relaxation alone. In three samples (Marks et al. 1991; Michelson et al. 1988; Öst et al. 1989), the patients were agoraphobic, whereas in the other four samples, the patients were characterized by no-to-moderate avoidance (Barlow et al. 1989; Clark et al. 1991; Öst 1988; Öst and Westling 1991). Again, the Marks et al. data were excluded from averages because of their unusual effect sizes.

An average of 13 sessions yielded very large effect sizes for generalized anxiety and panic attacks and a large effect for fear of fear (Table 12–4). An average of 14 months later, these results were well maintained (Table 12–5). An average of 61% of patients were panic-free at posttest and 64% at follow-up. Treatment was well tolerated, with an average dropout rate of 12%.

Cognitive Therapy

Tables 12–6 and 12–7 depict the effect sizes for studies conducted using the model of Beck's CT for panic disorder developed by Clark and Salkovskis (in press). CT trials in six studies (Beck et al. 1992; Clark et al. 1991; Margraf and Schneider 1991;

Table 12–4. Effects of relaxation training on panic disorder (PD) and agoraphobic (AG) patients: pretest to posttest

Study	Sample	No. of sessions	Effect sizes			% Panic-free
			Anxiety	No. of panic attacks	Fear of fear	
Barlow et al. 1989	PD	15	2.75	0.70	—	60
Clark et al. 1991	PD	12	1.07	1.56	0.85	50
Marks et al. 1991[a]	AG	6	4.50	4.14	—	47
Michelson et al. 1988	AG	12	1.28	—	—	75
Öst 1988	PD	14	—	—	—	100
Öst et al. 1989	AG	12	—	—	0.92	61
Öst and Westling 1991	PD	12	—	—	—	65
Weighted average[b]			1.62	1.27	0.88	61

[a]No applied relaxation component.
[b]Outlier (Marks et al. 1991) excluded.

Newman et al. 1990; Öst and Westling 1991; Sokol et al. 1989) conducted in four nations yielded very large effect sizes for all three variables; these were maintained or enhanced at follow-up. At both assessment points (posttreatment and follow-up), at least 85% of the patients were panic-free. The average dropout rate, 8%, was the lowest of the three psychosocial treatments we reviewed.

For three of these studies (Beck et al. 1992; Clark et al. 1991; Margraf and Schneider 1991), control group data were available either for a waiting-list period or for response to supportive psychotherapy (Table 12–8). Effect sizes contrasting the posttest scores of treatment groups to those of control groups were calculated with the formula

$$(M_{control} - M_{treatment}) / SD_{control}$$

These statistics provide a more rigorous evaluation of the effects of CT than do the uncontrolled data in Tables 12–6 and 12–7. The controlled effect sizes remain very large for all three variables, although somewhat smaller for generalized anxiety, than in the uncontrolled data. An average of 83% of CT patients were

Table 12–5. Effects of relaxation training on panic disorder (PD) and agoraphobic (AG) patients: pretest to follow-up

Study	Sample	Follow-up length (months)	Anxiety	Effect sizes No. of panic attacks	Fear of fear	% Panic-free
Clark et al. 1991	PD	15	1.70	1.71	1.08	47
Craske et al. 1991	PD	24	—	—	—	56
Marks et al. 1991[a]	AG	9	5.50	3.86	—	59
Michelson et al. 1988	AG	3	1.27	—	—	61
Öst 1988	PD	19	—	—	—	100
Öst et al. 1989	AG	12	—	—	0.91	—
Öst and Westling 1991	PD	12	—	—	—	82
Weighted average[b]			1.46	—	1.01	64

[a]No applied relaxation component.
[b]Outlier (Marks et al. 1991) excluded.

panic-free at posttest, compared with 12% of the control subjects. In other research, Newman et al. (1990) and Cottraux et al. (1986) demonstrated that CT can be successfully used to withdraw panic disorder patients from medication.

Combination Treatments

A general assumption made by clinicians and researchers alike is that combining elements of various effective treatments should lead to a more powerful treatment. Table 12–9 shows the results of six studies (Barlow et al. 1989; Chambless et al. 1986; Klosko et al. 1990; Margraf and Schneider 1991; Michelson et al. 1989, 1990) in which such an approach was followed. In all these studies, some form of in vivo exposure or exposure to interoceptive cues related to panic was used concurrently with a variety of cognitive strategies. Drawing meaningful conclusions from this set is made difficult by the heterogeneous interventions used and the sample variability. Table 12–10 provides four controlled effect sizes for combination treatment versus a waiting-list control period and one for combination treatment versus pill placebo. These effects are little changed from those for uncontrolled studies. An average of 72% of patients receiving combined treatment were panic-free at posttest versus 25% in control groups.

The combination treatments for agoraphobic patients appeared to yield no larger effect sizes than did exposure therapy alone, a finding reminiscent of the set

Table 12–6. Cognitive therapy for panic disorder: pretest to posttest effects of studies using the Beck and Emery/Clark and Salkovskis model

Study	No. of sessions	Effect sizes			% Panic-free
		Anxiety	No. of panic attacks	Fear of fear	
Beck et al. 1992	12	1.50	1.05	—	94
Clark et al. 1991	12	2.04	2.20	1.26	90
Margraf and Schneider 1991	15	1.18	1.00	1.00	90
Newman et al. 1990	12–16	1.62	0.51	2.29	83
Öst and Westling 1991	12	2.13	1.21	1.55	75
Sokol et al. 1989	15 (avg.)	1.69	0.80	—	100
Weighted average		1.68	0.98	1.75	88

of studies on avoidance behavior summarized above. For panic disorder patients, the combined findings looked no stronger than CT alone. These data suggest that our assumption that combined treatments are better may be wrong.

One exception to the general failure of combination treatments to boost treatment response was a study by Michelson et al. (1989) not included in these tables. Those investigators found that adding Beck's CT to exposure therapy for agoraphobia led to significantly better results on spontaneous (nonphobic) panic attacks and on a composite measure of high end-state functioning at follow-up. Of their combined group, 87.5% met criteria for high end-state functioning at 3-month follow-up versus 65% of those in the exposure-alone group. Michelson et al.'s data may be unique because they were the only investigators to combine Beck's CT with exposure therapy for agoraphobic patients. (All cognitive therapies may not be created equal!) Moreover, when investigators use combined treatment packages but hold the time in treatment constant, they may deprive patients of adequate time to learn any one treatment approach thoroughly. Following this rationale, Michelson et al. lengthened the patients' treatment to 16 sessions to allow patients time to incorporate changes in belief systems about panic and avoidance while also completing systematic homework assignments for in vivo exposure. Replication of this study is highly desirable.

We also need research that uses strategies for defining high end-state func-

Table 12–7. Cognitive therapy for panic disorder: pretest to follow-up effects of studies using the Beck and Emery/Clark and Salkovskis model

Study	Length of follow-up (months)	Effect sizes			% Panic-free
		Anxiety	No. of panic attacks	Fear of fear	
Beck et al. 1992	12	2.12	1.09	—	87
Clark et al. 1991	12	2.53	2.05	1.31	80
Margraf and Schneider 1991	1	1.33	1.08	1.00	90
Newman et al. 1990	12	1.65	0.49	2.13	80
Ost and Westling 1991	12	2.19	1.38	1.53	80
Sokol et al. 1989	12	1.69	0.80	—	100
Weighted average		1.73	1.00	1.53	85

tioning to examine how patients fare in a global sense (see Himadi et al. 1986; Mavissakalian and Michelson 1986b). It is conceivable that any advantages of combination treatments might be more apparent on such composite measures (e.g., Michelson et al. 1989). Given the very strong showing of CT in treating panic disorder without agoraphobia, it is possible that the development of combination treatments will be more important for patients with agoraphobia than for those with uncomplicated panic disorder.

Summary

Figures 12–1 through 12–4 summarize the effects of psychosocial treatment for panic, generalized anxiety, and fear of fear across types of psychosocial treatment. The number of studies is too small to permit formal statistical comparison, allowing only preliminary comparative statements about differential effectiveness.

All therapies showed large effect sizes for generalized anxiety, with applied relaxation and CT showing the best effects. Across studies, patients treated with psychosocial interventions averaged from a low of 54% panic-free with exposure therapy alone to a high of 88% panic-free with CT. These figures compare very favorably with posttest statistics for waiting-list and placebo treatments (averaging 12%–25% panic-free in our review) and for pharmacological treatment (e.g., 50%–59% for alprazolam [Ballenger et al. 1988; Klosko et al. 1990] and 55% for imipramine [Clark et al. 1991]). Even more impressive, the results of psychosocial

Table 12–8. Cognitive therapy (CT) for panic disorder: comparison with waiting-list (WL) or supportive therapy (ST) control groups in studies using the Beck and Emery/Clark and Salkovskis model

| | | Effect sizes | | | % Panic-free | |
Study	Contrast group	Anxiety	No. of panic attacks	Fear of fear	CT	Control
Beck et al. 1992	ST	0.86	0.66	—	71[a]	25
Clark et al. 1991	WL	1.63	1.68	1.89	90	7
Margraf and Schneider 1991	WL	0.94	1.00	1.50	90	5
Weighted average		1.15	1.12	1.71	83	12

[a]This figure differs from the 94% cited in Table 12–6 because the comparison in the present study was conducted after 8 sessions, whereas the statistic in Table 12–6 was computed on responses after 12 sessions.

treatment are well maintained at follow-up, which is typically not the case for pharmacotherapy after drug withdrawal (e.g., Clark et al. 1991; Fyer et al. 1987).

Examining effect sizes for average panic frequency, we found small to moderate effects for exposure therapy alone and in combination, but large effects for CT and applied relaxation. Effect sizes for measures of fear of fear are also presented, because fear of fear has been found to be an important factor in predicting the development of phobic avoidance among those with panic disorder, and of panic disorder among those with panic attacks. The effect sizes for exposure therapy alone and in combination and for applied relaxation are large and comparable, whereas the effect sizes for CT are extremely large. Figure 12–5 displays the relative effects of CT, combined exposure therapy plus cognitive modification techniques, and control groups at posttest. Only studies in which control groups were used are included in the averages depicted in this figure. Inspection of this graph shows that Beck's CT (Beck and Emery 1985), as developed for panic by Clark and Salkovskis (in press), shows very large effect sizes for all variables, whereas only small to modest changes are made with the passage of time or supportive therapy. The findings for combined treatments are more variable and never as great as for CT, suggesting that CT may be the most promising psychosocial treatment for panic disorder.

Table 12–9. Interoceptive or in vivo exposure plus various cognitive techniques: pretest to posttest effects

Study	Sample	No. of sessions	Effect sizes Anxiety	No. of panic attacks	Fear of fear	% Panic-free
Barlow et al. 1989	PD	15	1.11	0.20	—	87
Chambless et al. 1986	AG	10	—	0.33	0.52	43
Klosko et al. 1990	PD	15	1.31	—	—	87
Margraf and Schneider 1991	PD	15	0.90	0.88	1.77	75
Michelson et al. 1989	AG	16	1.22	.89	1.34	68
Michelson et al. 1990	PD	13	1.08	1.31	1.10	—
Weighted average			1.14	0.63	1.05	66

Note. PD = panic disorder patients; AG = agoraphobic patients.

Delivery of Services

The data reviewed in this chapter clearly demonstrate that effective psychosocial treatments for panic disorder have been developed; but how do we ensure that the public gets them? Can our society afford to provide these treatments to the millions of Americans who have panic disorder and agoraphobia? Given the personal, social, and economic costs of this disorder, can we afford *not* to provide them with treatment?

Perhaps because of the press for services in their National Health System (NHS), British researchers have been far more interested than those in the United States in containing costs and reducing the need for professional time in the treatment of agoraphobia. The research team at the University of Oxford devised a scheme for reducing therapist involvement by including the agoraphobic patient's spouse as a support person for in vivo exposure and by developing manuals for patients and spouses (Jannoun et al. 1980; Mathews et al. 1977). Although therapists' time was reduced to an average of 3.5 hours per patient, the gains were equivalent to those of prior trials of therapist-assisted exposure therapy. In further studies emphasizing the use of bibliotherapy, the amount of therapist

Table 12–10.   Combined psychosocial treatments versus waiting-list control condition

Study	Sample	No. of sessions	Effect sizes Anxiety	Effect sizes No. of panic attacks	Effect sizes Fear of fear	% Panic-free TG	% Panic-free WL
Barlow et al. 1989	PD	15	1.75	0.52	—	87	36
Chambless et al. 1986	AG	10	—	0.31	0.36	43	25
Klosko et al. 1990	PD	15					
versus waiting list			1.37	0.56	—	87	33
versus placebo[a]			0.63	0.42	—	87	36
Margraf and Schneider 1991	PD	15	0.57	0.86	1.09	75	5
Weighted average			1.07	0.49	0.57	72	25

Note.   PD = panic disorder patients. AG = agoraphobic patients. TG = treatment group.
WL = waiting-list control group.
[a]Not included in weighted average.

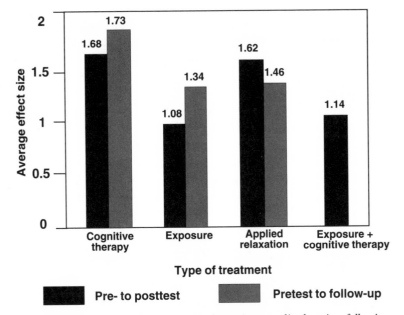

Figure 12–1. Average effect sizes depicting change in generalized anxiety following treatment with cognitive therapy, exposure, applied relaxation, or exposure plus cognitive modification techniques for patients with panic disorder.

time was reduced even further (Ghosh and Marks 1987). Studies of the effectiveness of treating housebound agoraphobic patients via bibliotherapy and telephone contact have yielded conflicting results (Holden et al. 1983; McNamee et al. 1989), but at least some of these very severely impaired patients can be helped in this way.

Marks and his colleagues at the Maudsley Hospital have explored a second way to reduce treatment costs. These researchers have studied the effectiveness of psychiatric nurses trained in behavior psychotherapy in a special 18-month curriculum. Nurse therapists have proved as effective as the more expensively trained psychiatrists and psychologists in treatment with exposure-based therapies and seem to be well accepted by patients (Marks et al. 1975). In a randomized trial of nurse therapists working in general practitioners' offices (Marks 1985), neurotic patients (including agoraphobic patients) treated by nurse therapists improved significantly more than those who received the usual treatment by general practitioners. The behaviorally treated patients reduced their use of general practitioners and other NHS resources and decreased their use of psychiatric drugs. Ginsberg et al. (1984) estimated that, for those patients who maintained their gains for a period of 2 years, as is typical with exposure treatments, the savings to the NHS would exceed the costs of treatment, with savings rising for each year of sustained improvement. Not only was treatment cost-effective, but providing therapy in general practitioners' offices also seemed to catch anxious patients an average of 3 years earlier than when they would have appeared in specialty clinics, and more patients found treatment at the general practitioners' office or at home preferable to visits in an outpatient psychiatric clinic.

These British studies indicate that, in an America increasingly concerned with health care cost containment and considering national health insurance, we could provide treatment for phobia earlier (thus reducing the likelihood of social and vocational disability) and more economically by placing specially trained master's level practitioners in primary health care settings where patients can be identified quickly and treated without the stigma of referral to a psychiatric facility. Although health maintenance organizations (HMOs), used by a growing number of Americans, as well as community mental health centers (CMHCs) would seem to provide ideal settings for replicating the British experience, we know of very few HMOs and CMHCs that provide specialized treatment for anxiety disorders.

Research on training and cost containment has so far been conducted only on exposure treatments for the phobic component of panic disorder. Research on training and dissemination of applied relaxation therapy and CT is greatly needed.

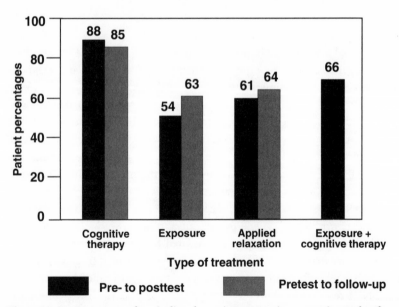

Figure 12–2.   Percentage of panic disorder patients reporting no panic attacks after treatment with cognitive therapy, exposure, applied relaxation, or exposure plus cognitive modification techniques.

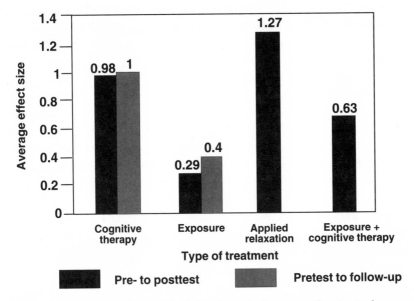

Figure 12–3.   Average effect sizes depicting change in frequency of panic attacks per week following treatment with cognitive therapy, exposure, applied relaxation, or exposure plus cognitive modification techniques for patients with panic disorder.

Although the growing body of research on these approaches emphatically substantiates their worth, practitioners outside specialty clinics remain largely ignorant of their use. The typical continuing education workshop, lasting from 3 hours to 2 days, is unlikely to provide adequate instruction in their application, especially where CT is concerned. We urgently need to develop more adequate retraining programs for those already in practice. The psychological cost of panic disorder aside, the economic effects of this problem alone argue for the probable cost effectiveness of having a properly trained person, at least part-time, in each community mental health/mental retardation center and HMO.

Conclusions

Additional research in psychosocial treatment of panic disorder should focus on increasing the global effectiveness of treatment, especially in raising the number of patients who achieve high-end state functioning on composite measures reflecting the variety of problems associated with this complex syndrome. In particular, we need to examine to what degree treatment normalizes panic, phobia, generalized anxiety, depression, and fear of fear, and how well patients are able to function in work and social spheres at follow-up. Additional research should focus on the treatment of panic disorder patients with comorbid disorders (e.g., major depression) that often lead to their exclusion from treatment trials.

Although such continued research on improvement of efficacy is very desirable, the data reviewed in this chapter convincingly demonstrate that current treatments are highly beneficial, especially exposure therapy for avoidance and CT for panic and fear of fear (both treatments are effective for generalized anxiety). More urgently required is research on dissemination of these findings as well as on methods of training. Demonstration projects should be funded to further these aims, and policymakers for publicly funded facilities and third-party payers should encourage providers to make these short-term therapies of documented efficacy available to all appropriate patients.

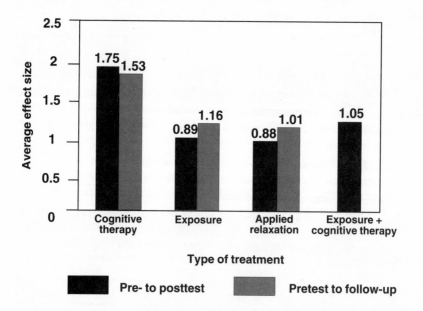

Figure 12–4.   Average effect sizes depicting change in fear of fear/anxiety sensitivity following treatment with cognitive therapy, exposure, applied relaxation, or exposure plus cognitive modification techniques for patients with panic disorder.

Type of treatment

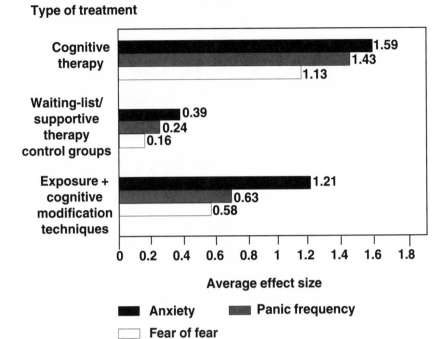

Figure 12–5. Average effect sizes for studies comparing panic disorder patients' response to treatment via cognitive therapy or exposure plus cognitive modification techniques with that of patients in waiting-list or supportive therapy control groups.

References

Arnow BA, Taylor CB, Agras WS, et al: Enhancing agoraphobia treatment outcome by changing couple communication patterns. Behavior Therapy 16:452–467, 1985

Ballenger JC, Burrows G, DuPont R, et al: Alprazolam in panic disorder and agoraphobia: results from a multicenter trial, I: efficacy in short-term treatment. Arch Gen Psychiatry 45:413–422, 1988

Barlow DH, O'Brien GT, Last CG: Couples treatment of agoraphobia. Behavior Therapy 15:41–58, 1984

Barlow DH, Craske MG, Cerny JA, et al: Behavioral treatment of panic disorder. Behavior Therapy 20:261–282, 1989

Beck AT, Steer RA: Manual for the Revised Beck Depression Inventory. San Antonio, TX, Psychological Corporation, 1987

Beck AT, Emery G: Anxiety Disorders and Phobias: A Cognitive Perspective. New York, Basic Books, 1985

Beck AT, Sokol L, Clark DA, et al: A cross-over study of focused cognitive therapy for panic disorder. Am J Psychiatry 149:778–783, 1992

Bibb J, Chambless DL: Alcohol use and abuse among diagnosed agoraphobics. Behav Res Ther 24:49–58, 1986

Bonn JA, Readhead CPA, Timmons BH: Enhanced adaptive behavioral response in agoraphobic patients pretreated with breathing retraining. Lancet 2:665–669, 1984

Cerny JA, Barlow DJ, Craske MG, et al: Couples treatment of agoraphobia: a two-year follow-up. Behavior Therapy 18:401–415, 1987

Chambless DL, Goldstein AJ, Gallagher R, et al: Integrating behavior therapy and psychotherapy in the treatment of agoraphobia. Psychotherapy 23:150–159, 1986

Clark DM, Salkovskis PM: Cognitive Therapy With Panic and Hypochondriasis. Oxford, England, Pergamon (in press)

Clark DM, Salkovskis PM, Hackman A, et al: A comparison of cognitive therapy, applied relaxation, and imipramine in the treatment of panic disorder. Paper presented at the meeting of the Association for the Advancement of Behavior Therapy, New York, November 1991

Cobb JP, Mathews AM, Childs-Clarke A, et al: The spouse as co-therapist in the treatment of agoraphobia. Br J Psychiatry 144:282–287, 1984

Cohen J: Statistical Power Analysis for the Behavioral Sciences, 2nd Edition. Hillsdale, NJ, Lawrence Erlbaum, 1988

Cottraux J, Mollard E, Duinat A, et al: Psychotropic medication suppression or reduction after behavior therapy in 81 agoraphobics with panic attacks. Paper presented at the annual meeting of the Association for the Advancement of Behavior Therapy, Chicago, IL, November 1986

Craske MG, Street L, Barlow DH: Instructions to focus upon or distract from internal cues during exposure treatment of agoraphobic avoidance. Behav Res Ther 27:663–672, 1989

Craske MG, Brown TA, Barlow DH: Behavioral treatment of panic disorder: a two-year follow-up. Behavior Therapy 22:289–304, 1991

de Ruiter C, Rijken H, Garssen B, et al: Breathing retraining, exposure and a combination of both, in the treatment of panic disorder with agoraphobia. Behav Res Ther 27:647–656, 1989

Emmelkamp PMG, Kuipers ACM: Agoraphobia: a follow-up study four years after treatment. Br J Psychiatry 134:352–355, 1979

Emmelkamp PMG, Mersch PP: Cognition and exposure in vivo in the treatment of agoraphobia: short-term and delayed effects. Cognitive Therapy and Research 6:77–90, 1982

Emmelkamp PMG, Kuipers A, Eggeraat J: Cognitive modification versus prolonged exposure in vivo: a comparison with agoraphobics. Behav Res Ther 16:33–41, 1978

Emmelkamp PMG, Brilman E, Kuiper H, et al: The treatment of agoraphobia: a comparison of self-instructional training, rational emotive therapy, and exposure in vivo. Behav Modif 10:37–53, 1986

Fyer A, Liebowitz M, Gorman J, et al: Discontinuation of alprazolam treatment in panic patients. Am J Psychiatry 144:303–308, 1987

Ghosh A, Marks IM: Self-directed exposure for agoraphobia: a controlled trial. Behavior Therapy 18:3–16, 1987

Ginsberg G, Marks IM, Waters H: Cost-benefit analysis of a controlled trial of nurse therapy for neuroses in primary care. Psychol Med 14:683–690, 1984

Gray J: Diazepam and in vivo exposure in the treatment of agoraphobia. Paper presented at the meeting of the British Association for Behavioural Psychotherapy, Oxford, England, July 1991

Hafner J, Marks I: Exposure in vivo of agoraphobics: contributions of diazepam, group exposure, and anxiety evocation. Psychol Med 6:71–88, 1976

Himadi WG, Boice R, Barlow DH: Assessment of agoraphobia, II: measurement of clinical change. Behav Res Ther 24:321–332, 1986

Holden AE, O'Brien GT, Barlow DH, et al: Self-help manual for agoraphobia: a preliminary report of effectiveness. Behavior Therapy 14:545–556, 1983

Jacobson NS, Wilson L, Tupper C: The clinical significance of treatment gains resulting from exposure-based interventions for agoraphobia: a reanalysis of outcome data. Behavior Therapy 19:539–554, 1988

Jannoun L, Munby M, Catalan J, et al: A home-based treatment program for agoraphobia: replication and controlled evaluation. Behavior Therapy 11:294–305, 1980

Jansson L, Öst L-G: Behavioral treatments for agoraphobia: an evaluative review. Clinical Psychology Review 2:311–336, 1982

Jansson L, Jerremalm A, Öst L-G: Follow-up of agoraphobic patients treated with exposure in vivo or applied relaxation. Br J Psychiatry 149:486–490, 1986

Kleiner L, Marshall WL, Spevack M: Training in problem-solving and exposure treatment for agoraphobics with panic attacks. Journal of Anxiety Disorders 1:313–323, 1987

Klosko JS, Barlow DH, Tassinari R, et al: A comparison of alprazolam and behavior therapy in treatment of panic disorder. J Consult Clin Psychol 58:77–84, 1990

Margraf J, Schneider S: Outcome and active ingredients of cognitive-behavioral treatments for panic disorder. Paper presented at the annual meeting of the Association for the Advancement of Behavior Therapy, New York, November 1991

Markowitz GS, Weissman MM, Ouellette R, et al: Quality of life in panic disorder. Arch Gen Psychiatry 46:984–992, 1989

Marks I: Controlled trial of psychiatric nurse therapists in primary care. BMJ 290:1181–1184, 1985

Marks IM, Mathews AM: Brief standard self-rating for phobic patients. Behav Res Ther 17:263–267, 1979

Marks IM, Hallam RS, Philpott R, et al: Nurse therapists in behavioral psychotherapy. BMJ 3:144–148, 1975

Marks IM, Grey S, Cohen SD, et al: Imipramine and brief therapist-aided exposure in agoraphobics having self exposure homework: a controlled trial. Arch Gen Psychiatry 40:153–162, 1983

Marks IM, Swinson RP, Basoglu M, et al: Alprazolam and exposure alone and combined in panic disorder with agoraphobia: a controlled study in London and Toronto. Paper presented at the meeting of the British Association for Behavioural Psychotherapy, Oxford, England, July 1991

Mathews AM, Teasdale J, Munby M, et al: A home-based treatment program for agoraphobia. Behavior Therapy 8:915–924, 1977

Mavissakalian M, Michelson L: Agoraphobia: relative and combined effectiveness of therapist-assisted in vivo exposure and imipramine. J Clin Psychiatry 47:117–122, 1986a

Mavissakalian M, Michelson L: Agoraphobia: Two year follow-up of exposure and imipramine treatment of agoraphobia. Am J Psychiatry 143:348–355, 1986b

McNamee G, O'Sullivan G, Lelliott P, et al: Telephone-guided treatment for housebound agoraphobics with panic disorder: exposure versus relaxation. Behavior Therapy 20:491–497, 1989

Michelson L, Mavissakalian M, Marchione K: Cognitive, behavioral, and psychophysiological treatments of agoraphobia: a comparative outcome investigation. Behavior Therapy 19:97–120, 1988

Michelson L, Marchione K, Greenwald M: Cognitive-behavioral treatments of agoraphobia. Paper presented at the annual meeting of the Association for the Advancement of Behavior Therapy, Washington, DC, November 1989

Michelson L, Marchione K, Greenwald M, et al: Panic disorder: cognitive-behavioral treatment. Behav Res Ther 28:141–151, 1990

Munby M, Johnston DW: Agoraphobia: the long-term follow-up of behavioral treatment. Br J Psychiatry 137:418–427, 1980

Newman CF, Beck JS, Beck AT, et al: Efficacy of cognitive therapy in reducing panic attacks and medication. Paper presented at the annual meeting of the Association for the Advancement of Behavior Therapy, San Francisco, CA, November 1990

Norcross JC, Prochaska JO: A national survey of clinical psychologists: affiliations and orientations. The Clinical Psychologist 35(3):1–7, 1982

Öst L-G: Applied relaxation in the treatment of panic disorder. Behav Res Ther 26:13–22, 1988

Öst L-G, Westling BE: Cognitive therapy versus applied relaxation in the treatment of panic disorder. Paper presented at the meeting of the European Association of Behavior Therapy. Oslo, Norway, September 1991

Öst L-G, Jerremalm A, Jansson L: Individual response patterns and the effects of different behavioral methods in the treatment of agoraphobia. Behav Res Ther 22:697–707, 1984

Öst L-G, Hellstrom K, Westling BE: Applied relaxation, exposure in vivo, and cognitive methods in the treatment of agoraphobia. Paper presented at the meeting of the Association for the Advancement of Behavior Therapy, Washington, DC, 1989

Rosenthal R: How are we doing in soft psychology? Am Psychol 45:775–778, 1990

Smith ML, Glass GV: Meta-analysis of psychotherapy outcome studies. Am Psychol 32:752–760, 1977

Sokol L, Beck AT, Greenberg RL, et al: Cognitive therapy of panic disorder: a non-pharmacological alternative. J Nerv Ment Dis 177:711–716, 1989

Taylor CB, King R, Margraf J, et al: Use of medication and in vivo exposure in volunteers for panic disorder research. Am J Psychiatry 145:1423–1426, 1989

Telch MJ, Agras WS, Taylor CB, et al: Combined pharmacological and behavioral treatment for agoraphobia. Behav Res Ther 23:325–335, 1985

Trull TJ, Nietzel MT, Main A: The use of meta-analysis to assess the clinical significance of behavior therapy for agoraphobia. Behavior Therapy 19:527–538, 1988

Williams SL, Rappoport A: Cognitive treatment in the natural environment for agoraphobics. Behavior Therapy 14:299–313, 1983

Zitrin CM, Klein DF, Woerner MG: Treatment of agoraphobia with group exposure in vivo and imipramine. Arch Gen Psychiatry 37:63–72, 1980

Combined Treatments of Panic Disorder

Chapter 13

Combined Pharmacological and Psychological Treatment of Panic Disorder: Current Status and Future Directions

Michael J. Telch, Ph.D.,
and Richard A. Lucas, M.A.

G iven the significant advances in both the pharmacological and psychological treatments for panic, it seems reasonable to consider the union of these
two approaches. Do combined treatments yield greater benefits to panic disorder
patients than either treatment administered alone?

The general enthusiasm generated for combination treatments is borne out by
data suggesting that most panic disorder patients in treatment receive both medication and psychotherapy (Taylor et al. 1989). Although it is not clear that the
particular singular treatments being combined in day-to-day clinical practice are
those with established efficacy, there appears to be a pervasive attitude that combined drug-psychological treatments are superior to singular treatments. A question of central import is whether this attitude is consistent with the scientific
evidence.

We organize our chapter around the following questions:

1. Why study combined treatments?
2. What is the current scientific knowledge base on combined treatments for
   panic disorder?
3. What is the clinical efficacy of combined treatments?
4. What implications do the research findings have for clinical practice?

177

5. What are the research priorities for advancing our understanding of combined treatments?

Rationales for Combined Treatments

The rationales for using a combined drug-psychological approach in treating panic disorder are inextricably linked to how one conceptualizes the disorder and the presumed efficacy and mechanisms of action of the singular treatments being combined. In this chapter, we do not review research on either the efficacy or mechanisms of action for psychological or pharmacological treatments, as that task is undertaken successfully in several other chapters. Rather, we briefly review a few of the most frequently discussed rationales for combining psychological treatment and medications. These include 1) treatment specificity, 2) facilitation of psychological treatment through pharmacotherapy, and 3) facilitation of pharmacotherapy through psychological treatment.

Treatment Specificity

The assumption that medications and psychological treatments exert their primary effect on different loci or facets of a disorder has been the subject of considerable debate. Originally, Klein (1980) stressed the specific action of certain classes of medications in blocking spontaneous panic. It was assumed that psychotherapies and benzodiazepines were ineffective for the spontaneous panic feature of the disorder, but that both could be helpful in treating the psychological complications of spontaneous panic, namely anticipatory anxiety and phobic avoidance. The assumption of treatment specificity for tricyclic antidepressants and the monoamine oxidase inhibitors (MAOIs), along with the recognition that panic disorder is a multifaceted syndrome, led to the recommendation of administering panic-blocking medication in conjunction with psychological treatment that encouraged patients to confront fear-provoking cues (Klein 1980). To the extent that medication and psychological treatments affect different symptom clusters within the panic syndrome, their combined use offers the advantage of treating multiple loci concurrently, and hence they may be more effective.

Facilitation of Psychological Treatment
Through Pharmacotherapy

A second rationale for a combined treatment approach is the facilitation of psychological treatment through pharmacotherapy. Even when a psychological approach is being used as the primary treatment for panic, there may be circumstances in which the addition of medication may be indicated. For example, panic disorder patients displaying marked depression while undergoing psychological treatment may possess insufficient energy or motivation to participate in an intensive cognitive-behavior treatment for panic. In such cases, the addition of an antidepressant may be desirable.

Another example of the potential facilitation of psychological treatment through pharmacotherapy is when the patient's extreme anxiety interferes with the psychological treatment. In these cases, short-term administration of benzodiazepines or some other anxiolytic may allow the patient to calm down sufficiently so that psychological treatment may be initiated.

Facilitation of Pharmacotherapy Through Psychological Treatment

A third rationale for combining medication and psychological treatments involves the potential facilitative effects that psychological interventions may have for patients undergoing drug treatments for panic. One such facilitative function may be increased compliance with medication. As noted in previous reviews of pharmacological treatments, many panic disorder patients display a fear of taking medications (Telch 1988; Telch et al. 1983). Although reassurance by the physician may be sufficient for some, psychological treatment specifically targeting medication fears may be needed for the more severely phobic patient.

Psychological treatments may also serve a facilitative role in assisting patients during medication withdrawal. Patients who are provided with psychological strategies aimed at enhancing their sense of mastery and control may be more likely to withdraw from medications successfully. Moreover, there is now evidence to suggest that patients displaying comorbid personality disorders may show a less favorable response to pharmacological treatment (Noyes et al. 1990; Reich and Green 1991) or have a higher probability of relapse (Green and Curtis 1988). Consequently, concurrent psychological intervention specifically addressing spheres such as personality dysfunction may help to reduce relapse.

Current Scientific Knowledge Base on Combined Treatments

The present review is limited to those controlled studies that have compared one or more drug-psychotherapy combination treatments with one or more singular treatments (drug or psychotherapy). Comparative studies of two or more singular treatments, whether drug or psychological, have been omitted because they do not directly address the issue of combined treatments. A total of 13 studies (11 published, 2 currently under editorial review) met the criteria for inclusion. Table 13–1 gives a breakdown of the types of combination treatments studied to date.

As seen in Table 13–1, the majority of combined drug-psychological treatment studies (8 of 13) used imipramine as the pharmacological treatment (Agras et al. 1991; Marks et al. 1983; Mavissakalian and Michelson 1986a, 1986b; Mavissakalian and Perel 1985; Sheehan et al. 1980; Telch et al. 1985; Zitrin et al. 1980, 1983). MAOIs were used in 3 of the combined studies (Lipsedge et al. 1973; Sheehan et al. 1980; Solyom et al. 1981), diazepam was used in one early study (Hafner and Marks 1976), and the high-potency benzodiazepine alprazolam was examined in one recently completed multicenter study (Marks and Swinson 1993). Finally, one study (Sheehan et al. 1980) included two separate combination treatments—imipramine plus supportive psychotherapy, and phenelzine plus supportive psychotherapy.

What are the psychological treatments employed in the combined studies? As was the case with imipramine and pharmacotherapy, exposure-based therapies were overly represented compared with the other two categories of psychological treatments—cognitive-behavior therapy and insight-oriented or supportive therapy. As is shown in Table 13–1, 11 of the 13 studies examined a medication combined with an exposure-based treatment, two studies (Sheehan et al. 1980; Zitrin et al. 1983) combined medication with nonbehavioral supportive psychotherapy, and one study (Zitrin et al. 1983) included two separate combined treatments: imipramine plus supportive psychotherapy and imipramine plus imaginal desensitization.

Table 13–1 highlights the limitations in our current knowledge. Of the 12 possible psychological-pharmacological treatment combinations, 6 have yet to be examined and several others have limited coverage. Indeed, with the exception of the combined treatment of imipramine and exposure therapy, our knowledge base of combined drug-psychological treatments is quite limited. For example, despite the widespread use of high-potency benzodiazepines in the treatment of panic, only one study (Marks and Swinson 1993) examined their efficacy in combination with a psychological treatment. Of particular importance is the absence of data on the combined effects of pharmacotherapy and the new genre of cognitive-behavior treatments for panic (see Chapters 9 and 10, this volume).

A more detailed description of study characteristics is presented in Table 13–2. Due to space limitations, a full summary of this information is not given here. However, a few remarks about the studies deserve highlighting. First, as seen in column 2, the patient samples are exclusively composed of agoraphobic patients. Patients with uncomplicated panic disorder or panic disorder with minimal avoidance are not represented. Only 4 of the studies (Agras et al. 1991; Mavissakalian et al. 1983; Solyom et al. 1981; Telch et al. 1985) included an active drug without psychological treatment as a comparison group. Moreover, none of the studies included a psychological treatment without placebo. As seen in the last column, 4 (Hafner and Marks 1976; Lipsedge et al. 1973; Sheehan et al. 1980; Solyom et al. 1981) of the 13 studies did not report outcome data for panic attacks. A discussion of these limitations and their implications for future research are presented later in this chapter.

Table 13–1. Combined treatment studies for panic disorder, classified by type of drug and type of psychological treatment

Psychological treatments	Drug treatments			
	Tricyclic antidepressants	Monoamine oxidase inhibitors	Low-potency benzodiazepines	High-potency benzodiazepines
Exposure-based therapy	Agras et al. 1991 Marks et al. 1983 Mavissakalian and Perel 1985 Mavissakalian et al. 1986a, 1986b Telch et al. 1985 Zitrin et al. 1980, 1983	Lipsedge et al. 1973 Solyom et al. 1981	Hafner and Marks 1976	Marks and Swinson 1993
Cognitive-behavior therapy	None	None	None	None
Insight-oriented/ supportive therapy	Sheehan et al. 1980 Zitrin et al. 1983	Sheehan et al. 1980		

Table 13–2. Studies of combined drug and psychological treatment for panic disorder

Study	Sample (no. of completers)	Design	No. per group	Assessment periods (weeks)	Duration of treatment (weeks)	Mean drug dosage (mg)	Assessment after drug withdrawal	Panic assessment
Agras et al. 1991	AG (87)	IM + EX IM + AEX PL + EX PL + AEX	24 23 20 20	0, 8, 16, 24	Drug: 24 EX: 8	Week 8: 142 Week 16: 168	Yes	Prospective self-monitoring
Hafner and Marks 1976	AG (57)	GE + DZ (waning) GE + DZ (peak) GE + PL IE (high anxiety) + PL IE (low anxiety) + PL	14 13 14 6 6	0, 2	2	0.1/kg body weight	No	None
Lipsedge et al. 1973	AG (60)	MSD + IZ SD + IZ IZ MSD + PL SD + PL PL	10 13 9 10 8 10	0, 8	8	IP: 50 BR 1% IV solution	No	None
Marks et al. 1983[a]	AG (45)	IM + EX or IM + RT PL + EX or PL + RT	23 22	0, 14, 28, 35, 52, 104	Drug: 24 EX: 12	Week 14: 158 Week 26: 110	Yes	Rating scales
Marks and Swinson 1993	AG (129)	AZ + EX AZ + RT PL + EX PL + RT	34 34 30 31	0, 8, 18, 23, 43	18	Week 8: 6	Yes	Prospective self-monitoring

Study	Sample	Treatment conditions	N	Assessment	Duration	Dose		Outcome measure
Mavissakalian et al. 1983	AG (15)	IM IM + PR	7 8	0, 12	12	125	No	Rating scales
Mavissakalian and Perel 1985; Mavissakalian et al. 1986a, 1986b	AG (62)	IM + FL IM + PR PL + FL PL + PR	14 17 17 14	0, 4, 8, 12	12	Month 1: 80 Month 2: 125 Month 3: 123	Yes	Rating scales
Sheehan et al. 1980	EA (57)	PH + SG IM + SG PL + SG	17 18 22	0, 6, 12	12	PH: 45 IM: 150	No	None
Solyom et al. 1981	AG (40)	PH + EX PH PL + EX PL	10 10 10 10	0, 8, 16	8	PH: 45	No	None
Telch et al. 1985	AG (29)	IM + EX IM + AEX PL + EX	10 10 9	0, 8, 26	Drug: 26 EX: 8	Week 8: 190 Week 26: 179	No	Prospective self-monitoring
Zitrin et al. 1980	AG (53)	IM + EX PL + EX	29 24	0, 14, 26	Drug: 26 EX: 10	200	No	Rating scales
Zitrin et al. 1983	AG, MP, SP (63)	IM + SD IM + ST PL + SD	18 24 21	0, 26	26	204	No	Rating scales

Note. **Treatment conditions:** IM = imipramine; EX = exposure therapy; AEX = anti-exposure instructions; PL = placebo; GE = group exposure; DZ = diazepam; IE = individual exposure; MSD = methohexitane-assisted systematic desensitization; IZ = iproniazid; SD = systematic desensitization; RT = relaxation training; AZ = alprazolam; PR = programmed practice; FL = flooding; PH = phenelzine; SG = support group; ST = supportive therapy. **Other:** AG = agoraphobic patients; EA = endogenous anxiety patients; MP = mixed phobic patients; SP = simple phobic patients; IV = intravenous.
[a]All groups received exposure homework.

Clinical Efficacy of Combined Treatments

Possible Outcomes When Evaluating Combined Treatments

In turning to the issue of efficacy, we should keep in mind that the combination of pharmacological and psychological treatments may result in one of several outcomes. These outcomes are illustrated in Figure 13–1. The first two outcomes, additivity and potentiation, are favorable in that the combination treatment outperforms either of the singular treatments. *Additivity* is displayed when the effects of the combined treatment resemble the sum of the effects of each singular treatment. *Potentiation* is demonstrated when the outcome of the combined treatment significantly surpasses the additive effects of the singular treatments.

Unfortunately, combining drug and psychological treatments does not always lead to additive or potentiation effects. Three additional outcomes are possible. *Inhibition* refers to a negative interaction between the treatments, resulting in a combined effect less than that from either treatment administered individually. Finally, two levels of *reciprocation*—combined treatment effects equivalent to the effects of either one or both of the singular treatments—are also possible.

Using real data from the panic disorder/agoraphobia literature, Figures 13–2 through 13–4 present a few possible outcomes. The figures show behavioral approach data at posttreatment from a recently completed treatment study of imipramine and exposure therapy (Agras et al. 1991). Note the additive effects of imipramine and exposure homework on the patient's behavioral approach test (BAT).

Figure 13–3 illustrates the potentiation of imipramine and exposure therapy reported by Telch et al. (1985). In this study the magnitude of change for the combination treatment exceeded the additive effects of the individual treatments. Agras et al. (1991) observed a significant negative interaction between imipramine and exposure therapy on agoraphobic patients' panic appraisals (Figure 13–4). Notice that imipramine appears to be inhibiting the effectiveness of exposure therapy on this measure of panic-related cognitions.

Short-Term Efficacy of Combined Treatments

How effective are combined treatments in the short term? To address this issue, we examined controlled studies comparing one or more combined treatments with one or more singular treatments. A series of meta-analyses were conducted to examine the relative efficacy of 1) combined treatments versus psychological treatments, and 2) combined treatments versus pharmacological treatments. Ef-

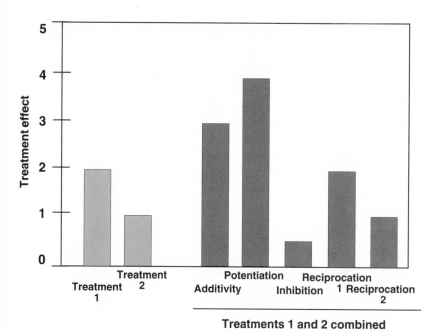

Figure 13–1. Possible drug-psychotherapy interactions. *Source.* Adapted from Uhlenhuth et al. 1969.

fect sizes for these two major sets of comparisons were calculated separately for each of the following five domains: 1) panic, 2) phobic anxiety, 3) phobic avoidance, 4) depression, and 5) global functioning or level of disability.

▮ **Combined versus psychological treatments.** Results of the eight studies (Agras et al. 1991; Marks and Swinson 1993; Marks et al. 1983; Mavissakalian and Perel 1985; Mavissakalian et al. 1986a, 1986b; Sheehan et al. 1980; Telch et al. 1985; Zitrin et al. 1980, 1983) that directly compared a combined treatment with a psychological treatment are presented in Table 13–3. Several studies were excluded from the meta-analysis for failing to report group means and standard deviations. The Sheehan et al. (1980) study is listed twice because it contributed two separate combined versus psychological comparisons to the analysis (imipramine plus supportive psychotherapy and phenelzine plus supportive psychotherapy). The row summaries represent the pooled effect size across the five assessment domains for each study, whereas the column summaries represent the average effect size for a particular assessment domain pooled across studies. Positive effect sizes signify an advantage for the combined treatment.

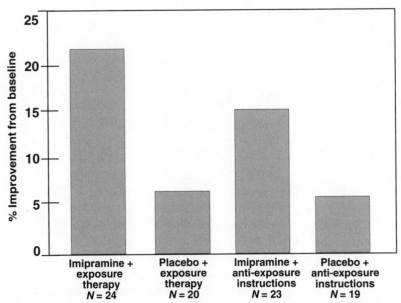

Figure 13–2.   Improvement in Behavioral Approach Test (BAT) scores from pre- to posttreatment.   *Source.* Data from Agras et al. 1991.

Results of this analysis reveal a significant overall advantage for the combined treatment for most of the studies. Moreover, inspection of the column summaries indicates that the short-term superiority of combined treatment was consistent across the five major assessment domains rather than being limited to one domain, such as panic. As seen in Table 13–3, a modest but significant overall advantage for combined treatments over psychological treatment alone was observed at posttreatment (overall pooled effect size = .45).

The data are at odds with a review by Clum (1989) in which he concluded that combined treatments were less effective than behavior therapies alone. It should be noted that Clum based this conclusion on comparisons of author-defined success rates for individual studies. Unfortunately, this analytical approach is flawed when one considers that the differences in success rates may simply reflect between-study differences in the criteria used to define successful outcome.

■   **Combined versus pharmacological treatments.**   A second set of analyses were conducted to examine the relative efficacy of combined versus pharmacological

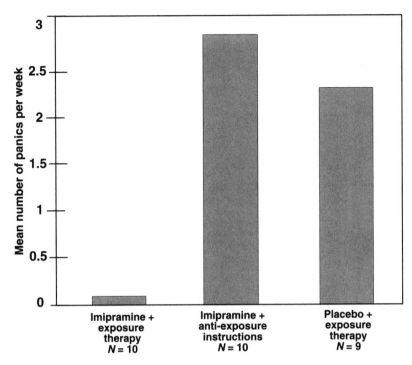

Figure 13–3. Mean number of panic attacks at 26 weeks posttreatment. *Source.* Data from Telch et al. 1985

treatments. Only three studies (Agras et al. 1991; Mavissakalian et al. 1983; Telch et al. 1985) included a direct comparison of a combined treatment with pharmacotherapy alone. In all three studies, the combined treatment was imipramine plus exposure-based therapy. These results are presented in Table 13–4.

Although limited by the small number of studies, this set of results reveals a clear short-term advantage for combined treatment over pharmacological treatment alone. As in the previous comparison, the advantage of the combined treatment over drug treatment alone was present across each of the major assessment domains, with the exception of panic (overall effect size = .39).

Long-Term Efficacy of Combined Treatments

Few studies have included an evaluation of the longer term effects of combined treatments. In a follow-up study of the patients originally treated in the Marks et al. (1983) study, Cohen et al. (1984) reported that approximately two-thirds of the patients interviewed (90% of the original cohort) at 2-year follow-up were im-

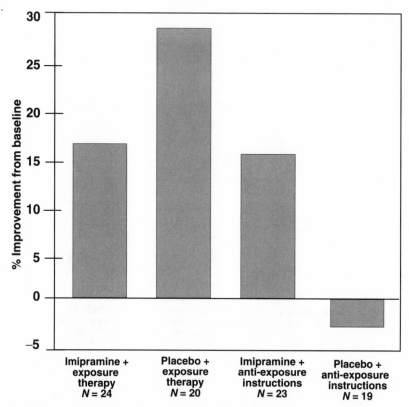

Figure 13–4. Improvement in panic appraisals from pre- to posttreatment. *Source.*
Agras et al. 1991.

proved or much improved from their pretreatment level of functioning. No
significant advantage of the combined treatment was observed on any of the major
clinical outcome measures. Mavissakalian and Michelson (1986b) conducted a
2-year follow-up of agoraphobic patients treated in their original study, comparing the singular and combined efficacy of imipramine and therapist-assisted exposure therapy. All subjects received a systematic program of self-directed exposure
therapy. Seventy-six percent of the original cohort were interviewed. The overall
improvement was maintained throughout follow-up. However, the superiority of
the combined treatment over exposure therapy alone, which was present at week
12, was no longer present at follow-up because of higher relapse among the
imipramine-treated patients and the continued improvement for patients in the
self-directed exposure therapy control group. Consistent with the follow-up find-

Table 13–3. Posttreatment effect sizes for combined treatment versus psychological treatment

Study	Weeks	Assessment domain					Pooled effect sizes across assessment domains
		Panic	Phobic anxiety	Phobic avoidance	Depression	Functioning/ disability	
Agras et al. 1991	8	.30 (.10)	−.22 (.03)	.38 (.05)*	.18 (.09)	.10 (.05)	−.08 (.01)
Marks et al. 1983	14	NR	NR	.13 (.04)	.01 (.09)	.39 (.09)	.16 (.02)
Marks and Swinson 1993	8	.41 (.06)	.37 (.06)	0.00 (.06)	.37 (.06)	.36 (.03)*	.31 (.01)**
Mavissakalian and Perel 1985; Mavissakalian et al. 1986a, 1986b	12	.30 (.07)	.52 (.01)**	.05 (.03)	.23 (.06)	.36 (.03)*	.36 (.01)**
Sheehan et al. 1980 (imipramine)	12	NR	.81 (.04)**	.76 (.11)**	.97 (.06)**	.55 (.10)*	.81 (.02)**
Sheehan et al. 1980 (phenelzine)	12	NR	1.10 (.04)**	1.19 (.12)**	1.26 (.06)**	1.30 (.13)**	1.19 (.02)**
Telch et al. 1985	8	.18 (.21)	.67 (.11)*	.83 (.06)**	.04 (.07)	NR	.48 (.02)**
Zitrin et al. 1980	14	.65 (.05)**	NR	.66 (.04)**	NR	.65 (.03)**	.65 (.01)**
Zitrin et al. 1983	26	.48 (.02)**	.56 (.04)**	.53 (.03)**	.41 (.11)	.51 (.03)**	.51 (.01)**
Pooled effect sizes across studies	—	.45 (.01)**	.52 (.01)**	.34 (.001)**	.48 (.01)**	.47 (.01)**	.45 (.001)**

Note. Numbers in parentheses refer to the variance of the effect size. Positive effect sizes signify an advantage for the combined treatment. NR = no means reported for this domain.
*$P \le .05$. **$P \le .01$.

Table 13–4. Posttreatment effect sizes for combined treatment versus drug treatment

| Study | Weeks | Assessment domain | | | | | Pooled effect sizes across assessment domains |
		Panic	Phobic anxiety	Phobic avoidance	Depression	Functioning/disability	
Agras et al. 1991	8	−.37 (.09)	.12 (.03)	.19 (.04)	.23 (.09)	.40 (.04)	.16 (.01)
Mavissakalian et al. 1983	12	.30 (.09)	.45 (.27)	.87 (.15)*	.93 (.15)**	1.05 (.30)*	.65 (.03)**
Telch et al. 1985	8	.14 (.20)	.94 (.11)**	1.23 (.06)**	.17 (.07)	NR	.71 (.02)**
Pooled effect sizes across studies		−.003 (.04)	.30 (.02)*	.66 (.02)**	.35 (.03)*	.48 (.04)**	.39 (.006)**

Note. Numbers in parentheses refer to the variance of the effect size. Positive effect sizes signify an advantage for the combined treatment. NR = no means reported for this domain.
*$P \le .05$; **$P \le .01$.

ings from the Marks et al. (1983) study, approximately two-thirds of the patients assessed cross-sectionally at the 2-year follow-up were markedly improved.

Preliminary data on the long-term effects of combined alprazolam and exposure therapy are now available from the recently completed multicenter trial conducted in London and Toronto (Marks and Swinson 1993). These data are of particular interest because they represent the only available information on the efficacy of a combined alprazolam plus exposure treatment. Our effect size analyses presented earlier suggested a slight advantage of the combined alprazolam-exposure treatment over exposure therapy plus placebo at the posttreatment assessment. In contrast to the short-term results, data on the combined treatment's long-term efficacy after medication withdrawal revealed that patients receiving the combination treatment evidenced a significantly poorer outcome at follow-up, compared with those patients treated with exposure therapy plus placebo. The poorer long-term outcome for the combined alprazolam-exposure group was due to a markedly higher relapse rate among those treated with alprazolam, rather than further gains made by the placebo plus exposure therapy group. These findings are consistent with early reports suggesting that tranquilizing medication may interfere with the therapeutic effects of exposure therapy (Chambless et al. 1979).

Conclusions Regarding the Efficacy of Combined Treatments

▌ **Short-term efficacy.** From the data just presented, several conclusions about the short-term efficacy of combined treatments seem warranted:

1. Approximately 66%–75% of patients displaying panic disorder with agoraphobia achieved marked improvement when treated with a combination of imipramine plus exposure therapy or alprazolam plus exposure therapy.
2. For patients displaying panic disorder with agoraphobia, the combination of imipramine and exposure therapy offers a short-term advantage over either imipramine alone or exposure therapy alone.
3. For patients displaying panic disorder with agoraphobia, the combination of alprazolam and exposure therapy offers a slight short-term advantage over exposure therapy alone, and a marked short-term advantage over alprazolam alone.

▌ **Long-term efficacy.** Based on the limited data available, conclusions concerning the long-term effects of combined treatments are as follows:

1. Between one-half and two-thirds of agoraphobic patients treated with exposure therapy and imipramine will evidence marked improvement at follow-
   ups ranging from 12 to 24 months.
2. For patients displaying panic disorder with agoraphobia, the combination of
   imipramine and exposure therapy is no more effective than exposure therapy
   alone.
3. For patients displaying panic disorder with agoraphobia, the use of alprazolam
   in combination with exposure therapy results in higher relapse and poorer
   long-term outcome than exposure therapy treatment without alprazolam.

Recommendations for Clinical Practice

What are our recommendations for clinical practice with respect to combining
treatment of panic disorder using a combined pharmacological and psychological
approach? The gaps in the current knowledge base severely limit prescriptions for
clinical practice. Despite our conclusion that the combination of imipramine and
exposure therapy confers a short-term advantage over either treatment administered individually, the failure of the combined treatment to show an advantage in
the long term argues against its routine use as a first-line treatment. Similarly, the
combined use of exposure therapy plus alprazolam cannot be recommended,
given the recent findings from the London-Toronto multicenter study (Marks and
Swinson 1993) showing that alprazolam plus exposure therapy was less effective in
the long term than placebo plus exposure therapy.

Considering the current state of knowledge on combined treatments and the
recent data supporting the efficacy of cognitive-behavior therapy administered
without medications (see Chapters 12 and 16, this volume), we cannot recommend any combined treatment as the first line of attack for the panic disorder
patient. Rather, we recommend that either an antidepressant (such as imipramine) or a high-potency benzodiazepine (such as alprazolam) be administered in
conjunction with a psychological treatment that includes a systematic program of
self-directed exposure to feared cues under the following conditions:

1. When an 8- to 12-week trial of cognitive-behavior therapy is either unavailable
   or unacceptable to the patient
2. When an adequate trial of cognitive-behavior therapy has proved unsuccessful
3. When other clinical considerations (e.g., the presence of severe depression or
   substance abuse) suggest that the patient may be unsuitable for cognitive-
   behavior therapy

Critique and Future Directions

Despite the interest in combined treatments for panic disorder, research on them has lagged behind that for single treatments. Previous reviews of the combined treatment literature on panic disorder have enumerated many design and measurement deficiencies (Telch 1988; Telch et al. 1983). The more significant of these included 1) the confounding of drug and exposure therapy, 2) the inappropriate use of placebo plus psychotherapy to represent psychotherapy alone, 3) the measurement deficiencies in the assessment of panic, and 4) the failure to assess the long-term effects of combined treatments. Most of these deficiencies are still with us today, although there are some promising developments.

Priorities for Future Research on Combined Treatments

Where do we go from here? The gaps in our current knowledge base and the conceptual and methodological limitations in the research to date suggest a tentative listing of recommended research. (The order of the following listing in no way implies a ranking of importance.)

1. *Clinical trials examining the efficacy of pharmacotherapy in conjunction with the new genre of psychological treatments.* As discussed in Chapters 9 and 10 (this volume), there are now compelling data that support the effectiveness of a new genre of cognitive-behavior treatments that target panic directly. However, as seen in Table 13–1, there are as yet no data on the efficacy of cognitive-behavior therapy plus pharmacotherapy. Efficacy studies are clearly indicated.
2. *Clinical trials evaluating the efficacy of combined treatments for patients displaying panic disorder without agoraphobia.* As noted in Table 13–2, research on the efficacy of combined treatments for panic disorder have been restricted to patients displaying agoraphobia. The generalizability of these findings to uncomplicated panic disorder has not been examined. This is a particular concern given that approximately two-thirds of panic disorder patients in the general population have little or no agoraphobia (see Chapter 3, this volume).
3. *Use of experimental designs that correct for 1) the confounding of drug effects and psychological treatment effects and 2) the inappropriate use of placebo plus psychotherapy to represent psychotherapy alone.* We need to move beyond the 2×2 factorial study in which active drug versus placebo is crossed with the presence or absence of an active psychological treatment. None of the studies reviewed included a "pure" psychological treatment without pill placebo. The problems associated with using pill placebo plus psychotherapy to represent

psychotherapy alone have been cogently discussed (Hollon and Beck 1978; Hollon and DeRubeis 1981). In short, designs that rely on placebo-plus-psychotherapy comparisons, although useful in illuminating the mechanisms governing the interaction of medication and psychotherapy, are inadequate for drawing valid inferences about differential outcome. The scant empirical evidence directly comparing placebo plus psychotherapy with psychotherapy alone suggests it is misguided to assume equivalence. For example, Klerman et al. (1974) found that depressed patients receiving placebo plus interpersonal psychotherapy had twice the relapse rate (i.e., 28% versus 14%) of a similar group receiving interpersonal psychotherapy alone.

4. *Research aimed at identifying optimal sequencing and dosing of combined treatments.* We have yet to scratch the surface in understanding how best to sequence combination treatments. Systematic examination of sequencing variations is needed to deliver combined treatment in an optimal fashion. In addition to sequencing, the dosing of psychological treatments deserves study. For instance, it is not uncommon for pharmacological studies to continue medication for 6 months, yet the dosing of psychological treatments in the combined treatment studies has been relatively low.

5. *Research aimed at identifying patient subtypes for whom combined treatments are indicated and those for whom combined treatments are contraindicated.* Moderator analyses aimed at identifying patient variables that predict response to combined treatment are critical for attaining an effective system of matching treatment modality and patient characteristics. The presence of severe depression, Axis II psychopathology, or obsessive-compulsive symptomatology are just a few of the factors that deserve careful study and that may assist the clinician in determining whether a combination treatment is indicated. To assist in meeting the sample size requirements for moderator analyses, outcome data from several research centers might be pooled and reanalyzed.

6. *The development of a standardized panic assessment battery to facilitate cross-study comparisons.* Panic researchers continue to employ idiosyncratic methods for assessing panic attacks. Moreover, recent data (Telch et al. 1989) point to the importance of moving beyond panic attack and symptom counts and toward a more comprehensive assessment of the meaning that patients give to their attacks. Panic appraisal dimensions, including 1) beliefs in the likelihood of panic, 2) beliefs in the negative consequences of panic, and 3) the perceived capacity to cope with panic, should be routinely assessed in treatment outcome studies.

7. *Need for a broader assessment of treatment utility that integrates information along several evaluative dimensions.* The evaluation of treatments for panic,

whether singular or combined, has been too limited in scope. We need to move beyond unitary indices of treatment effectiveness (e.g., percentage panic-free) to a more multidimensional mapping of treatment utility that integrates information from several evaluative dimensions, such as 1) degree of symptom improvement, 2) clinical significance of improvements, 3) quickness of action, 4) attrition, 5) adverse effects, and 6) treatment durability. The development of evaluative algorithms for integrating diverse information into a composite index of treatment utility would be a major advance. Preliminary work along these lines has recently appeared (see Chapter 16, this volume).

Concluding Remarks

Research and clinical management of panic disorder have been plagued by a biology-versus-psychology polarization (Middleton 1991; Telch 1991). This polarization impedes advancement of the field by fostering a defensive posture among investigators and consequently inhibiting the disconfirmatory process so important in the practice of good science. Can this sundered state of affairs be improved? As with the integration of disparate psychosocial treatments (Goldfried 1982), the integration of biological and psychological perspectives can occur at several levels of analysis, including the study of common change mechanisms and integration at the procedural level. The National Institute of Mental Health has recently funded a four-site multicenter panic treatment study to investigate the singular and combined effects of imipramine and cognitive-behavior therapy for panic disorder. In addition to its methodological advances (e.g., inclusion of a psychological treatment without placebo, the long-term follow-up of patients following medication withdrawal), the study is noteworthy because it attests to the feasibility of collaborative research between biologically and psychologically minded investigators. Demonstration of such cooperation provides hope that in the years to come depolarization between the two disciplines will occur and with it a deeper understanding of combined treatments.

References

Agras WS, Telch MJ, Taylor CB, Roth WT, Brouillard M: Imipramine and exposure therapy in agoraphobia: untangling the actions and interactions. Unpublished data, 1991

Chambless DL, Foa EB, Groves GA, et al: Flooding with Brevital in the treatment of agoraphobia: countereffective? Behav Res Ther 17:243–251, 1979

Clum GA: Psychological interventions versus drugs in the treatment of panic. Behavior Therapy 20:429–457, 1989

Cohen SD, Monteiro W, Marks IM: Two-year follow-up of agoraphobics after exposure and imipramine. Br J Psychiatry 144:276–281, 1984

Goldfried MR: On the history of therapeutic integration. Behavior Therapy 13:572–593, 1982

Green MA, Curtis GC: Personality disorders in panic patients: response to termination of anti-panic medication. Journal of Personality Disorders 2:303–314, 1988

Hafner J, Marks IM: Exposure in vivo of agoraphobics: contributions of diazepam, group exposure, and anxiety evocation. Psychol Med 6:71–88, 1976

Hollon SD, Beck AT: Psychotherapy and drug therapy: comparison and combinations, in Handbook of Psychotherapy and Behavior Change: An Empirical Analysis, 2nd Edition. Edited by Garfield SL, Bergin AE. New York, Wiley, 1978, pp 473–490

Hollon SD, DeRubeis RJ: Placebo-psychotherapy combinations: inappropriate representation of psychotherapy in drug-psychotherapy comparative trials. J Consult Clin Psychol 90:467–477, 1981

Klein DF: Anxiety reconceptualized. Compr Psychiatry 21:411–427, 1980

Klerman GL, DiMascio A, Weissman M, et al: Treatment of depression by drugs and psychotherapy. Am J Psychiatry 131:186–191, 1974

Lipsedge MS, Hajioff J, Huggins P, et al: The management of severe agoraphobia: a comparison of iproniazid and systematic desensitization. Psychopharmacologia 32:667–680, 1973

Marks IM, Swinson RP: Alprazolam and exposure alone and combined in panic disorder with agoraphobia. Br J Psychiatry 162:776–787, 1993

Marks IM, Gray S, Cohen D, et al: Imipramine and brief therapist-aided exposure in agoraphobics having self-exposure homework. Arch Gen Psychiatry 40:153–162, 1983

Mavissakalian M, Michelson L: Agoraphobia: relative and combined effectiveness of therapist-assisted in vivo exposure and imipramine. J Clin Psychiatry 47:117–122, 1986a

Mavissakalian M, Michelson L: Two-year follow-up of exposure and imipramine treatment of agoraphobia. Am J Psychiatry 143:1106–1112, 1986b

Mavissakalian M, Perel J: Imipramine in the treatment of agoraphobia: dose-response relationships. Am J Psychiatry 142:1032–1036, 1985

Mavissakalian M, Michelson L, Dealy RS: Pharmacological treatment of agoraphobia: imipramine versus imipramine with programmed practice. Br J Psychiatry 143:348–355, 1983

Middleton HC: Psychology and pharmacology in the treatment of anxiety disorders: cooperation or confrontation? Journal of Psychopharmacology 5:281–285, 1991

Noyes R, Reich J, Christiansen J, et al: Outcomes of panic disorder: relationship to diagnostic subtypes and comorbidity. Arch Gen Psychiatry 47:809–818, 1990

Reich JH, Green AF: Effect of personality disorders on outcome of treatment. J Nerv Ment Dis 179:74–82, 1991

Sheehan DV, Ballenger J, Jacobsen G: Treatment of endogenous anxiety with phobic, hysterical, and hypochondriacal symptoms. Arch Gen Psychiatry 37:51–59, 1980

Solyom C, Solyom L, LaPierre Y, et al: Phenelzine and exposure in the treatment of phobias. Biol Psychiatry 16:239–247, 1981

Taylor CB, King R, Margraf J, et al: Use of medication and in vivo exposure in volunteers for panic disorder research. Am J Psychiatry 146:1423–1426, 1989

Telch MJ: Combined pharmacological and psychological treatments for panic sufferers, in Panic: Psychological Perspectives. Edited by Rachman S, Maser J. Hillsdale, NJ, Lawrence Erlbaum, 1988, pp 167–187

Telch MJ: Beyond sterile debate. Journal of Psychopharmacology 5:296–298, 1991

Telch MJ, Tearnan BH, Taylor CB: Antidepressant medication in the treatment of agoraphobia: a critical review. Behav Res Ther 21:505–517, 1983

Telch MJ, Agras WS, Taylor CB, et al: Combined pharmacological and behavioral treatment for agoraphobia. Behav Res Ther 23:325–335, 1985

Telch MJ, Brouillard M, Telch CF, et al: Role of cognitive appraisal in panic-related avoidance. Behav Res Ther 27:373–383, 1989

Zitrin CM, Klein DF, Woerner MG: Treatment of agoraphobia with group exposure in vivo and imipramine. Arch Gen Psychiatry 37:63–72, 1980

Zitrin CM, Klein DF, Woerner MG, et al: Treatment of phobias, I: comparison of imipramine hydrochloride and placebo. Arch Gen Psychiatry 40:125–133, 1983

Chapter 14

Critique of the Research Literature on Combined Treatment of Panic Disorder

Gerald L. Klerman, M.D.

In the process of establishing the efficacy of the combination of psychological treatments and medication, important theoretical, methodological, and clinical issues are raised. In this area, clinical practice in panic disorder is ahead of the research activities. Clinicians have been "experimenting" with giving various combinations of psychological treatments and medications, either concurrently or sequentially, for more than two decades. Only recently have systematic studies been undertaken to evaluate the efficacy of such combinations and to assess their place in the treatment strategy for panic disorder.

In my discussion of Telch and Lucas's chapter (Chapter 13), initial attention is given to methodology and design. Then problems related to ideology and professional relations are discussed. Finally, recommendations for the future are offered.

Issues in Methodology and Design

Ideally, studies of combined treatment should follow investigations of the safety and efficacy of the individual component treatments, whether they are medication or psychological treatments. This is best accomplished by randomized placebo-controlled parallel group designs in which the new treatment (pharmacological or

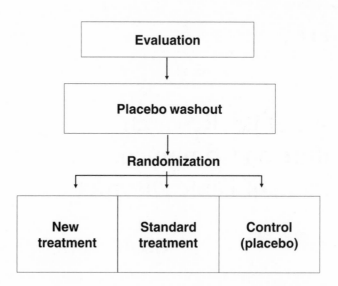

Figure 14–1. Three-group design for evaluating efficacy of new medication or psychological treatment.

psychological) is compared with a placebo or other control condition and with standard treatment (see Figure 14–1). The combined treatments may be administered concurrently or sequentially.

Designs for Evaluating Concurrent Treatment

As shown in Figure 14–2, the optimal design for studying concurrent treatments is the four-group, "No-by-Mo," factorial design. This design allows the use of analysis of variance (or analysis of covariance) as the appropriate statistical test, and further allows for the detection of interactions that may be interpreted as synergistic effects (see Figure 14–3). At a minimum, it is hoped that each of the components will have an independent main effect, in which case the combination should provide an additive effect. It is also hoped that there will be positive interaction (i.e., that the combined treatment has synergistic effects). This possibility rarely has been demonstrated with data from available studies.

In designs for testing concurrent combined treatments, patients are randomized early in the treatment to one of the four treatment groups shown in Figure 14–2 after initial evaluation and possibly a placebo washout period.

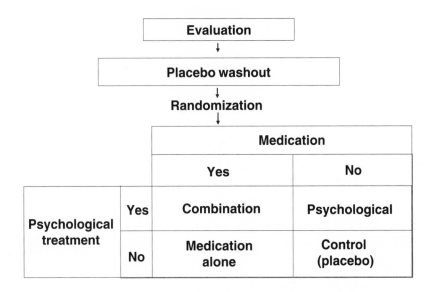

Figure 14–2. Four-cell design for evaluating combined medication and psychological treatment.

Sequential Designs

In clinical practice, sequential prescription of treatment is common. The order of this sequence is heavily influenced by the patient's attitudes, expectations, and therapeutic experience, which then interact in some complex way with the training, expertise, and ideological commitments of the therapist or investigator. The most common sequences are 1) psychological treatment first, followed by medication or combination, or 2) medication first, followed by psychological treatment or combination.

In research designs used to test the efficacy of sequential treatments (see Figure 14–4), the point of randomization is later—4–8 weeks after the effectiveness of the initial treatment has been judged—than it is for concurrent treatments. Patients who meet specific criteria for improvement or remission are not randomized but usually are continued on the initial medication; randomization is afforded to patients who, by whatever criteria, are judged to have not adequately responded to the initial treatment and who are then offered the sequential treatment.

In designs to evaluate the efficacy of sequential treatments (sometimes called

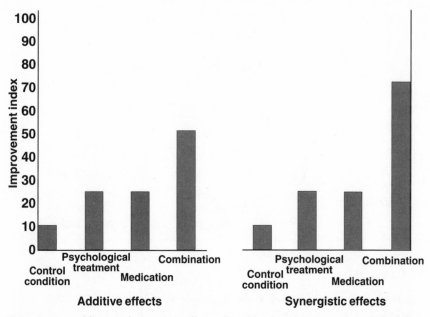

Figure 14–3. Additive and synergistic effects of combined medication and psychological treatment.

crossover designs), it is important that there be no carryover effect between the initial treatment and randomization phase to the second treatment. This may be a particular problem if the initial treatment was with a medication of the benzodiazepine type, because discontinuation and dosage tapering must be prolonged over a considerable amount of time to avoid withdrawal reactions. Patients may be reluctant to discontinue medication if they feel they will experience a period of distress with possible relapse, recurrence, and rebound.

Issues of Ideology and Professional Relations

Thus far, the discussion has centered on scientific issues of methodology and design. Closely aligned to the scientific issues are matters related to ideologies and professional commitment. The choice between psychological treatments and medication seldom occurs in a vacuum of values.

There is a long-standing background of conflict and disputes over the relative merits of psychological and pharmacological treatments for mental disorders. This ideological issue is confounded by the professional loyalty of the investigators. Investigators or clinicians using psychological techniques tend to be doctorate-level psychologists and tend to emphasize learning cognitive and psychological theories as well as their expertise in the delivery of various forms of individual and group psychotherapy. In contrast, most investigators of psychopharmacology are physicians, usually psychiatrists, committed to biological approaches to the causes and treatments of panic disorder. These two groups have, at times, experienced polemic and hostile interactions with each other, and relatively few investigators are able to avoid being caught up in the struggles for professional and scientific loyalty.

Prospects for the Future

As Telch and Lucas (Chapter 13) point out, we have relatively few systematic studies of combined treatment. In most of these studies, tricyclic antidepressants

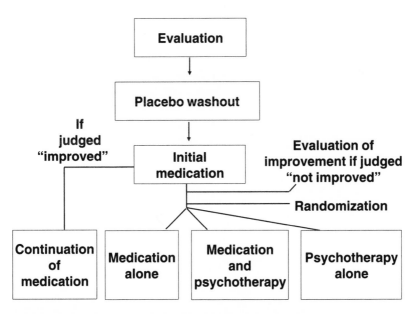

Figure 14–4. Research design for sequential treatment with medication and psychological treatments.

have been compared with other medication techniques in combination with psychological techniques (usually exposure). Only recently have systematic studies of alprazolam appeared. A number of cognitive relearning and retraining of breathing tasks have been developed in the United States, United Kingdom, and Western Europe for specific application to panic symptoms, independent of agoraphobic avoidance. The early results of these studies are promising, but relatively few conclusions can be drawn.

Conclusion

Combined psychological and psychopharmacological treatment of panic disorder has considerable clinical and theoretical appeal. However, further studies are needed to assess the place of combined treatments in the overall treatment strategy for panic disorder.

Bibliography

Cox DJ, Ballenger JC, Laraia M, et al: Different rates of improvement of different symptoms in combined pharmacological and behavioral treatment of agoraphobia. J Behav Ther Exp Psychiatry 19:119–126, 1988

Mavissakalian M: Agoraphobia, in Integrating Pharmacotherapy and Psychotherapy. Edited by Beitman BD, Klerman GL. Washington, DC, American Psychiatric Press, 1991, pp 165–181

Shear MK: Panic disorder, in Integrating Pharmacotherapy and Psychotherapy. Edited by Beitman BD, Klerman GL. Washington, DC, American Psychiatric Press, 1991, pp 143–164

Telch MJ: Combined pharmacological and psychological treatments for panic sufferers, in Panic: Psychological Perspectives. Edited by Rachman S, Maser JD. Hillsdale, NJ, Lawrence Erlbaum, 1991, pp 167–187

Section VI

Risk-Benefit Issues in Treatment of Panic Disorder

Chapter 15

Risk-Benefit Issues in Pharmacological Treatment of Panic Disorder

Karl Rickels, M.D., and Edward Schweizer, M.D.

Over the past decade, researchers have established the efficacy of three classes of compounds for the treatment of panic disorder: 1) the tricyclic antidepressants (TCAs), with the most evidence reported for imipramine, although other compounds such as clomipramine and desipramine have also been shown to be effective; 2) the monoamine oxidase inhibitor (MAOI) antidepressants, with the most evidence reported for phenelzine; and 3) the high-potency benzodiazepines, with the most evidence reported for alprazolam, although clonazepam and lorazepam have also been shown to be effective.

Demographic and illness variables have not been identified that clearly predict differential response to one versus any other class of compound. As a result, the choice of which medication to use in treating panic disorder depends on a more generic estimation of the relative risk-benefit ratios of each. The risk-benefit assessment can be considered separately for *acute treatment*, arbitrarily defined as ≤ 12 weeks of treatment, and *chronic or maintenance treatment*, defined as > 12 weeks.

This chapter was supported in part by USPHS Research Grant MH08957.

Benefits of Pharmacological Treatment of Panic Disorder

At least four components should be considered in judging the benefit of acute antipanic treatment. These include the ability of a compound to 1) reduce or block panic attacks, 2) reduce anticipatory and nonpanic anxiety, 3) reduce phobic avoidance, and 4) reduce miscellaneous associated (but much less frequently reported) features such as hypochondriasis, medical help seeking, and social and occupational disability. Table 15–1 summarizes the relative efficacy of acute and long-term treatment of panic disorder with TCAs, MAOIs, and the high-potency benzodiazepines.

Table 15–1. Pharmacological treatments of panic disorder: benefits

| | Drug class | | |
| | MAOIs (phenelzine) | Tricyclic antidepressants (imipramine) | Benzodiazepines (alprazolam) |
Condition			
Acute treatment			
Reduction/blockade of panic attacks	+++	+++	+++
Rapidity of antipanic response	+	+	+++
Reduction in anticipatory/ nonpanic anxiety	++	+	+++
Reduction in phobic avoidance	++	++	++
Long-term treatment			
Antipanic efficacy (sustained)	+++	+++	+++
Antidepressant efficacy	+++	+++	+
Lack of tolerance	+++	+++	+++
Prophylactic benefit (postdiscontinuation)	—	—	—

Note. MAOIs = monoamine oxidase inhibitors. + = mild; ++ = moderate; +++ = marked; — = no data available.

Acute Treatment

All three drugs appear to have comparable acute efficacy in achieving blockade of panic attacks, although the benzodiazepines achieve this antipanic response much faster (Ballenger et al. 1988; Sheehan et al. 1980).

Surprisingly few fixed-dosage studies, including plasma level determinations, have been reported (Mavissakalian and Perel 1989; Uhlenhuth et al. 1989). As a result, not enough information exists about either minimal or maximal effective dosages for these three classes of drugs. The wide range of dosages that have been found to be effective in flexible-dosage studies is hard to interpret for at least two reasons. First, a good response at a low dosage of an active drug early in treatment is likely to be a placebo response in up to one-third of all cases (Dager et al. 1990; Quitkin et al. 1987). Conversely, response at a higher dosage does not preclude the possibility that a patient might have responded to a longer period of treatment at a lower dosage. Because adverse effects are, to a certain extent, correlated with daily dose, and because attrition due to adverse effects ranges from 15%–20% for benzodiazepines to 30%–35% for the TCAs, more research should be devoted to these dosage-response issues.

Besides an advantage in rapidity of response, benzodiazepines appear to be more effective than TCAs or MAOIs in reducing both anticipatory and generalized anxiety. More than 50% of panic disorder patients have substantial subsyndromic levels of nonpanic generalized anxiety, and at least 25% actually meet criteria for comorbid generalized anxiety disorder (Barlow et al. 1986; Breier et al. 1985), so the extent to which nonpanic anxiety complicates the clinical picture of panic disorder must be taken into consideration.

Finally, all three classes of medications appear to have significant, and comparable, efficacy in reducing phobic avoidance, although this clinical effect may be somewhat less robust than the panic-blockade effect, suggesting that adjunctive cognitive-behavior treatment might be beneficial.

Long-Term Treatment

With long-term treatment (Table 15–1), panic efficacy appears to be sustained. There is no evidence either from controlled prospective studies or from naturalistic studies that tolerance develops to the antipanic efficacy of benzodiazepines. Consistent with this finding is that dosage escalation with long-term benzodiazepine use is not commonly reported. It should be noted, however, that there is no evidence for a protective antipanic effect continuing after discontinuation of medication. In fact, for the benzodiazepines there is even a concern that medication discontinuation, especially if it is too rapid, may result in a withdrawal syndrome that might trigger a recrudescence of panic attacks.

An important clinical concern in long-term treatment is the prior presence or later development of a comorbid illness, especially major depression, which is reported in more than 50% of panic disorder patients (Breier et al. 1985, 1986). The TCAs and MAOIs may offer a therapeutic advantage in panic disorder patients with major depression but, again, more research must be conducted to address this issue, especially regarding combinations of drugs (e.g., benzodiazepines and antidepressants) and regarding the combination of drug therapy and cognitive-behavior therapy.

Risks of Pharmacological Treatment of Panic Disorder

Table 15–2 summarizes the relative risks associated with acute and long-term treatment of panic disorder with the three classes of drugs, again as exemplified by phenelzine, imipramine, and alprazolam.

Acute Treatment

For acute treatment, the main risk is the symptom constellation of sedation and cognitive and psychomotor impairment. Although generalizations are difficult, these effects appear to be greatest with the benzodiazepines, less prominent with the TCAs, and least prominent with the MAOIs, at least in the initial phases of acute treatment. After 4–6 weeks at a stable daily dose, tolerance appears to develop to the adverse effects of benzodiazepines more completely than to the adverse effects of the antidepressants. Even after long-term treatment, some patients treated with the TCAs and MAOIs continue to complain of persistent, albeit milder, side effects (e.g., anticholinergic, sedative, and orthostatic effects, and, for the MAOIs in particular, problems with initial and middle insomnia in at least one-third of patients) (Rabkin et al. 1984). In addition, both short- and long-term use of MAOIs always carry the risk of hypertensive reactions, even crises, if tyramine-rich or otherwise monoamine-active foodstuffs or medications are inadvertently consumed. The availability in Europe, and eventually in the United States, of reversible and selective monoamine oxidase inhibitor–A (MAOI-A) compounds may provide an effective alternative, although more controlled research is needed.

Long-Term Treatment

Long-term therapy with the TCAs and MAOI antidepressants also leads to weight gain and, particularly with the MAOIs, to sexual dysfunction. Both of these side effects are frequently cited as reasons for discontinuing long-term therapy (Noyes et al. 1989; Robinson et al. 1986).

Long-term therapy with benzodiazepines (e.g., alprazolam), and to some extent short-term therapy (6–8 weeks), involves the risk of panic rebound and physical dependence, which necessitates a slow tapering from the treatment dose. There is the risk that a certain percentage of patients will be unable to taper off their benzodiazepine completely. Mild withdrawal reactions after abrupt discontinuation may be present even after phenelzine and imipramine therapy, but,

Table 15–2. Pharmacological treatments of panic disorder: risks

| | Drug class | | |
| | MAOIs | Tricyclic antidepressants | Benzodiazepines |
Condition	(phenelzine)	(imipramine)	(alprazolam)
Acute treatment			
Sedation	+	++	++
Psychomotor impairment	+	+	++
Cognitive or other central nervous system effects	+	+	++
Anticholinergic effects	+	++	0
Orthostatic hypotension	++	++	0
Interaction with alcohol	++	+	+++
Hypertensive reactions	+ to +++	0	0
Hyperstimulation	+	++	0
Dietary restrictions	+++	0	0
Long-term treatment			
Physical dependence	0	0	++
Withdrawal reaction	+	+	+ to +++[a]
Risk of abuse	0	0	+ −
Risk of adverse medical effects	+	+	0
Weight gain	++	++	0
Sexual dysfunction	+++	++	+ −

Note. MAOIs = monoamine oxidase inhibitors. + = mild severity/frequency; ++ = moderate severity/frequency; +++ = marked severity/frequency; + − = minimal severity/frequency; 0 = not present.
[a]Depends on such factors as rate of taper, dosage of drug, and half-life.

depending on taper speed, withdrawal reactions are much more marked for the benzodiazepines. It should be pointed out here that adequate antipanic therapy with alprazolam, for example, often requires fairly aggressive dosing in the range of 2–6 mg/day or occasionally up to 10 mg/day. Even at these dosages, there is only minimal risk of abuse (Woods et al. 1987). The risk of adverse medical effects, particularly hypertensive or cardiovascular effects, is mild for the MAOIs and TCAs and is not present for the benzodiazepines. Weight gain, which occurs frequently with imipramine or phenelzine treatment, is particularly a problem for women. Finally, the occurrence of sexual dysfunction is more marked for phenelzine and TCAs than for the benzodiazepines.

Given comparable levels of acute efficacy, patient acceptance of drug therapy can be taken as a measure of the relative degree of adverse effects. Attrition rates for phenelzine range around 30% or higher for fixed-dosage studies (Sheehan et al. 1980; Tyrer et al. 1973). Aggregate attrition rates for imipramine average about 30% (Andersch et al. 1991; Charney et al. 1986; Cross-National Collaborative Panic Study 1992; Mavissakalian and Perel 1989; Schweizer et al. 1993; Sheehan et al. 1980; Uhlenhuth et al. 1989). In contrast, attrition rates for alprazolam average around 15% in well-controlled, double-blind studies (Ballenger et al. 1988; Cross-National Collaborative Panic Study 1992; Schweizer et al. 1993; Uhlenhuth et al. 1989).

The main concern with long-term benzodiazepine therapy of panic disorder—a condition that is frequently chronic—is the development of physical dependence and the resulting withdrawal syndrome during tapered drug discontinuation. This is a definite risk for patients on long-term benzodiazepine therapy, particularly with the short half-life drugs such as alprazolam (Fyer et al. 1987; Noyes et al. 1991; Pecknold et al. 1988; Rickels et al. 1993), but also to a lesser degree with the long half-life benzodiazepine diazepam (Roy-Byrne et al. 1989).

Choosing Among the Three Classes of Medication

As there are several different classes of medication to choose from, all of which have demonstrated acute efficacy, the unanswered question for clinical research remains, Which treatment offers the best long-term outcome with the smallest risk?

Very few studies have systematically assessed the risk of physical dependence, as evidenced by withdrawal symptomatology, when panic disorder patients are gradually tapered from benzodiazepines. The study by Rickels et al. (1993) was one of the few in which the effects of tapered withdrawal from a benzodiazepine were considered. In that study, alprazolam, imipramine, and placebo were prescribed for an 8-month period and were then tapered over 3–5 weeks. The results clearly showed a significant rebound of panic attacks and significant occurrence of withdrawal symptomatology in the majority of patients on alprazolam, but not in those patients on imipramine or placebo. Thirty percent of patients were either unable to complete the taper or resumed treatment to counter withdrawal symptomatology after 1–3 days without alprazolam therapy (Rickels et al. 1993). The percentage of taper success rates was 100% for the 11 imipramine patients who were treated with 175 mg/day for 8 months, 100% for the 10 placebo patients, but only 67% for the 27 alprazolam patients who were treated with a mean daily dosage of 5.8 mg/day. In this particular study, the percentage of patients experiencing withdrawal phenomena ranged anywhere from 41% for alprazolam and 0% for imipramine and placebo patients, to 89% for alprazolam and 9% for imipramine and placebo patients, depending on the criterion used. Clearly, then, only alprazolam caused withdrawal symptoms.

Rickels et al. (1988) conducted a multiple search regression analysis for 39 patients who were treated with imipramine, alprazolam, or placebo; who were available at 15-month follow-up posttreatment; and also who had completed a Minnesota Multiphasic Personality Inventory (MMPI; McKinley and Hathaway 1943) at intake. They observed that patients felt improved and panic-free at 15-month follow-up if they had started with a lower phobia score, were younger, had more frequent and more intense initial panic attacks, but, most interestingly, were significantly lower in the MMPI dependence subscale (a scale reflecting feelings of inadequacy, low self-confidence, conformity, and passivity associated with overdependency). In other words, the more ego strength a patient possessed, the greater improvement he or she experienced at follow-up. Rickels et al. (1988) also used the Eysenck Neuroticism Scale (Eysenck and Eysenck 1964) as a personality measure and found it predictive of poor taper outcome, but at a slightly lower level of significance than the MMPI dependence scale.

Assessing the Need for Continued Pharmacological Treatment

Because panic disorder is a chronic illness whose symptoms may be intermittently present, it is important to interrupt therapy at certain intervals to see whether patients are still in need of therapy. This reassessment can be done relatively easily with MAOIs or imipramine, but it is more difficult to do with benzodiazepines such as alprazolam. In tapering alprazolam, it is therefore important to stress to the patient that he or she has to be able to taper the alprazolam down to zero. Moreover, the patient must remain drug-free for at least 3 weeks to allow the physician to differentiate with at least some degree of certainty between a return of original symptomatology and the occurrence of withdrawal symptoms and rebound panic attacks. The latter two are only transient events, whereas relapse or recurrence of symptoms occurs more gradually and symptom levels do not return to normal levels. Patients should be informed that tapering will prevent patients from experiencing seizures or convulsions or becoming psychotic, but will not necessarily help them to be free of withdrawal symptoms. Even a slow withdrawal will produce low levels of symptomatology in some patients. If gradual tapering is being conducted over several months, then it might be very difficult to separate any withdrawal symptoms that are still present from a relapse or recurrence of the original illness.

Summary

In summary, a risk-benefit comparison for the three major classes of drugs discussed clearly shows a benefit for the benzodiazepine alprazolam in terms of early onset of panic relief and relief of concurrent symptoms of phobia and anxiety; alprazolam also is effective over the long term without the risk of developing tolerance. Its major negative feature is the taper problem and the development of physical dependence, especially if prescribed in dosages of 6–10 mg/day. Advantages for imipramine and phenelzine are that, although their onset of panic attack relief is more gradual, they seem to be slightly more antiphobic agents, and discontinuation of therapy with them produces no clinically significant withdrawal problems. Both drugs, however, have a disturbing side effect potential. Interestingly enough, panic disorder patients seem to be more sensitive to the agitation and similar early side effects of imipramine than are anxious patients with generalized anxiety (Rickels et al., in press).

More follow-up data are needed to establish clearly for how long panic disorder patients need to be treated with either one of the three classes of drugs discussed. Similar to the course of depression, it may be that, once a panic episode is terminated, patients remain symptom-free for months or even years, but then, for whatever reason, reexperience panic symptoms and need treatment again.

We are sure that, in the future, other drugs, possibly various serotonin reuptake blockers or drugs that are either agonists or antagonists of particular serotonin subtype receptors, may prove effective in the treatment of panic disorder. These compounds would not have the problem of producing physical dependence. Until better drugs do become available, the physician has to discuss the risk-benefit issues for each of the three compounds with his or her patients prior to initiating therapy.

One final point should be mentioned. Once patients have been treated for 8 months or longer with a benzodiazepine for panic disorder, it is important they be gradually tapered and kept medication-free for about 3–5 weeks. This is important because, by that time, many panic disorder patients might not be in need of further therapy, at least for a significant time interval. In addition, we (Rickels et al. 1990; Schweizer et al. 1990) have found that, following discontinuation of therapy, patients who have been treated with benzodiazepines for a mean of over 8 years frequently feel better and have lower anxiety and depression levels than prior to drug discontinuation. In fact, in a 3-year follow-up of such patients, Rickels et al. (1991) found that those patients who stayed off their benzodiazepine had significantly lower scores in both anxiety and depression factors of the Hopkins Symptom Checklist—90 (Derogatis et al. 1974) than did patients who were unable to discontinue benzodiazepine therapy.

Experience has also shown that panic disorder patients treated with alprazolam, and probably also with other benzodiazepines such as clonazepam and lorazepam, do decrease their daily medication intake significantly over time. Rickels et al. (1993) found this to be true in a 15-month follow-up study of patients treated for 8 months with alprazolam at a dosage of 5.8 mg/day. This dosage was reduced for those patients who were still taking or who had resumed taking alprazolam up to 1.5 mg/day at time of follow-up. Whether this phenomenon indicates that in the acute or chronic treatment phases patients were treated with dosages of alprazolam that were too high, or whether patients treated for 8 months simply are in need of lower levels of medications, or whether patients are panic-free and need a low daily dose of alprazolam simply to treat their emerging withdrawal symptomatology, cannot be determined from data presently available in the literature.

References

Andersch S, Rosenberg NK, Kullingsjo H, et al: Efficacy and safety of alprazolam, imipramine and placebo in treating panic disorder: a Scandinavian multicenter study. Acta Psychiatr Scand 365 (suppl):18–27, 1991

Ballenger JC, Burrows GD, DuPont RL Jr, et al: Alprazolam in panic disorder and agoraphobia: results from a multicenter trial, I: efficacy in short-term treatment. Arch Gen Psychiatry 45:413–422, 1988

Barlow DH, Di Nardo PA, Vermilyea BB, et al: Co-morbidity and depression among the anxiety disorders: issues in diagnosis and classification. J Nerv Ment Dis 174:63–72, 1986

Breier A, Charney DS, Heninger GR: The diagnostic validity of anxiety disorders and their relationship to depressive illness. Am J Psychiatry 142:787–817, 1985

Breier A, Charney DS, Heninger GR: Agoraphobia with panic attacks: development, diagnostic stability, and course of illness. Arch Gen Psychiatry 43:1029–1036, 1986

Charney DS, Woods SW, Goodman WK, et al: Drug treatment of panic disorder: the comparative efficacy of imipramine, alprazolam and trazodone. J Clin Psychiatry 47:580–586, 1986

Cross-National Collaborative Panic Study, Second Phase Investigators: Drug treatment of panic disorder: comparative efficacy of alprazolam, imipramine, and placebo. Br J Psychiatry 160:191–202, 1992

Dager SR, Khan A, Cowley D, et al: Characteristics of placebo response during long-term treatment of panic disorder. Psychopharmacol Bull 26(3):273–278, 1990

Derogatis LR, Lipman RS, Rickels K, et al: The Hopkins Symptom Checklist (HSCL): a self-report symptom inventory. Behav Sci 19:1–15, 1974

Eysenck HJ, Eysenck SBG: The Manual of the Eysenck Personality Inventory. London, England, University of London Press, 1964

Fyer AJ, Liebowitz MR, Gorman JM, et al: Discontinuation of alprazolam treatment in panic patients. Am J Psychiatry 144:303–308, 1987

Mavissakalian MR, Perel JM: Imipramine dose-response relationship in panic disorder with agoraphobia: preliminary findings. Arch Gen Psychiatry 46(2):127–131, 1989

McKinley JC, Hathaway SR: The identification and measurement of the psychoneuroses in medical practice: the Minnesota Multiphasic Personality Inventory. JAMA 122:161–167, 1943

Noyes R Jr, Garvey MJ, Cook BL, et al: Problems with tricyclic use in patients with panic disorder or agoraphobia: results of a naturalistic follow-up study. J Clin Psychiatry 50:163–169, 1989

Noyes R Jr, Garvey MJ, Cook B, et al: Controlled discontinuation of benzodiazepine treatment for patients with panic disorder. Am J Psychiatry 148(4):517–523, 1991

Pecknold JC, Swinson RP, Kuch K, et al: Alprazolam in panic disorder and agoraphobia: results from a multicenter trial, III: discontinuation effects. Arch Gen Psychiatry 45:429–436, 1988

Quitkin FM, Rabkin JD, Markowitz JM, et al: Use of pattern analysis to identify true drug response: a replication. Arch Gen Psychiatry 44(3):259–264, 1987

Rabkin J, Quitkin F, Harrison W, et al: Adverse reactions to the monoamine oxidase inhibitors, part I: a comparative study. J Clin Psychopharmacol 4:270–278, 1984

Rickels K, Schweizer E, Case WG, et al: Benzodiazepine dependence, withdrawal severity, and clinical outcome: effects of personality. Psychopharmacol Bull 24(3):415–420, 1988

Rickels K, Schweizer E, Case WG, et al: Long-term therapeutic use of benzodiazepines, I: effects of abrupt discontinuation. Arch Gen Psychiatry 47:899–907, 1990

Rickels K, Case WG, Schweizer E, et al: Long-term benzodiazepine users 3 years after participation in a discontinuation program. Am J Psychiatry 148(6):757–761, 1991

Rickels K, Schweizer E, Weiss S, et al: Maintenance drug treatment for panic disorder, II: short- and long-term outcome after drug taper. Arch Gen Psychiatry 50:61–68, 1993

Rickels K, Downing R, Schweizer E, et al: Antidepressants for the treatment of generalized anxiety disorder: a placebo-controlled comparison of imipramine, trazodone, and diazepam. Arch Gen Psychiatry (in press)

Robinson DS, Kayser A, Bennett B, et al: Maintenance phenelzine treatment of depression: an interim report. Psychopharmacol Bull 22:12–15, 1986

Roy-Byrne PP, Dager SR, Cowley DS, et al: Relapse and rebound following discontinuation of benzodiazepine treatment of panic attacks: alprazolam versus diazepam. Am J Psychiatry 146(7):860–865, 1989

Schweizer E, Rickels K, Case WG, et al: Long-term therapeutic use of benzodiazepines, II: effects of gradual taper. Arch Gen Psychiatry 47:908–915, 1990

Schweizer E, Rickels K, Weiss S, et al: Maintenance drug treatment for panic disorder, I: results of a prospective, placebo-controlled comparison of alprazolam and imipramine. Arch Gen Psychiatry 50:51–60, 1993

Sheehan DV, Ballenger JC, Jacobsen G: Treatment of endogenous anxiety with phobic, hysterical and hypochondriacal symptoms. Arch Gen Psychiatry 37:51–59, 1980

Tyrer P, Candy J, Kelly D: Phenelzine in phobic anxiety: a controlled trial. Psychopharmacologia 32:237–254, 1973

Uhlenhuth EH, Matuzas W, Glass RM, et al: Response of panic disorder to fixed doses of alprazolam or imipramine. J Affective Disord 17:261–270, 1989

Woods JH, Katz JL, Winger G: Abuse liability of benzodiazepines. Pharmacol Rev 39:251–419, 1987

Chapter 16

Risk-Benefit Issues in Psychosocial Treatment of Panic Disorder

Larry K. Michelson, Ph.D.

Anxiety disorders are among the most prevalent and debilitating clinical dysfunctions in the United States. Panic disorder with or without agoraphobia exhibits high incidence and prevalence, and is associated with myriad sequelae, including depression; suicide; alcohol and substance abuse; minor tranquilizer addiction; generalized anxiety disorder; social, simple, and sexual phobias; and impaired social, marital, and occupational functioning. Although panic disorders represent the leading reason patients seek outpatient services and psychotropic medications, fewer than 25% of panic disorder individuals seek out treatment (Dryman and Weissman 1991). Hence, the prevalence, severity, and long-term effects of panic disorder emphasize the importance of developing effective, safe, and tolerable treatments.

The primary aim of this chapter is to review psychotherapeutic and pharmacological treatments of panic disorder with and without agoraphobia. Also examined are the overarching conceptual, methodological, and clinical research issues pertaining to these treatments and their relative strengths, limitations, and possible interactions.

Review of Psychological and Pharmacological Treatments of Panic Disorder Table 16–1 presents a hypothetical cohort of 100 panic disorder patients with agoraphobia receiving alternative psychosocial and pharmacological treatments, and delineates the percentages of patients who drop out, achieve clinically significant improvement, or relapse, as well as the overall long-term efficacy rate of these treatments. These data represent estimates based on literature reviews, recent meta-analyses, and current clinical research (cf., Michelson and Marchione 1991). The efficacy index was derived from using the criteria of "clinically significant

Table 16–1. Hypothetical cohort of 100 panic disorder patients with agoraphobia

| | Beta-blockers | | Low-potency benzo-diazepines | | High-potency benzo-diazepines | | Mono-amine oxidase inhibitors | | Tricyclic anti-depressants | | Pro-grammed practice | | Relaxa-tion training | | Graded exposure | | Imipra-mine + graded exposure | | Cognitive therapy + graded exposure | | Cognitive-behavior treatment of panic disorder without agora-phobia | |
Measure	%	n_{rem}	%	n_{rem}	%	n_{rem}	%	n_{rem}	%	n_{rem}	%	n_{rem}	%	n_{rem}	%	n_{rem}	%	n_{rem}	%	n_{rem}	%	n_{rem}
Attrition	20	80	15	85	15	85	35	65	25	75	15	85	15	85	15	85	25	75	15	85	5	95
Clinically significant improvement	10	8	15	13	60	51	45	29	60	45	25	21	55	47	65	55	70	53	87	74	90	86
Relapse	90	1	85	2	90	5	40	17	35	29	15	18	15	40	15	47	25	39	10	67	5	81
Long-term overall efficacy index	1		2		5		17		29		18		40		47		39		67		81	

Note. n_{rem} = number remaining. Because of the routine use of exposure instructions in many pharmacotherapeutic studies of panic disorder patients with agoraphobia, the unitary effectiveness of these medications awaits future research. However, the efficacy rates of these agents might be reduced if administered in the absence of behavior counseling.

Source. Adapted from Michelson L, Marchione K: "Behavioral, Cognitive and Pharmacological Treatments of Panic Disorder With Agoraphobia: Critique and Synthesis." *Journal of Consulting and Clinical Psychology* 59:100–114, 1991. Copyright 1991 American Psychological Association. Reprinted by permission.

improvement" (50% or greater) or remission at posttreatment.

The *beta-blockers* exhibited a moderate attrition rate, a low improvement rate, and a high relapse rate, yielding an overall efficacy index of 1%. The *low-potency benzodiazepines* showed modest attrition and improvement rates, a high relapse rate, and a long-term efficacy index of 2%. The *high-potency benzodiazepines* exhibited a low attrition rate, a moderate improvement rate, and a high relapse rate (90%), resulting in an overall efficacy index of 5%. The *monoamine oxidase inhibitors* had a high attrition rate and moderate levels of improvement and relapse, resulting in an efficacy index of 17%. The *tricyclic antidepressants,* regarded as the gold standard of pharmacotherapy, also had a relatively high attrition rate (25%), with similar outcome and relapse rates generating an efficacy rate of 29%.

The *programmed practice* column reveals low attrition, moderate improvement, and low relapse rates, yielding an 18% efficacy index. *Relaxation training paired with programmed practice* exhibited low attrition and relapse rates and moderate outcome, generating an overall efficacy index of 40%. Regarding *graded exposure,* the attrition rate was low, with 65% of patients achieving clinically significant improvement, and the relapse rate was low, resulting in an efficacy index of 47%. *Imipramine plus graduated exposure* evinced a relatively high attrition rate, a slightly elevated outcome (compared with the effects of these treatments separately), and a moderate relapse rate, which resulted in an efficacy rate of 39%. *Cognitive therapy plus graded exposure,* which was derived from the Michelson et al. (1993) panic disorder with agoraphobia outcome study, revealed a low attrition rate and high posttreatment efficacy (85%), with a 10% relapse rate, resulting in an overall efficacy rate of 67%. (This latter treatment is the most effective treatment the authors tested to date for panic disorder with agoraphobia.) Finally, for comparative purposes, estimates were also computed for recent studies on *cognitive treatments of panic disorder with no or mild phobic avoidance.* These studies indicated negligible attrition and relapse rates, a high (90%) improvement rate, and an overall efficacy index of 81%. Although these data are hypothetical, they are representative of the extant studies and indicate that cognitive therapy combined with graded exposure for panic disorder with agoraphobia, and cognitive-behavior treatments for panic disorder foster optimal short- and long-term outcomes.

Overarching Conceptual, Methodological, and Clinical Research Issues

Potential Risks of Psychosocial Treatments

As seen in the data in Table 16–1, the benefits of psychosocial treatments include their relatively high public acceptance, low attrition rates, safety, negligible side effects, and relative effectiveness. There are several potential risks, which apply equally across all treatments.

∎ **Lack of consideration of concurrent disorders.** One of the most common potential pitfalls concerns the failure to address concomitant dysfunctions and disorders, both Axis I disorders (e.g., generalized anxiety disorder, posttraumatic stress disorder) and Axis II disorders, all of which may influence the effectiveness of panic disorder treatment. For example, conservative estimates suggest that 50%–75% of panic disorder patients with or without agoraphobia meet diagnostic criteria for concurrent disorders. Because these phenomena have not been empirically examined in the context of comparative outcome studies, their possible influence and whether they are a cause, correlate, or consequence of panic disorder (or possibly all of these) remain a mystery. Hence, more integrative theories and psychotherapies are needed. Future research should study comorbidity issues more programmatically in the context of psychotherapy investigations.

∎ **Incomplete emotional processing.** Greater attention should be paid to ensuring that complete emotional processing has been achieved, as described by Jack Rachman in his classic (1980) article and in the Foa and Kozak (1986) article on the same topic. This could be accomplished using a multimatrix assessment paradigm that would encompass information and psychophysiological processing of threat or phobic cues, and clinical, behavioral, and self-report indexes of emotional processing.

∎ **Need for more advanced training for mental health professionals in cognitive-behavior treatments.** Therapists working with panic disorder patients should develop proficiency in the various cognitive-behavior treatments by attending workshops, reading relevant books and journals, and obtaining clinical consultation.

∎ **Inadequate graduate-level training.** Advanced degree training programs in psychology, psychiatry, and social work should include specific courses and supervised clinical experiences in treating panic disorder patients.

These endeavors should modulate potential risks and promote advances in the effective treatment of panic disorder.

Optimal Treatment Regimens

Overall, this review indicates that the treatment of choice for panic disorder with no or mild phobic avoidance is cognitive-behavior therapy aimed at panic cessation. Treatment should include panic management, breathing retraining, exposure to interoceptive cues, and applied relaxation training. For those patients requiring additional therapy, alternative psychological or pharmacological treatments can be considered. For patients experiencing panic disorder with agoraphobia, more comprehensive, multimodal treatments are needed to address the disorder's complex nature. Programmed practice instructions should be routinely given as well as therapist-assisted graded exposure when necessary. In-depth cognitive therapy of panic disorder with agoraphobia, as described by Marchione et al. (1987) and Michelson et al. (1993), should also be provided to address complex, dysfunctional schema and core beliefs that maintain the disorder (Michelson and Ascher 1989).

Panic disorder patients with agoraphobia who decline, drop out, or do not fully respond to these interventions or who are severely depressed may benefit from a trial of tricyclic antidepressants or high-potency benzodiazepines combined with cognitive-behavior therapy. However, it is still unknown how much additional benefit can be expected from such a combination. Further studies examining the relative and combined effects of psychosocial and pharmacological treatments will, it is hoped, illuminate issues concerning treatment mechanisms, differential pathways, individual differences, tripartite outcome, and longitudinal adjustment. Pharmacotherapy can be helpful in the treatment of panic disorders. However, future investigations will need to address issues concerning enhancing compliance, long-term maintenance, patient attributions of improvement, and optimal strategies to promote additive or synergistic effects when combined with psychosocial therapies.

Conclusions

Although major strides have been made in the treatment of panic disorder, many unresolved theoretical and clinical issues that require further research remain. First, different psychotherapeutic models should be explored as potential complementary or alternative approaches for treatment, particularly as multi-axis disorders appear to be frequently superimposed on panic disorder.

Second, it is hoped that the theoretical and clinical advances in panic disorder will be extended to include largely unexplored and related phenomena that may later masquerade as panic disorder, such as posttraumatic stress disorder, dissociative disorders, or trauma resulting from psychological, physical, or sexual abuse. Prevention studies should be supported to identify strategies to reduce the incidence and prevalence of panic disorder. Both retrospective and prospective studies would be helpful in identifying developmental links among child, adolescent, and adult anxiety disorders. Prevention research should include early intervention with individuals experiencing initial panic attacks to provide rapid resolution of emerging symptoms. These humanitarian and scientific endeavors could directly reduce the long-term effects of the untreated, incipient panic disorder.

Finally, an important methodological issue concerns the need for continued dialogue to develop a consensus definition of "clinically significant change." Investigators will need to adopt conceptually coherent, clinically salient, psychometrically sound, and normatively based indexes of improvement and end-state functioning. This will permit cross-study comparisons, elucidate outcome effects, and inform theoretical advances.

References

Dryman A, Weissman M: Panic and phobia, in Psychiatric Disorders in America. Edited by Robins L, Regier D. New York, Free Press, 1991

Foa E, Kozak M: Emotional processing of fear: exposure to corrective information. Psychol Bull 99:20–35, 1986

Marchione K, Michelson L, Greenwald M, et al: Cognitive-behavioral treatments of agoraphobia. Behav Res Ther 25:319–328, 1987

Michelson L, Ascher LM: Anxiety and Stress Disorders: Cognitive-Behavioral Assessment and Treatment. New York, Guilford, 1989

Michelson L, Marchione K: Behavioral, cognitive and pharmacological treatments of panic disorder with agoraphobia: critique and synthesis. J Consult Clin Psychol 59:100–114, 1991

Michelson L, Marchione K, Greenwald M, Testa S, Marchione N: A comparative outcome follow-up investigation of panic disorder with agoraphobia: the relative and combined efficacy of cognitive therapy, relaxation training and therapist-assisted exposure. Pennsylvania State University. Unpublished manuscript, May 1993

Rachman J: Emotional processing. Behav Res Ther 18:51–60, 1980

Issues for the Future

Chapter 17

Panic Disorder:
Directions for Future Research

M. Katherine Shear, M.D.,
Andrew Leon, Ph.D., and Lisa Spielman, Ph.D.

The current era of panic disorder research began with the seminal work of Donald Klein, whose studies led directly to the designation of panic disorder as a syndrome. A series of pharmacological treatment studies (Klein 1964; Klein and Fink 1962) conducted 3 decades ago provided a major impetus for identifying panic as a distinct form of anxiety, and for the elaboration of the panic-centered conceptualization of the pathogenesis of agoraphobia (Klein 1981). Klein's view of panic's nosology is now generally accepted by both psychopharmacologists and cognitive-behavior therapists. In Klein's etiologic model, panic is thought to involve a pathologically lowered threshold for firing of a hard-wired neuronal pattern in the central nervous system that mediates an ethologically important survival function, such as separation or perhaps suffocation anxiety (Klein 1993). This model has informed the large-scale neurobiological research effort reviewed by other participants at the National Institutes of Health's Consensus Development Conference on Panic. Klein's work has also been a stimulus for the thus far mostly successful search for treatments focused on blocking the occurrence of panic. (Some of this work has been reviewed in other chapters of this volume.)

The current status of treatment outcome research indicates that 1) there are high rates (70%–90%) of full remission of panic episodes with a range of treatments; 2) there are treatments that have statistically and clinically significant effects on panic disorder symptomatology; 3) several different pharmacological agents are effective in treating panic disorder; 4) the efficacy of specific cognitive-behavior techniques is as good as or better than that of pharmacological treatments; and 5) there is continued overall improvement from pretreatment status on long-term follow-up by panic disorder patients. A large-scale multicenter study (Shalomskas et al. 1990) is under way to answer some of the crucial remaining questions about the relative efficacy of medication and cognitive-behavior treatments separately and in combination.

Do these successes mean we can reach a consensus that panic disorder, like scarlet fever, will be under control if only we can ensure that a "panic penicillin" is widely available? Unfortunately, they do not. Certainly, information about effective interventions needs to be disseminated, but enthusiasm for short-term focused treatments must be tempered by more sober consideration of what remains to be done. In this chapter we focus on four of these problems:

1. The lack of standardized methodology for assessing treatment outcome makes generalizations and comparative outcome assessment difficult.
2. Data are available regarding efficacy of different interventions, but not regarding optimal treatment.
3. Cognitive-behavior studies have focused on the treatment of panic or agoraphobia; little is known about the efficacy of an integrated approach to the treatment of panic and agoraphobia.
4. There is insufficient information about the origins and vicissitudes of comorbidity, which is the rule rather than the exception in panic disorder patients.

Consideration of these problems, as we hope to illustrate, leads to the conclusion that there is a need to broaden the working model of the panic-agoraphobic syndrome to incorporate data on residual symptoms, discontinuity between panic and phobic avoidance, and the prevalence and impact of comorbidity. We suggest that a set of highly interesting, if preliminary, studies by Kagan et al. (1990a), Rosenbaum et al. (1988), and Biederman et al. (1990) of behaviorally inhibited children and by Suomi (1991) of high-reactive rhesus monkeys provide the basis for an extended model. This model predicts that at least a subgroup of panic patients might be conceptualized as having a lifelong, perhaps inherited, anxiety diathesis in the form of heightened physiological reactivity and behavioral inhibition. We elaborate on these ideas below.

Lack of Standardized Assessment Methodology

A central problem in evaluating treatment outcome research is the lack of standardized assessment methodology. The original plan for this chapter was to review reports of controlled treatment studies to assess the degree of residual symptoms that occur with treatments of documented efficacy. However, because there is no uniformity in reporting treatment outcome, this goal could not be achieved. Outcome criteria are not defined consistently across studies, and outcome measures are not standardized. Different dimensions are assessed in different studies, and different measures are used to assess the same dimensions. The main outcome measures vary; they may be defined as change in panic or phobic state or clinical global improvement. Even when the main outcome is the same in two studies, the units in which that outcome is reported may differ. Panic status may be reported as the percentage of patients panic-free (sometimes with an unspecified time frame), mean percentage of decrease in panic frequency, or mean change in panic frequency. In some cases, only the statistical significance of the pre- to posttreatment change is noted. Finally, there is a lack of operational criteria for different types of successful outcomes. The term *responder* is used to indicate either some response to treatment or achievement of remission; recovery and remission are not differentiated and relapse criteria vary. For example, Clark (Chapter 10, this volume) used a criterion of full reemergence of the DSM-III-R (American Psychiatric Association 1987) syndrome to rate relapse and trigger a referral for further treatment. Sheehan (1986) considered recurrence of limited symptom episodes an indication for further treatment. This means that subjects will vary in intervening treatment received and in reported relapse rates.

Given these limitations, we still tried to construct a composite picture to assess the degree of overall success in treating a wide range of symptoms. Our literature review, derived from subsets that reported each symptom, suggests mean percentage changes in panic disorder symptomatology as follows: panic attacks, 78%; anticipatory anxiety, 58%; and phobic fear, 69%. These percentages provide a rough indication of the degree of responsiveness of the different symptoms to current treatment and indicate that residual symptoms are often present after short-term treatment.

We used two other strategies to approximate the percentages of subjects who might be expected to achieve full and lasting treatment effects. First, we analyzed a data set of 110 subjects who met DSM-III-R criteria for panic disorder as the predominant diagnosis and who participated in either a medication trial ($n = 65$) or a psychological treatment study ($n = 45$) at the Payne Whitney Anxiety Disorders Clinic. Sixty-four percent of the patients in these two studies became panic-free, a rate comparable with that of most other existing studies. We then divided the group into those who did or did not reach criteria for full remission of associated symptoms. We used a remitted criterion for anticipatory anxiety of less than 10% of the day spent worrying about panic, and a remitted criterion for phobic distress of a score of less than 4 on a 0–10 rating scale. This analysis revealed that 20% of the subjects showed full remission of panic, anticipatory anxiety, and phobic avoidance, whereas another 27% achieved remission of panic and one of the other two symptoms. Seventeen percent achieved panic remission with residual phobic and anxiety symptoms still present. In the group of subjects who were not panic-free, 50% (19% of the overall sample) did achieve remission of anticipatory anxiety and/or phobic symptoms, with only 19% of the overall sample still symptomatic in all three areas. In addition to providing a novel perspective on treatment outcome, these analyses suggest that panic remission, although important, is neither necessary nor sufficient to ensure remission of other panic disorder symptoms in a brief treatment intervention.

The second strategy we used was based on Michelson and Marchione's (1991) hypothetical predicted outcomes for a variety of different treatment modalities, based on their clinical studies, a literature review, and existing meta-analytic papers. (For these analyses we omitted treatments, such as beta-blockers, that are generally believed to be less effective modalities for panic disorder patients.) Based on these predictions, 68% of subjects would achieve a successful clinical outcome. When predicted dropouts are considered, the success rate would fall to 49%, and when predicted relapse (31%) is also included, the expected success rate would fall to 18%. It is important to note that the relapse rate of 31% is actually somewhat lower than that estimated by considering data from available long-term follow-up studies. For example, Nagy et al. (1989) showed residual symptoms in 56% of patients in their long-term follow-up. In the Harvard naturalistic follow-up study (Pollack et al. 1990), only 54% of patients reported full symptom remission at 2 months and 35% at 6 months. These rates are similar to those reported in the naturalistic follow-up study by Noyes et al. (1989), those presented in a review by Brown and Barlow (1992) of long-term follow-up of cognitive-behavior studies (when high end-state functioning is the criterion of success), and the data presented by Katschnig and Amering (Chapter 6, this volume). It is important to note that these data refer to persistent residual symptoms rather than to full recurrence of the panic disorder syndrome.

In summary, we believe there is a need for agreement on a uniform battery of assessments, a uniform set of assessment instruments, and a uniform format for reporting results, and a need for a consensus on definitions of response categories. Workers in the field of panic disorder also need to develop a battery of posttreatment interval assessments to help identify and treat relapse vulnerability. In addition, the field would be well served by a careful study of dropouts, with strategies for minimizing their numbers and a focus on improving rates and maintaining stability of full remission.

Lack of an Integrated Approach in Treating Panic and Agoraphobia

Two subjects that may provide insight into the problem of incomplete remission are the degree of phobic avoidance and the occurrence of comorbid symptomatology. The original, elegant, and influential model elaborated by Klein focused attention on the role of panic in the genesis of agoraphobic fear and avoidance. This generally supported model predicts a causal relationship between panic, fear of panic, duration of panic, and degree of phobic avoidance. The idea that panic causes the development of agoraphobia has led to a focus on unidimensional antipanic treatment approaches.

Studies confirm that panic precedes the onset of agoraphobia in the majority of cases. Variables related to panic and fear of panic show a statistically significant relationship to the degree of phobic avoidance. However, the timing, course, and intensity of anticipatory anxiety and phobic avoidance are highly variable. There is a considerable range of phobic avoidance for any given panic frequency or intensity and for any given duration of panic symptomatology (Craske et al. 1988). In addition, the treatments currently used for panic disorder have not been well studied in agoraphobic patients. It appears that for some patients treatment of panic is accompanied by complete remission of phobic symptoms, but for others this is not the case (Muskin and Fyer 1981).

The strongest predictor of phobia related to fear of panic is the fear of social consequences (Telch et al. 1989). Chambless (1985) reported that comorbid social phobia, fear of negative evaluation, and assertiveness inhibition are all predictors of higher levels of avoidance, as are depression, high neuroticism scores on the Eysenck Personality Questionnaire (Eysenck and Eysenck 1964), and social class. Recent work by Pollack and co-workers at Massachusetts General Hospital (M. W. Otto, M. H. Pollack, J. F. Rosenbaum, G. S. Sachs, and R. H. Asher, unpublished manuscript, 1993) further indicated that comorbid social phobia is related to childhood anxiety disorders and high levels of anxiety sensitivity, raising the possibility of an early anxiety diathesis in the more severe agoraphobic patients.

Comorbidity in Panic Disorder

In addition to agoraphobia, the presence of other comorbid disorders is the rule for panic disorder patients. We estimate from a review of existing literature that roughly 70% of these patients have Axis I comorbidity (Brier et al. 1984; Bowen et al. 1984; DiNardo and Barlow 1990) and 50% (perhaps overlapping with the 70% of patients) have Axis II comorbidity (Friedman et al. 1987; Mavissakalian and Hamann 1986; Reich 1988). This important area is only beginning to be addressed in treatment studies. Investigators in one study (Mellman and Uhde 1987) indicated that patients with comorbid obsessive-compulsive disorder have a poorer treatment outcome with medication. Several studies (Klerman 1990; Lesser et al. 1988; Maddock and Blacker 1991) have suggested that comorbid affective disorder is associated with more severe panic disorder symptomatology, but not with differential treatment outcome. Several other studies (Reich and Green 1991; Pollack et al. 1992) have documented poorer outcome in patients with comorbid Axis II disorders. Little more is known of the vicissitudes of comorbid symptoms in treatment studies.

Comorbidity is potentially of importance in teasing apart the heterogeneous group of panic disorder patients with agoraphobia. Comorbidity may be an indicator of overall illness severity or of different underlying psychological or biological processes. Some types of comorbidity may contribute to difficulties in achieving full remission, and may indicate a need for a different treatment approach, either combined with or instead of standard treatment.

In summary, more attention should be given to phobic symptoms as possible indicators of an underlying psychological or physiological disturbance. Treatment interventions targeted at alleviating phobic symptoms are needed. Also, more attention should be given to comorbid Axis I disorders, with assessments being conducted posttreatment as well as pretreatment. Patients with Axis II disorders need to be better characterized and treatment strategies need to be developed to incorporate interventions directed at ameliorating these disorders.

Insights Into Panic Disorder Provided by Temperament Research

We conclude with a brief review of work conducted by infant (Kagan) and primate (Suomi) temperament researchers, and a discussion of the possible relevance of this work to panic disorder. Kagan and Suomi, each interested in infant temperament and individual differences in stress reactivity, independently identified a subgroup of seemingly normal individuals with high levels of reactivity to novel phenomena and exaggerated reactions to separation stress. High-reactive young humans, like rhesus monkey infants, showed low levels of exploratory behavior and high levels of physiological arousal on exposure to novel situations (Kagan et al. 1990b). This trait is identifiable early in life (Kagan et al. 1989) and apparently present in a stable way through development. These children are at high risk for childhood anxiety disorders (Biederman et al. 1990) and their parents have an increased prevalence of panic disorder with agoraphobia (Rosenbaum et al. 1988) and of social phobia (Rosenbaum et al. 1991).

Suomi (1991) has reported that high-reactive infants have ongoing marked reactivity to life stress. This investigator also has indicated that nurturing parenting can mitigate the development of social phobia in monkeys (Suomi 1987). Several studies have indicated that parents of panic disorder patients are typically remembered as being overcontrolling or uncaring (Faravelli et al. 1991; Silove 1986; Solyom et al. 1976), a type of parenting not expected to mitigate phobic symptoms. Thus, a possible model for at least a subgroup of panic disorder patients might include early neurophysiological diathesis for anxiety, combined with suboptimal parental attitudes and behaviors, leading to a high prevalence of early problems with anxiety regulation, social insecurities, development of social phobia, and, finally, to panic disorder.

Conclusions

We have come far in developing methodologies for conducting treatment studies and demonstrating efficacy of specific interventions in panic disorder. However, the direct translation of these results to recommendations for optimal clinical care remains problematic. We should be particularly wary of drawing premature conclusions about relative effectiveness of treatments that have not yet been properly compared, and in patient populations that may not have been fully characterized.

Although there have been major insights into panic, it is clear that residual symptomatology is common and that persistent long-term symptoms occur in patients treated with effective short-term interventions. Moreover, a number of studies have documented that preexisting anxiety disorders (e.g., overanxious disorder, social phobia, generalized anxiety disorder, or even agoraphobia) are present in a substantial subgroup before the onset of the first panic episode. The postulated central neurophysiological deficit in panic disorder has not yet been identified and the nature of the relationship between phobic avoidance and panic episodes has not been fully elucidated. Comorbidity of panic with other anxiety disorders, substance abuse, depression, and personality disorders is the rule. We are left with the concern that identification and treatment of panic *episodes* may not be sufficient to understand and treat panic *disorder,* and that we should consider the possibility that there are predisposing psychological or biological traits that still need to be identified and addressed.

References

American Psychiatric Association: Diagnostic and Statistical Manual of Mental Disorders, 3rd Edition, Revised. Washington, DC, American Psychiatric Association, 1987

Biederman J, Rosenbaum JF, Hirschfeld DR: Psychiatric correlates of behavioral inhibition in young children of parents with and without psychiatric disorders. Arch Gen Psychiatry 47:21–26, 1990

Bowen RC, Cipywynk D, D'Arcy C, et al: Alcoholism, anxiety disorders and agoraphobia. Alcohol Clin Exp Res 8:48–50, 1984

Brier A, Charney DS, Heninger GR: Major depression in patients with agoraphobia and panic disorder. Am J Psychiatry 143:1569–1574, 1984

Brown TA, Barlow DH: Long-term clinical outcome following cognitive behavioral treatment of panic disorder and panic disorder with agoraphobia, in Principles and Practice of Relapse Prevention. Edited by Wilson PH. New York, Guilford, 1992, pp 191–212

Chambless DL: The relationship of severity of agoraphobia to associated psychopathology. Behav Res Ther 23:305–310, 1985

Craske MG, Rapee RM, Barlow DH: The significance of panic expectancy for individual patterns of avoidance. Behavioral Therapy 19:577–592, 1988

DiNardo PA, Barlow DH: Syndrome and symptom comorbidity in the anxiety disorders, in Comorbidity in the Anxiety and Mood Disorders. Edited by Maser JD, Cloninger CR. Washington, DC, American Psychiatric Press, 1990

Eysenck HC, Eysenck SBG: Manual of the Eysenck Personality Inventory. London, University of London Press, 1964

Faravelli C, Panichi C, Rivilli S, et al: Perception of early parenting in panic and agoraphobia. Acta Psychiatr Scand 84:6–8, 1991

Friedman K, Shear MK, Frances AJ: Prevalence of personality disorder in panic disorder patients. Journal of Personality Disorders 1:132–135, 1987

Kagan J, Reznick JS, Gibbons J: Inhibited and uninhibited types of children. Child Dev 60:838–845, 1989

Kagan J, Reznick JS, Snidman N, et al: Origins of panic disorder, in Neurobiology of Panic Disorder: Frontiers of Clinical Neuroscience. Edited by Ballenger JC. New York, Alan R Liss, 1990a, pp 71–87

Kagan J, Reznick JS, Snidman N: Biological basis of childhood shyness. Science 240:167–171, 1990b

Klein DF: Delineation of two drug-responsive anxiety syndromes. Psychopharmacology 5:397–408, 1964

Klein DF: Anxiety reconceptualized, in Anxiety: New Research and Changing Concepts. Edited by Klein DF, Rabkin JG. New York, Raven, 1981, pp 235–263

Klein DF: False suffocation alarms, spontaneous panics, and related conditions. Arch Gen Psychiatry 50:306–317, 1993

Klein DF, Fink M: Psychiatric reaction patterns to imipramine. Am J Psychiatry 119:432–438, 1962

Klerman GL: Depression and panic anxiety: the effect of depressive co-morbidity on response to drug treatment of patients with panic disorder and agoraphobia. J Psychiatr Res 24:27–41, 1990

Lesser IM, Rubin RT, Pecknold JC: Secondary depression in panic disorder and agoraphobia. Arch Gen Psychiatry 45:437–443, 1988

Maddock RJ, Blacker KH: Response to treatment in panic disorder with associated depression. Psychopathology 24:1–6, 1991

Mavissakalian M, Hamann MS: DSM-III personality disorder in agoraphobia. Compr Psychiatry 27:471–479, 1986

Mellman TA, Uhde TW: Obsessive-compulsive symptoms in panic disorder. Am J Psychiatry 144:1573–1576, 1987

Michelson L, Marchione K: Behavioral, cognitive and pharmacological treatments of panic disorder with agoraphobia: critique and synthesis. J Consult Clin Psychol 59:100–114, 1991

Muskin P, Fyer A: Treatment of panic disorder. J Clin Psychopharmacol 1 (suppl):81–90, 1981

Nagy LM, Krystal JH, Woods SW, et al: Clinical and medication outcome after short-term alprazolam and behavioral group treatment in panic disorder: 2.5 year naturalistic follow-up study. Arch Gen Psychiatry 46:993–999, 1989

Noyes R, Garvey MJ, Cook BL: Follow-up study of patients with panic disorder and agoraphobia with panic attacks treated with tricyclic antidepressants. J Affective Disord 16:249–257, 1989

Pollack MH, Otto MW, Rosenbaum JF, et al: Longitudinal course of panic disorder: finding from the MGH naturalistic study. J Clin Psychiatry 51 (suppl 12A):12–16, 1990

Pollack MH, Otto MW, Rosenbaum JF, et al: Personality disorders in patients with panic disorder: association with childhood anxiety disorders, early trauma comorbidity and chronicity. Compr Psychiatry 33:78–83, 1992

Reich J: DSM-III personality disorders and outcome of treated panic disorder. Am J Psychiatry 145:1149–1152, 1988

Reich JH, Green AI: Effect of personality disorders on outcome to treatment. J Nerv Ment Dis 179:74–82, 1991

Rosenbaum J, Biederman J, Gersten M, et al: Behavioral inhibition in children of parents with panic disorder and agoraphobia. Arch Gen Psychiatry 45:463–470, 1988

Rosenbaum JF, Biederman J, Hirshfeld MA: Further evidence of an association between behavioral inhibition and anxiety disorders: results from a family study of children from a non-clinical sample. J Psychiatr Res 25:49–65, 1991

Shalomskas DE, Barlow DH, Cohen J, et al: Drug/behavior treatment of panic: study design. Paper presented at the annual meeting of the American Psychiatric Association, New York, 1990

Sheehan D: One-year follow-up of patients with panic disorder and withdrawal from long-term antipanic medications. Paper presented at the Upjohn Panic Disorder Biological Research Workshop, Washington, DC, April 1986

Silove D: Perceived parental characteristics and reports of early parental deprivation in agoraphobic patients. Aust N Z J Psychiatry 20:365–369, 1986

Solyom L, Silberfeld M, Solyom C: Maternal overprotection in the etiology of agoraphobia. Canadian Psychiatric Association Journal 21:109–113, 1976

Suomi S: Genetic and maternal contributions to individual differences in rhesus monkeys: a biobehavioral perspective, in Perinatal Development: A Psychobiologic Perspective. Edited by Krasnegor NA, Blass EM, Hofer MA, et al. New York, Academic Press, 1987, pp 397–417

Suomi SJ: Early stress and adult emotional reactivity in rhesus monkeys, in Ciba Foundation Symposium: The Childhood Environment and Adult Disease. Edited by Bock GR, Whelan J. Chichester, England, Wiley, 1991, pp 171–188

Telch MJ, Brouillard M, Telch CF, et al: The role of cognitive appraisal in panic-related avoidance. Behav Res Ther 27:273–384, 1989

Chapter 18

Treatment of Panic Disorder: Consensus Statement

Panic disorder with and without agoraphobia is a debilitating condition that will afflict at least 1 out of every 75 people in this country and worldwide during their lifetime. Panic attacks are characterized by sudden and unexpected discrete periods of intense fear or discomfort associated with shortness of breath, dizziness, palpitations, nausea, or abdominal distress. During an attack people often believe that they are having a heart attack or, alternately, that they are losing their mind. Panic sufferers often develop agoraphobia secondary to the occurrence of these unexpected panic attacks. Consequently, they begin to avoid places where they fear a panic attack may occur or where help would be difficult to obtain. If the agoraphobia becomes severe enough, a person may become housebound.

A growing body of knowledge indicates that some medications and selected psychosocial treatments are effective for panic disorder with and without agoraphobic avoidance. Two classes of antidepressants (i.e., tricyclics and monoamine oxidase inhibitors) as well as certain high-potency benzodiazepines (e.g., alprazolam, lorazepam, and clonazepam) have been found to be effective in reducing or eliminating panic attacks associated with the various forms of panic disorder. Substantial research efforts continue the search for other medications useful in the treatment of these conditions. Initial indications are that some of these other agents, particularly the serotonin uptake blockers, may be effective panic medications. The pharmacological agents may present problems such as undesirable side effects, the risk of dependence, and a significant relapse rate once medication is discontinued.

Several variations and combinations of behavior and cognitive treatment approaches also have demonstrated efficacy in the reduction and/or elimination of panic attacks and agoraphobia. Early reports of research specifically targeting panic attacks indicate that significant numbers of patients are panic-free at the end

This chapter was originally published as *Panic: Consensus Statement*. NIH Consensus Development Conference, September 25–27, 1991. Volume 9, Number 2.

of cognitive-behavior treatment and remain so at a 2-year follow-up.

Information is sparse on such issues as 1) the effectiveness of combined psychosocial and pharmacological treatments, 2) the mechanisms of therapeutic action, 3) demographic and other patient factors that may predict responsiveness to either class of treatment, 4) the long-term effectiveness of treatments for panic disorder once treatment stops, and 5) the value of these treatments for those patients who suffer from panic disorder in combination with other psychological and psychiatric disorders. The latter group represents a significant segment of those people suffering from panic disorder.

To help resolve questions surrounding these and other issues, the Office of Medical Applications of Research of the National Institutes of Health in conjunction with the National Institute of Mental Health convened a Consensus Development Conference on the Treatment of Panic Disorder on September 25–27, 1991. Following a day and a half of presentations by experts in the relevant fields and discussion from the audience, a consensus panel comprising experts in psychology, psychiatry, cardiology, internal medicine, and methodology, as well as members of the general public, considered the scientific evidence and formulated a consensus statement that addressed the following five questions:

■ What are the epidemiology, natural history, and course of panic disorder with and without agoraphobia? How is it diagnosed?
■ What are the current treatments? What are the short-term and long-term effects of acute and extended treatment of this disorder?
■ What are the short-term and long-term adverse effects of these treatments? How should they be managed?
■ What are considerations for treatment planning?
■ What are the significant questions for future research?

What Are the Epidemiology, Natural History, and Course of Panic Disorder With and Without Agoraphobia? How Is It Diagnosed?

What Is Panic Disorder?

Beginning in the 1960s, investigators and clinicians began to differentiate patients who had unexpected anxiety attacks from patients with other anxiety disorders. The diagnostic category of panic disorder was first officially recognized with the publication of the *Diagnostic and Statistical Manual of Mental Disorders* (Third Edition) of the American Psychiatric Association in 1980 (DSM-III). These criteria were modified slightly with the 1987 publication of the revised version of the diagnostic manual, DSM-III-R.

Fundamental to the diagnosis of panic disorder is the occurrence of panic attacks. These attacks consist of discrete periods of intense fear or discomfort in which at least four of the symptoms noted below develop abruptly and reach a crescendo within 10 minutes, typically lasting 10 minutes or so. Attacks may recur repeatedly and rapidly; however, once these symptoms abate, severe anxiety may last for many hours. The symptoms include

∎ Shortness of breath (or smothering sensations)
∎ Dizziness, unsteady feelings, or faintness
∎ Palpitations or accelerated heart rate (tachycardia)
∎ Trembling or shaking
∎ Sweating
∎ Choking
∎ Nausea or abdominal distress
∎ Depersonalization or derealization
∎ Numbness or tingling sensations (paresthesias)
∎ Flushes (hot flashes) or chills
∎ Chest pain or discomfort
∎ Fear of dying
∎ Fear of going crazy or doing something
  uncontrolled

Panic attacks may occur as rare isolated incidents that cause little or no sustained impact on the individual's functioning or as clusters of attacks with adverse effects. They also occur during sleep.

To satisfy the diagnostic criteria for panic disorder, at least some of the panic attacks must occur unexpectedly or spontaneously, that is, in the absence of specific environmental or situational triggers such as elevators, public speaking, snakes, closed spaces, or other situations that evoke fearful avoidance in some people. Further, the diagnostic criteria require either a clustering of at least four attacks spread over a 4-week period or one or more attacks followed by at least 1 month of fearful anticipation of experiencing more such attacks.

Although research is under way to test and refine these criteria, there is a broad consensus that panic disorder, as currently defined, is a distinct condition with a specific presentation, course, positive family history, complications, and response to treatment.

Panic disorder must be differentiated from other disorders that may share similar clinical features. At this time, diagnosis is dependent on a detailed clinical assessment of the presenting complaints and history because there are no specific laboratory tests. A medical workup is recommended to rule out other conditions. At the same time, the risk of misdiagnosis leading to costly medical investigations and delays in treatment for panic disorder must also be guarded against.

Currently, two main subtypes of panic disorder are widely recognized and codified in DSM-III-R. These subtypes vary in the severity and extensiveness of phobic avoidance: panic disorder without agoraphobia and panic disorder with agoraphobia. In cases of panic disorder with agoraphobia, there is avoidance of places or situations from which escape might be difficult or embarrassing or in which help might not be available in the event of a panic attack. The degree of avoidance may vary from mild to moderate or, at the extreme, to a constricted life-style imposed by severe avoidance, resulting in the individual's being nearly or completely housebound or otherwise severely dysfunctional.

Investigators are seeking to develop additional ways of subtyping panic disorder based on the phenomenology, age at onset, response to treatment, and so on, that may have implications for etiology, diagnosis, and treatment.

Differential Diagnosis: Separating Panic Disorders From Other Disorders

There are many other disorders in which panic attacks may occur. The more common are simple phobia (in which the panic occurs immediately before or upon exposure to the feared situation and nowhere else) and social phobias (in which they occur only when individuals feel they are the focus of others' attention [e.g., while eating]). Other disorders that should be considered in differential diagnosis include claustrophobia, severe depression, dissociative disorders, generalized anxiety without panic, alcohol or drug withdrawal, stimulant abuse (caffeine, cocaine, amphetamines), and physical disorders such as cardiac, adrenal, vestibular, thyroid, or seizure disorders.

Epidemiology and Course

Panic disorder is relatively common; similar rates have been found in many countries in international studies. Approximately one-third of the individuals with panic disorder also have agoraphobia, although in clinical settings, the majority present with some agoraphobia. Panic disorder with agoraphobia is diagnosed about twice as frequently in females as in males.

The most common age at onset is middle teens and early adulthood; however, panic disorder may onset at any time. A common pattern of onset is the occurrence of occasional unexpected panic attacks that then increase in frequency and are associated with mounting fears of having subsequent attacks. Over time there is often a pattern of spreading fearful avoidance.

Little is known about the long-term course of this disorder. The limited findings to date suggest that in most cases it is a chronic disorder that waxes and wanes in severity. However, some people may have a limited period of dysfunction that never recurs, while others may experience a severe chronic form of the disorder. Those with agoraphobia tend to have a more severe and complicated course. Treatment early in the development of this disorder may shorten the duration and may prevent complications, including agoraphobia and depression.

Comorbidity: Associated Disorders

Certain conditions have been found to be associated with panic disorder, particularly in those individuals with long-standing panic attacks and agoraphobia. These conditions include abuse of alcohol and drugs, depression, and other anxiety and personality disorders. Other medical disorders that occur more commonly in patients with panic disorder may include atypical chest pain, irritable bowel syndrome, asthma, and migraine.

What Are the Current Treatments? What Are the Short-Term and Long-Term Effects of Acute and Extended Treatment of This Disorder?

Panic disorder is a treatable condition. The effectiveness of treatment should be evaluated on a number of dimensions: 1) acceptance and tolerance by patients; 2) reduction or elimination of panic attacks, reduction of clinically significant anxiety and disability secondary to phobic avoidance, amelioration of other common comorbid conditions such as depression; and 3) long-term prevention of relapse.

Several different classes of treatment have been shown to be clinically effective, including cognitive and behavior, pharmacological, and combinations of the two. The most commonly used behavior approach is graduated exposure, aimed primarily at reducing phobic avoidance and anticipatory anxiety. Cognitive-behavior approaches, developed more recently, also treat panic attacks directly.

These treatments involve cognitive restructuring, that is, changing of maladaptive thought processes, and are generally used in combination with a variety of behavior techniques, including breathing retraining and activities that target exposure to bodily sensations and external phobic situations. Ongoing assignments to practice the techniques are made by the therapist. These treatments seem to be well accepted by patients and typically involve weekly sessions for 8 to 12 weeks. Initial improvement is noted in many patients within 3 to 6 weeks of beginning treatment. Among the various psychotherapeutic approaches, combined treatments that include cognitive therapy in addition to other techniques appear to be most effective, especially in reducing panic attacks. Longer term follow-up of these interventions suggests a low relapse rate.

Pharmacological treatments include tricyclic antidepressants, monoamine oxidase inhibitors (MAOIs), and high-potency benzodiazepines. A significant proportion of patients do not easily tolerate certain of the tricyclics, whereas benzodiazepines are better accepted. Patients who tolerate tricyclics show significant improvement, with a reduced number of panic attacks during the period of treatment, ranging from 8 to 32 weeks in controlled trials. Benzodiazepines have a rapid onset of action with immediate reduction of panic symptoms, whereas antidepressants require 3 to 6 weeks to achieve therapeutic effect. In addition, the action of benzodiazepines in reducing anxiety between attacks is thought advantageous by some clinicians. Careful titration of medication to effective therapeutic doses with gradual increase in dosage is necessary. Very gradual increases may be particularly important with tricyclics in order to reduce attrition. Longer term duration of treatment probably increases clinical response. Gradual tapering of all medications when treatment ends is strongly indicated. The relapse rate following termination of medication for antidepressants is moderate but is probably higher for benzodiazepines. The relatively high response rate to the control conditions (placebo) needs further examination.

Few studies have examined combined behavior and pharmacological methods. There is some evidence that a combination of tricyclics and exposure therapy may have additive effects in the short term, but there is no evidence for long-term advantage over either method alone. Currently, there are few published studies available that assess the combined effect of cognitive and pharmacological intervention, nor has the optimal sequence of combined methods been examined satisfactorily. Whether using a combination of two effective methods improves upon the effectiveness of either alone or is less effective than either alone is not a settled issue. There are no controlled data on efficacy of treatment for panic disorder or other widely used approaches, such as psychodynamic psychotherapy.

What Are the Short-Term and Long-Term Adverse Effects of These Treatments? How Should They Be Managed?

Adverse effects can be classified in a number of categories, including drug-related disturbances and other physical effects, adverse psychological and behavioral side effects, rebound effects (i.e., worsening of the disorder when treatment is removed), and misplaced confidence in unproven treatments that may preclude other treatments with a better chance of effectiveness.

The adverse effects discussed in this section are based on clinical research studies of panic disorder. It is unclear how and on what dimensions research patients may differ from the general clinical population; thus, the research samples may not be representative of the group of patients that present for treatment in a nonresearch, clinical setting.

In programs offering pharmacotherapy, individuals are not admitted to studies if they have preexisting medical conditions (including pregnancy) that would contraindicate the use of the medications under study. In both pharmacotherapy and cognitive-behavior studies, individuals are typically referred elsewhere if the individual meets criteria for substance abuse.

Cognitive and Behavior Treatments

Cognitive and behavior treatments are ordinarily well tolerated when applied by skilled therapists. Dropout rates in controlled studies range from 5% to 8% in the cognitive-behavior therapies and between 12% and 16% in the relaxation and in vivo exposure-based treatments. Therapies that include cognitive techniques may also address accompanying depression. Although very few adverse effects of these treatments have been reported, there have been some instances of panic attacks induced by relaxation. This can be counteracted by a more gradual approach to relaxation and teaching the patient techniques for controlling the relaxation procedure. No other adverse effects have been reported.

Other Psychotherapies

In the absence of any empirical studies examining the effectiveness of treatments other than cognitive and behavior therapies, no conclusions can be drawn about adverse effects. However, given that recent research results have identified useful pharmacotherapy and psychotherapy approaches, one risk of maintaining individuals in nonvalidated treatments of panic disorder is that misplaced confidence in the therapy's potential effectiveness may preclude application of more effective treatment. This can be particularly problematic with psychotherapy treatments if the nature of the therapeutic relationship makes it difficult for the patient to seek additional or alternate treatment. Psychotherapies without demonstrated effectiveness in panic, such as psychodynamic psychotherapy, however, may be helpful for other difficulties that the patient presents. Thus, when progress in the reduction of panic disorder is not apparent within 6 to 8 weeks, ancillary pharmacotherapy or cognitive-behavior treatment or a brief break in psychotherapy for these treatments should be considered.

Pharmacological Treatments

With three effective classes of pharmacological agents now available in the treatment of panic disorder, risks and benefits of each need to be considered.

Tricyclic antidepressants offer the benefit of once-a-day dosing, a low risk of dependence, and no dietary restrictions. They also have a concomitant antidepressant effect that is frequently helpful. Adverse effects include anticholinergic side effects, low blood pressure, overstimulation, and weight gain. Taken together, these effects may cause up to 35% of patients to discontinue treatment before therapeutic benefits occur.

The benefits of MAOIs include, as with the tricyclics, an antidepressant effect and a low risk of dependence. However, the anticholinergic effects may be lower than for the tricyclics. Sexual difficulties, particularly problems in orgasm, may occur as do hypotension and weight gain. One added complication that may be difficult for some patients is the need to follow a low-tyramine diet.

One benefit of the benzodiazepines, because they have a rapid onset of action, is that they can be used to treat surges of anticipatory anxiety or panic. This "as needed" use of benzodiazepines should not replace the use of sufficient daily doses when that is indicated. Risks include sedation and psychomotor impairment. Benzodiazepines will interact with alcohol if its intake is not restricted. Although some of these adverse side effects largely subside after 4 to 6 weeks of treatment, subjective cloudiness may remain. The most serious risk with this class of medication is that of physical dependence. Withdrawal symptoms or a recurrence of panic symptoms during drug tapering is a definite risk with long-term treatment.

The attrition rate in pharmacological studies varies with the drug under investigation. It is approximately 25% for the tricyclics, slightly lower for the MAOIs, and approximately 15% for the high-potency benzodiazepines. Many of these dropouts appear directly related to the drug side effects. With imipramine, starting with a low dose and building up slowly may significantly reduce the risk of premature treatment termination. Similarly, the potential excessive use of benzodiazepines requires caution in their use in individuals who have a history or risk of drug dependence. Care must be exercised in prescribing the tricyclic and the MAOI medications for individuals with cardiovascular disease; if acute relief is needed in such patients, high-potency benzodiazepines are the treatment of choice.

What Are Considerations for Treatment Planning?

The practicing clinician does not usually see panic disorder in its pure form. Further, because there are a number of different treatment strategies with similar treatment efficacy in the acute phase, the central question becomes not What is the treatment of choice? but, What factors need to be considered in choosing optimum treatment? Decisions need to be made regarding choice of single modality, concurrent, or sequential interventions.

Primary care physicians or other clinicians who identify patients with panic disorder will need to address the issue of potential referral for treatments specific to panic disorder with or without agoraphobia.

The factors that need to be considered by any clinician include degree of urgency, comorbid conditions, history, and patient fit and compliance issues.

Each of these groups of factors will be examined independently both in terms of the assessment data required and their implications for strategic interventions.

Degree of Urgency

There are emergency cases, such as medical complications secondary to the phobic fears (e.g., fear of swallowing leading to dehydration and weight loss), imminent loss of job or relationship, inability to undergo necessary medical procedures, children's welfare at risk, or acute and rapid generalization of phobic behavior. In such cases, mobilization of family resources or high-potency benzodiazepines may be the starting point for treatment once the patient has received basic educational information. This may be accompanied by cognitive-behavior treatment, alternative medications, and other follow-up care. The patient's own subjective sense of urgency may or may not indicate a need for urgent intervention. A panic attack in and of itself is not an emergency. Common obsessive fears of losing control need to be carefully distinguished from actual imminent loss of control.

History

The history of the patient and his or her family will yield critical information for treatment planning. Is this the first episode or one in a lifetime series? Has the patient ever received the diagnosis before? What treatments have been tried in the past, and were they successful in some or any measure? Is there a family history of psychiatric disorder or substance abuse? Did the patient or the family engage in or respond to any treatment? Were there recent events that may have triggered the current onset of symptoms, such as surgery, illness, childbirth, miscarriage, trauma, loss, or external stressors? Are there any known developmental vulnerabilities such as a history of abuse or a dysfunctional family? The need for and advisability of including family or significant others in the educational and treatment process should be assessed.

Comorbid Conditions

There are three kinds of medical conditions that may affect treatment planning and may need to be treated concurrently. These are 1) conditions that may affect the safety or efficacy of psychopharmacological treatments (such as some specific cardiovascular, pulmonary, gastrointestinal, or endocrine disorders; pregnancy; or lactation); 2) conditions with a prominent component of anxiety (such as thyroid disease, polycythemia, lupus, and pulmonary insufficiency); and 3) conditions requiring treatment with medications such as vasoconstrictors, bronchodilators, or steroids, which may cause or exacerbate anxiety.

The necessity for a complete psychological assessment in addition to the medical workup cannot be overemphasized. Up to 70% of patients with panic disorder may have a comorbid psychological or psychiatric condition that will need to be included in the treatment planning, and perhaps be addressed therapeutically concomitantly or at a later point. A high percentage are depressed or demoralized secondary to suffering panic attacks but should be treated for panic first. Other conditions such as major depression, posttraumatic stress disorder, bipolar mood disorder, dissociative disorders, other anxiety disorders such as obsessive-compulsive disorder or social phobia, eating disorders, or complex personality disorders may require concurrent treatment.

Finally, individuals need to be assessed explicitly regarding substance abuse, including alcohol, marijuana, opiates, hallucinogens, cocaine, over-the-counter drugs such as nasal sprays and diet pills, caffeine, or benzodiazepines. Patients in current withdrawal or active abuse must be treated for substance abuse before or concurrent with specific panic disorder treatment.

Patient Fit and Compliance Issues

The clinician, in consultation with the patient, should select one of the treatments with demonstrated efficacy or a combination as the initial treatment. Selection should be based on patient preference in the context of a comprehensive assessment of urgency, history, and comorbidity. It may be the case that the selected treatment will require referral, consultation, or supervision.

The individual with panic disorder needs to be an active, fully informed participant in the treatment planning process. Education and demystification are frequently needed. This means advising the patient not only of the short-term benefits and risks but also of long-term benefits and risks where known and addressing the issue of long-term relapse prevention. The patient's initial degree of relief and motivation following education may give direction to the next step. Attitudes and concerns regarding various treatment options must be explored and negotiated. The patient's request in presenting for treatment must be kept in mind. Answering questions such as "Why me?" or "Why now?" or "What is this about?" may establish a better foundation for treatment.

Patients should be given education about the disorder and encouragement to re-enter phobic situations gradually when medication alone is chosen as the initial treatment. Current research suggests that an absence of any noticeable improvement after about 6 to 8 weeks of any treatment should suggest a reassessment, consultation, or change of modality.

Particularly for those patients for whom there has been a chronic course or a history of multiple episodes of acute symptomatology, recovery, and relapse, longer term strategies need to be considered following the acute phase of treatment. Unfortunately, at this time, little is known regarding the relative long-term efficacy of maintenance doses of medication, other psychotherapies, changes in life-style aimed at stress reduction, or participation in ongoing self-help groups. These current practices have been shown to be of value in other disorders and may in the future be shown to be so in panic disorder as well. As with many other treatable disorders, access to effective care is at times limited by regulatory decisions, lack of financial resources, inadequate third-party coverage, and stigma.

What Are the Significant Questions for Future Research?

As would be expected in a relatively new field, many research questions remain, and each new finding is likely to stimulate further questions. Among the most important questions are the following.

Identifying Those at Risk

Although onset is known to be most frequent in adolescence and young adulthood, little is known about who is more likely to have an isolated attack, and, of those persons, who will go on to develop the full disorder, and what sequence of events may influence this. In this area, promising leads to follow are the investigation of temperament and personality, family and genetic patterns, developmental growth characteristics, and other biological, psychological, and environmental factors. Thus, both high-risk studies (e.g., children of high-risk families) and population studies are needed to answer these questions.

Course of Disorder

Much of the information currently available is derived from cross-sectional studies and from short-term follow-up. Also needed are long-term prospective studies that track episodes and the context in which they occur over time, assessment of the development of comorbid conditions, treatment-seeking behavior, medical care utilization, and costs with and without treatment for panic disorder, as well as changes in functioning and the quality of life.

Methodological Studies

Currently, different measures, often idiosyncratic and some of undocumented quality, make comparison of subjects and results across studies difficult. More reliable, valid measures of all clinical features of panic disorder must be developed and standardized for general use. Similarly, there is a need for standardized methodologies for measuring all facets of outcome, including operational definitions of response, remission, recovery, and relapse.

Although field studies of diagnostic boundaries and criteria are ongoing, further research is required on the clinical definition of panic disorder, including the validity of the diagnostic criteria and possible subtyping or variations of the disorder, which may have different natural histories or responses to treatment. Sensitive screening diagnostic instruments will be needed for population and genetic studies, prevention programs, and general clinical use.

Treatment Research

It is essential that recruitment strategies, success rates, and inclusion and exclusion criteria be very carefully and fully documented in each clinical research study.

Current information does not permit satisfactory comparison of the effectiveness and value of cognitive-behavior and pharmacological treatments. Not only are multisite studies and comparable control groups needed, but cross-disciplinary studies within sites will facilitate interprofessional exchange of knowledge and skills. Multisite studies should be done in which psychosocial and pharmacological therapies are compared with each other and with combinations of the two. Further research is needed on optimal duration of treatment and on strategies to maintain treatment response. Studies are also needed to ascertain the type and extent of training of clinicians necessary for effective intervention. Studies are needed to assess patient match with treatment methods, including the sequencing of treatments.

Patients who drop out of clinical trials should be carefully followed. Some clinical drug trials also have revealed a high placebo response, suggesting that there are nonspecific, psychosocial, unsystematic exposure instructions or other unspecified factors that may have a potential influence on therapeutic outcomes.

Finally, new emphasis should be placed on prevention research programs for individuals at risk.

Basic Research

Current evidence supports familial prevalence, but there is only preliminary evidence for genetic transmission. Larger studies are needed to separate the genetic from the environmental contribution and to identify the most salient milieu influences (life events, family functioning, etc.). In such studies, there should be a focus on identification of which diagnostic criteria are most likely to identify a genetic form of the disorder. Segregation studies should be done to determine likely patterns of transmission and to obtain estimates of genetic parameters necessary for the successful analysis of linkage studies.

Further basic studies of the biological and psychological underpinnings, as well as the influence of environmental factors, associated with the disorder are needed to understand its nature. Neurobiological studies, including molecular approaches, and experimental studies of basic cognitive and behavior processes will yield information and contribute to more effective treatment.

Conclusions and Recommendations

❚ Panic disorder is a distinct condition with a specific presentation, course, and positive family history and for which there are effective pharmacological and cognitive-behavior treatments.

■ Treatment that fails to produce benefit within 6 to 8 weeks should be reassessed.
■ Patients with panic disorder often have one or more comorbid conditions that require careful assessment and treatment.
■ The most critical research needs are
  ■ The development of reliable, valid, and standard measures of assessment and outcome;
  ■ The identification of optimal choices and structuring of treatments designed to meet the varying individual needs of patients; and
  ■ The implementation of basic research to define the nature of the disorder.
■ Barriers to treatment include awareness, accessibility, and affordability.
■ An aggressive educational campaign to increase awareness of these issues should be mounted for clinicians, patients and their families, the media, and the general public.

Consensus Development Panel

Layton McCurdy, M.D.
Panel and Conference Chairperson, Vice President for Medical Affairs;
Dean, Medical University of South Carolina, Charleston, South Carolina

Frank A. DeLeon-Jones, M.D.
Professor of Psychiatry, University of California at Los Angeles,
Olive View Medical Center, Los Angeles, California

Susan Dime-Meenan
Executive Director, National Depressive and Manic Depressive Association,
Chicago, Illinois

Jean Endicott, Ph.D.
Chief, Department of Research Assessment and Training,
New York State Psychiatric Institute, New York, New York

Raquel E. Gur, M.D., Ph.D.
Professor of Psychiatry and Neurology, Department of Psychiatry,
University of Pennsylvania, Philadelphia, Pennsylvania

Helena Chmura Kraemer, Ph.D.
Professor of Biostatistics in Psychiatry, Department of Psychiatry
and Behavioral Sciences, Stanford University, Stanford, California

Marsha M. Linehan, Ph.D.
Professor of Psychology, Psychology Department, University of Washington, Seattle, Washington

Carl I. Margolis, M.D.
Internal Medicine/Psychiatry Private Practice, Rockville, Maryland

Charles R. Marmar, M.D.
Associate Professor of Psychiatry, University of California at San Francisco; Director, Post-Traumatic Stress Disorder Program, San Francisco Veterans Administration Medical Center, San Francisco, California

Susan Mineka, Ph.D.
Professor of Psychology, Department of Psychology, Northwestern University, Evanston, Illinois

Jeanne S. Phillips, Ph.D.
Professor of Psychology, Department of Psychology, University of Denver, Denver, Colorado

Ray H. Rosenman, M.D.
Director of Cardiovascular Research (Ret.), SRI International, Menlo Park; Associate Chief of Medicine, Mt. Zion Hospital and Medical Center, San Francisco, California

Peter C. Whybrow, M.D.
Professor and Chairman, Department of Psychiatry, University of Pennsylvania School of Medicine, Philadelphia, Pennsylvania

Sally M. Winston, Psy.D.
Director, Anxiety Disorders Program, Sheppard and Enoch Pratt Hospital, Baltimore, Maryland

Speakers

James C. Ballenger, M.D.
"Acute Pharmacological Treatment of Panic Disorder: Standard Medications"

David H. Barlow, Ph.D.
"Behavioral Treatment of Panic Disorder"

Dianne L. Chambless, Ph.D.
"Discussion of Psychotherapy Treatments"

David M. Clark, D.Phil.
"Cognitive Therapy for Panic Disorder"

Allen Frances, M.D.
"Psychodynamic Treatment of Panic Disorders"

Jack M. Gorman, M.D.
"New and Experimental Pharmacological Treatments for Panic Disorder"

George R. Heninger, M.D.
"Mechanism of Action in the Pharmacotherapy of Panic Disorder"

Wayne Katon, M.D.
"Primary Care Panic Disorder Management Model"

Heinz Katschnig, M.D.
"The Long-Term Course of Panic Disorder"

Gerald L. Klerman, M.D.[1]
"A Critique of the Research Literature on Combined Treatment of Panic Disorder Discussion"

Michael R. Liebowitz, M.D.
"Diagnosis and Clinical Course of Panic Disorder With and Without Agoraphobia"

Larry K. Michelson, Ph.D.
"Risk-Benefit Issues in Psychosocial Treatment of Panic Disorders"

S. Rachman, Ph.D.
"Mechanisms of Action in Psychosocial Treatments of Panic Disorder"

Karl M. Rickels, M.D.
"Risk-Benefit Issues in Pharmacological Treatment of Panic Disorders"

M. Katherine Shear, M.D.
"The Future"

---

[1] Deceased.

Michael J. Telch, Ph.D.
"A Critique of the Research Literature on Combined Treatment of Panic Disorder"

Thomas W. Uhde, M.D.
"Discussion of Pharmacotherapy"

Myrna M. Weissman, Ph.D.
"The Epidemiology and Genetics of Panic Disorder"

Planning Committee

Robert M. A. Hirschfeld, M.D.
Planning Committee Chairperson; Chairman, Department of Psychiatry and
Behavioral Science, University of Texas Medical Branch at Galveston, Galveston,
Texas

James C. Ballenger, M.D.
Professor and Chairman, Department of Psychiatry and Behavioral Sciences;
Director, Institute of Psychiatry, Medical University of South Carolina,
Charleston, South Carolina

David H. Barlow, Ph.D.
Distinguished Professor of Psychology, University at Albany, State University
of New York, Albany, New York

Lynn Cave
Information Office, National Institute of Mental Health, Alcohol, Drug Abuse,
and Mental Health Administration, Rockville, Maryland

Marsha Corbett
Director, Office of Scientific Information, National Institute of Mental Health,
Alcohol, Drug Abuse, and Mental Health Administration, Rockville, Maryland

Jerry M. Elliott
Program Analyst, Office of Medical Applications of Research, National Institutes
of Health, Bethesda, Maryland

Paul Emmelkamp, Ph.D.
Professor of Clinical Psychology and Psychotherapy, Academic Hospital,
Department of Clinical Psychology, Groningen, The Netherlands

John H. Ferguson, M.D.
Director, Office of Medical Applications of Research, National Institutes
of Health, Bethesda, Maryland

William H. Hall
Director of Communications, Office of Medical Applications of Research,
National Institutes of Health, Bethesda, Maryland

Lewis L. Judd, M.D.
Professor and Chairman, Department of Psychiatry, School of Medicine,
University of California at San Diego, La Jolla, California

Martin B. Keller, M.D.
Professor and Chairman, Department of Psychiatry and Human Behavior,
Brown University, Butler Hospital, Providence, Rhode Island

Donald F. Klein, M.D.
State University of New York, College of Medicine at New York City;
Director of Psychiatric Research, New York State Psychiatric Institute; Professor
of Psychiatry, College of Physicians and Surgeons of Columbia University, New
York, New York

Gerald L. Klerman, M.D.[2]
Professor of Psychiatry, Associate Chairman for Research, Cornell University
Medical College, Payne Whitney Clinic, New York, New York

Jack D. Maser, Ph.D.
Chief, Anxiety and Somatoform Disorders Program, Division of Clinical and
Treatment Research, National Institute of Mental Health, National Institutes
of Health, Rockville, Maryland

S. Rachman, Ph.D.
Professor, Psychology Department, University of British Columbia, Vancouver,
British Columbia, Canada

Darrel A. Regier, M.D., M.P.H.
Director, Division of Epidemiology and Services Research, National Institute
of Mental Health, National Institutes of Health, Rockville, Maryland

---

[2] Deceased.

Morton Reiser, M.D.
School of Medicine, Yale University, New Haven, Connecticut

Thomas W. Uhde, M.D.
Chief, Section on Anxiety and Affective Disorders, Biological Psychiatry Branch, Intramural Research Program, National Institute of Mental Health, National Institutes of Health, Rockville, Maryland

Barry E. Wolfe, Ph.D.
Chief, Psychosocial Treatment Research Program, Division of Clinical and Treatment Research, National Institute of Mental Health, National Institutes of Health, Rockville, Maryland

Conference Sponsors

National Institute of Mental Health
Alan Leshner, Ph.D., Acting Director

Office of Medical Applications of
Research, National Institutes of Health
John H. Ferguson, M.D., Director

Bibliography

January 1985 through July 1991
1,448 Citations

Prepared by
Karen Patrias, M.L.S.,
National Library of Medicine
Barry E. Wolfe, Ph.D.,
National Institute of Mental Health

P anic disorder in all of its various manifestations (e.g., with and without agoraphobia) is increasingly recognized as a serious and prevalent mental disorder. It has been estimated that over 3 million people in the United States may suffer from some form of panic disorder in the course of a lifetime. Because panic disorder is so often mistaken for a large number of physical and emotional disorders, it has become a significant public health issue that demands the development of procedures for accurate diagnosis and effective treatment.

Emergency room and primary care physicians, in particular, are in need of the best information available regarding the diagnosis and treatment of panic disorder, because they are usually the first to see such patients who believe themselves to be suffering from some cardiovascular crisis. Data are now available on the diagnosis and treatment of panic disorder, but controversy exists about the interpretation of these data and their implications for patient management.

This bibliography was prepared in support of the National Institutes of Health Consensus Development Conference titled "Treatment of Panic Disorder," which was held in Bethesda, Maryland on September 25–27, 1991. The citations cover various aspects of panic disorder, including its epidemiology, etiology, and diagnosis and classification, and its psychological and pharmacological methods of treatments as well as their mechanisms of action. The bibliography relies primarily

Originally published as *Treatment of Panic Disorder With and Without Agoraphobia* (Current Bibliographies in Medicine Publication Number CBM 91-8). Prepared by Patrias K, Wolfe BE. Rockville, MD, U.S. National Institutes of Health, 1991.

on journal articles, conference proceedings, and books and book chapters. Only English;language materials have been included. There are a few case reports to illustrate various approaches to the treatment of panic disorder with and without agoraphobia. Letters and abstracts have been excluded. Finally, there is a special section on studies of agoraphobia that do not specifically discuss panic disorder. With the exception of the pharmacological treatment section, a citation appears under only one category.

Search Strategy

A variety of online data bases are usually searched in preparing bibliographies in the Current Bibliographies in Medicine series. To assist you in updating or otherwise manipulating the material in this search, the strategy used for the National Library of Medicine's (NLM's) MEDLINE data base is given below. Please note that the search strategies presented here differ from individual demand searches in that they are generally broadly formulated and irrelevant citations are edited out prior to printing.

SS 1 = *PANIC OR PANIC (TF) OR PANIC/DRUG EFFECTS OR
        *AGORAPHOBIA
SS 2 = (TW) PANIC
SS 3 = TS (AB) :PANIC DISORDER:
SS 4 = ANXIETY DISORDERS OR PHOBIC DISORDERS OR MENTAL
        DISORDERS OR AGORAPHOBIA
SS 5 = 2 AND EXP TRANQUILIZING AGENTS
SS 6 = 2 AND EXP ANTIDEPRESSIVE AGENTS
SS 7 = 2 AND EXP MONOAMINE OXIDASE INHIBITORS
SS 8 = 2 AND EXP F4
SS 9 = EXP CLINICAL TRIALS OR COMBINED MODALITY
        THERAPY OR COMORBIDITY
SS10 = (TW) ACUTE AND PANIC AND INVENTORY
SS11 = 2 AND 4 OR 2 AND 9
SS12 = 1 OR 3 OR 5 OR 6 OR 7 OR 8 OR 10 OR 11
SS13 = 12 AND NOT LETTER (TF)
SS14 = 13 AND NOT FOR (LA)

Grateful Med

To make online searching easier and more efficient, the Library offers GRATEFUL MED, microcomputer-based software that provides a user-friendly interface to most NLM data bases. This software was specifically developed for health professionals and features multiple-choice menus and "fill in the blank" screens for easy search preparation. GRATEFUL MED runs on an IBM (or IBM-compatible) personal computer with DOS 2.0 or on a Macintosh personal computer, and requires a Hayes (or Hayes-compatible) modem, which may be purchased from the National Technical Information Service in Springfield, Virginia, for $29.95 (plus $3.00 per order for shipping).

Sample Citations

Citations in this bibliographic series are formatted according to the rules established for *Index Medicus®*. Sample journal and monograph citations appear below. For journal articles written in a foreign language, the English translation of the title is placed in brackets; for monographs, the title is given in the original language. In both cases the language of publication is shown by a three letter abbreviation appearing at the end of the citation. Note also that a colon (:) may appear within an author's name or article title. The NLM computer system automatically inserts this symbol in the place of a diacritical mark.

Journal Article:

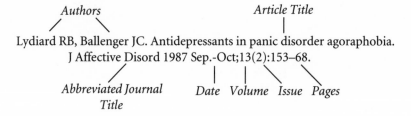

Monograph:

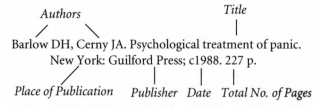

Contents

Diagnosis and Classification

Albus M, Maier W, Shera D, Bech P. Consistencies and discrepancies in self- and observer-rated anxiety scales. A comparison between the self- and observer-rated Marks-Sheehan scales. Eur Arch Psychiatry Clin Neurosci 1990;240(2):96–102.

Alnaes R, Torgersen S. DSM-III personality disorders among patients with major depression, anxiety disorders, and mixed conditions. J Nerv Ment Dis 1990 Nov;178(11):693–8.

Alnaes R, Torgersen S. Major depression in combination with panic and non-panic anxiety: Childhood memories and precipitating events. J Anxiety Disord 1990;4(3):191–9.

Alnaes R, Torgersen S. MCMI personality disorders among patients with major depression with and without anxiety disorders. J Pers Disord 1990;4(2):141–9.

Anastasiades P, Clark DM, Salkovskis PM, Middleton H, Hackman A, Gelder MG, Johnston DW. Psychophysiological responses in panic and stress. J Psychophysiology 1990;4(4):331–8.

Argyle N, Deltito J, Allerup P, Maier W, Albus M, Nutzinger D, Rasmussen S, Ayuso JL, Bech P. The Panic-Associated Symptom Scale: measuring the severity of panic disorder. Acta Psychiatr Scand 1991 Jan;83(1):20–6.

Argyle N, Roth M. The definition of panic attacks, Part I. Psychiatr Dev 1989 Autumn;7(3):175–86.

Argyle N, Roth M. The phenomenological study of 90 patients with panic disorder, Part II. Psychiatr Dev 1989 Autumn;7(3):187–209.

Aronson TA. A follow-up of two panic disorder-agoraphobic study populations. The role of recruitment biases. J Nerv Ment Dis 1987 Oct;175(10):595–8.

Aronson TA. Is panic disorder a distinct diagnostic entity? A critical review of the borders of a syndrome. J Nerv Ment Dis 1987 Oct;175(10):584–94.

Aronson TA, Carasiti I, McBane D, Whitaker-Azmitia P. Biological correlates of lactate sensitivity in panic disorder. Biol Psychiatry 1989 Sep;26(5):463–77.

Aronson TA, Logue CM. Phenomenology of panic attacks: a descriptive study of panic disorder patients' self-reports. J Clin Psychiatry 1988 Jan;49(1):8–13.

Austin LS, Lydiard RB, Fossey MD, Zealberg JJ, Laraia MT, Ballenger JC. Panic and phobic disorders in patients with obsessive compulsive disorder. J Clin Psychiatry 1990 Nov;51(11):456–8.

Ayuso Mateos JL, Bayon Perez C, Santo-Domingo Carrasco J, Olivares D. Atypical chest pain and panic disorder. Psychother Psychosom 1989;52(1-3):92–5.

Balon R, Ortiz A, Pohl R, Yeragani VK. Heart rate and blood pressure during placebo-associated panic attacks. Psychosom Med 1988 Jul-Aug;50(4):434–8.

Balon R, Pohl R, Yeragani V, Rainey J, Oxenkrug GF. Platelet serotonin levels in panic disorder. Acta Psychiatr Scand 1987 Mar;75(3):315–7.

Balon R, Pohl R, Yeragani VK, Rainey JM Jr, Berchou R. Follow-up study of control subjects with lactate- and isoproterenol-induced panic attacks. Am J Psychiatry 1988 Feb;145(2):238–41.

Balon R, Pohl R, Yeragani VK, Rainey JM, Weinberg P. Lactate- and isoproterenol-induced panic attacks in panic disorder patients and controls. Psychiatry Res 1988 Feb;23(2):153–60.

Balon R, Rainey JM, Pohl R, Yeragani VK, Oxenkrug GF, McCauley RB. Platelet monoamine oxidase activity in panic disorder. Psychiatry Res 1987 Sep;22(1):37–41.

Balon R, Yeragani VK, Pohl R. Phenomenological comparison of dextrose, lactate, and isoproterenol associated panic attacks. Psychiatry Res 1988 Oct;26(1):43–50.

Balon R, Yeragani VK, Pohl R, Muench J, Berchou R. Somatic and psychological symptoms during isoproterenol-induced panic attacks. Psychiatry Res 1990 May;32(2):103–12.

Barlow DH, Vermilyea J, Blanchard EB, et al. The phenomenon of panic. J Abnorm Psychol 1985;94(3):320–8.

Barreto E, Amado H. Identifying panic disorders. New Dir Ment Health Serv 1986 Winter;(32):31–44.

Basha I, Mukerji V, Langevin P, Kushner M, Alpert M, Beitman BD. Atypical angina in patients with coronary artery disease suggests panic disorder. Int J Psychiatry Med 1989;19(4):341–6.

Bass C, Chambers JB, Kiff P, Cooper D, Gardner WN. Panic anxiety and hyperventilation in patients with chest pain: a controlled study. Q J Med 1988 Dec;69(260):949–59.

Bass C, Gardner WN. Respiratory and psychiatric abnormalities in chronic symptomatic hyperventilation. Br Med J [Clin Res] 1985 May 11;290(6479):1387–90.

Bass C, Lelliott P, Marks I. Fear talk versus voluntary hyperventilation in agoraphobics and normals: a controlled study. Psychol Med 1989 Aug;19(3):669–76.

Baumbacher GD. Signal anxiety and panic attacks. Psychother Theory Res Pract Train 1989;26(1):75–80.

Beck JG, Berisford MA, Taegtmeyer H, Bennett A. Panic symptoms in chest pain without coronary artery disease: A comparison with panic disorder. Behav Ther 1990;21(2):241–52.

Beck JG, Scott SK. Frequent and infrequent panic: a comparison of cognitive and autonomic reactivity. J Anxiety Disord 1987;1(1):47–58.

Beck JG, Taegtmeyer H, Berisford MA, Bennett A. Chest pain without coronary artery disease: An exploratory comparison with panic disorder. J Psychopathol Behav Assess 1989;11(3):209–20.

Beitman BD, Basha I, Flaker G, DeRosear L, Mukerji V, Lamberti J. Non-fearful panic disorder: panic attacks without fear. Behav Res Ther 1987;25(6):487–92.

Beitman BD, Basha I, Flaker G, DeRosear L, Mukerji V, Lamberti JW. Major depression in cardiology chest pain patients without coronary artery disease and with panic disorder. J Affective Disord 1987 Jul-Aug;13(1):51–9.

Beitman BD, Basha I, Flaker G, DeRosear L, Mukerji V, Trombka L, Katon W. Atypical or nonanginal chest pain. Panic disorder or coronary artery disease? Arch Intern Med 1987 Sep;147(9):1548–52.

Beitman BD, Kushner M, Lamberti JW, Mukerji V. Panic disorder without fear in patients with angiographically normal coronary arteries. J Nerv Ment Dis 1990 May;178(5):307–12.

Beitman BD, Kushner MG, Basha I, Lamberti J, Mukerji V, Bartels K. Follow-up status of patients with angiographically normal coronary arteries and panic disorder. JAMA 1991 Mar 27;265(12):1545–9.

Beitman BD, Lamberti JW, Mukerji V, DeRosear L, Basha I, Schmid L. Panic disorder in patients with angiographically normal coronary arteries. A pilot study. Psychosomatics 1987 Sep;28(9):480–4.

Beitman BD, Mukerji V, Alpert M, Peters JC. Panic disorder in cardiology patients. Psychiatr Med 1990;8(2):67–81.

Beitman BD, Mukerji V, Lamberti JW, Schmid L, DeRosear L, Kushner M, Flaker G, Basha I. Panic disorder in patients with chest pain and angiographically normal coronary arteries. Am J Cardiol 1989 Jun 1;63(18):1399–403.

Beitman BD, Mukerji V, Lamberti JW, Schmid L, Kushner M. Major depression and agoraphobia in patients with angiographically normal coronary arteries and panic disorder. Can J Psychiatry 1990 May;35(4):298–304.

Bell CC, Hildreth CJ, Jenkins EJ, Carter C. The relationship of isolated sleep paralysis and panic disorder to hypertension. J Natl Med Assoc 1988;80(3):289–94.

Black B, Robbins DR. Panic disorder in children and adolescents. J Am Acad Child Adolesc Psychiatry 1990 Jan;29(1):36–44.

Blowers GH, McClenahan KL, Roth WT. Panic-disordered subjects' perceptions of film: a repertory grid study. Percept Mot Skills 1986 Dec;63(3):1119–28.

Borden JW, Turner SM. Is panic a unique emotional experience? Behav Res Ther 1989;27(3):263–8.

Borkovec TD. "Relaxation-induced panic (RIP): When resting isn't peaceful": Commentary. A. Integr Psychiatry 1987 Jun;5(2):104–6.

Bradley S, Wachsmuth R, Swinson R, Hnatko G. A pilot study of panic attacks in a child and adolescent psychiatric population. Can J Psychiatry 1990 Aug;35(6):526–8.

Bradley SJ. Panic disorder in children and adolescents: a review with examples. Adolesc Psychiatry 1990;17:433–50.

Bradwejn J, Koszycki D. Comparison of the panicogenic effect of cholecystokinin 30-33 and carbon dioxide in panic disorder. Prog Neuropsychopharmacol Biol Psychiatry 1991;15(2):237–9.

Bradwejn J, Koszycki D, Meterissian G. Cholecystokinin-tetrapeptide induces panic attacks in patients with panic disorder. Can J Psychiatry 1990 Feb;35(1):83–5.

Breier A, Charney DS, Heninger GR. Agoraphobia with panic attacks. Development, diagnostic stability, and course of illness. Arch Gen Psychiatry 1986 Nov;43(11):1029–36.

Breier A, Charney DS, Heninger GR. Major depression in patients with agoraphobia and panic disorder. Arch Gen Psychiatry 1984;41(12):1129–35.

Breier A, Charney DS, Heninger GR. The diagnostic validity of anxiety disorders and their relationship to depressive illness. Am J Psychiatry 1985 Jul;142(7):787–97.

Brooks RB, Baltazar PL, Munjack DJ. Co-occurrence of personality disorders with panic disorder, social phobia, and generalized anxiety disorder: A review of the literature. J Anxiety Disord 1989;3(4):259–85.

Brown TA, Cash TF. The phenomenon of nonclinical panic: Parameters of panic, fear, and avoidance. J Anxiety Disord 1990;4(1):15–29.

Buller R, Maier W, Benkert O. Clinical subtypes in panic disorder: their descriptive and prospective validity. J Affective Disord 1986 Sep-Oct;11(2):105–14.

Buller R, Maier W, Goldenberg IM, Lavori PW, Benkert O. Chronology of panic and avoidance, age of onset in panic disorder, and prediction of treatment response. A report from the Cross-National Collaborative Panic Study. Eur Arch Psychiatry Clin Neurosci 1991;240(3):163–8.

Buller R, von Bardeleben U, Maier W, Benkert O. Specificity of lactate response in panic disorder, panic with concurrent depression and major depression. J Affective Disord 1989 Mar-Jun;16(2-3):109–13.

Cameron OG, Kuttesch D, McPhee K, Curtis GC. Menstrual fluctuation in the symptoms of panic anxiety. J Affective Disord 1988 Sep-Oct;15(2):169–74.

Cameron OG, Lee MA, Kotun J, McPhee KM. Circadian symptom fluctuations in people with anxiety disorders. J Affective Disord 1986 Nov-Dec;11(3):213–8.

Carr DB, Fishman SM, Kasting NW, Sheehan DV. Vasopressin response to lactate infusion in normals and patients with panic disorder. Funct Neurol 1986 Apr-Jun;1(2):123–7.

Carson SW, Halbreich U, Yeh CM, Goldstein S. Altered plasma dexamethasone and cortisol suppressibility in patients with panic disorders. Biol Psychiatry 1988 May;24(1):56–62.

Casat CD. Childhood anxiety disorders: A review of the possible relationship to adult panic disorder and agoraphobia. Special Issue: Perspectives on panic-related disorders. J Anxiety Disord 1988;2(1):51–60.

Cassano GB, Perugi G, Musetti L, Akiskal HS. The nature of depression presenting concomitantly with panic disorder. Compr Psychiatry 1989 Nov-Dec;30(6):473–82.

Cassano GB, Petracca A, Perugi G, Toni C, Tundo A, Roth M. Derealization and panic attacks: a clinical evaluation on 150 patients with panic disorder/agoraphobia. Compr Psychiatry 1989 Jan-Feb;30(1):5–12.

Castellani S, Quillen MA, Vaughan DA, Hund MA, Ho L, Ziegler MG, Le Vine WR. TSH and catecholamine response to TRH in panic disorder. Biol Psychiatry 1988 May;24(1):87–90.

Charney DL. "Relaxation-induced panic (RIP): When resting isn't peaceful": Commentary. Integr Psychiatry 1987 Jun;5(2):108–9.

Charney DS, Heninger GR, Price LH, Breier A. Major depression and panic disorder: diagnostic and neurobiological relationships. Psychopharmacol Bull 1986;22(2):503–11.

Clark DB, Taylor CB, Hayward C, King R, Margraf J, Ehlers A, Roth WT, Agras WS. Motor activity and tonic heart rate in panic disorder. Psychiatry Res 1990 Apr;32(1):45–53.

Clum GA, Broyles S, Borden J, Watkins PL. Validity and reliability of the panic attack symptoms and cognitions questionnaires. J Psychopathol Behav Assess 1990;12(3):233–45.

Comings DE, Comings BG. A controlled study of Tourette syndrome. III. Phobias and panic attacks. Am J Hum Genet 1987 Nov;41(5):761–81.

Conti S, Savron G, Bartolucci G, Grandi S, Magelli C, Semprini F, Saviotti FM, Trombini G, Fava GA, Magnani B. Cardiac neurosis and psychopathology. Psychother Psychosom 1989;52(1-3):88–91.

Cook BL, Noyes R Jr, Garvey MJ, Beach V, Sobotka J, Chaudhry D. Anxiety and the menstrual cycle in panic disorder. J Affective Disord 1990 Jul;19(3):221–6.

Coryell W. Panic disorder and mortality. Psychiatr Clin North Am 1988 Jun;11(2):433–40.

Coryell W, Endicott J, Andreasen NC, Keller MB, Clayton PJ, Hirschfeld RM, Scheftner WA, Winokur G. Depression and panic attacks: the significance of overlap as reflected in follow-up and family study data. Am J Psychiatry 1988 Mar;145(3):293–300.

Coryell W, Noyes R Jr, Clancy J, Crowe R, Chaudhry D. Abnormal escape from dexamethasone suppression in agoraphobia with panic attacks. Psychiatry Res 1985 Aug;15(4):301–11.

Coryell W, Noyes R Jr, House JD. Mortality among outpatients with anxiety disorders. Am J Psychiatry 1986 Apr;143(4):508–10.

Coryell W, Noyes R Jr, Reich J. The prognostic significance of HPA-axis disturbance in panic disorder: a three-year follow-up. Biol Psychiatry 1991 Jan 15;29(2):96–102.

Cottraux JA, Gebuhrer L, Bardi R, Betuel H. HLA system and panic attacks. Biol Psychiatry 1989 Feb;25(4):505–8.

Cowley DS, Arana GW. The diagnostic utility of lactate sensitivity in panic disorder. Arch Gen Psychiatry 1990 Mar;47(3):277–84.

Cowley DS, Dager SR, Dunner DL. Lactate-induced panic in primary affective disorder. Am J Psychiatry 1986 May;143(5):646–8.

Cowley DS, Dager SR, Foster SI, Dunner DL. Clinical characteristics and response to sodium lactate of patients with infrequent panic attacks. Am J Psychiatry 1987 Jun;144(6):795–8.

Cowley DS, Dunner DL. Response to sodium lactate in panic disorder: relationship to presenting clinical variables. Psychiatry Res 1988 Sep;25(3):253–9.

Cowley DS, Hyde TS, Dager SR, Dunner DL. Lactate infusions: the role of baseline anxiety. Psychiatry Res 1987 Jun;21(2):169–79.

Cowley DS, Jensen CF, Johannessen D, Parker L, Dager SR, Walker RD. Response to sodium lactate infusion in alcoholics with panic attacks. Am J Psychiatry 1989 Nov;146(11):1479–83.

Cowley DS, Roy-Byrne PP. Hyperventilation and panic disorder. Am J Med 1987 Nov;83(5):929–37.

Cowley DS, Roy-Byrne PP. Panic disorder during pregnancy. J Psychosom Obstet Gynecol 1989;10(3):193–210.

Cox BJ, Endler NS, Swinson RP. Clinical and nonclinical panic attacks: An empirical test of a panic-anxiety continuum. J Anxiety Disord 1991;5(1):21–34.

Cox BJ, Norton GR, Swinson RP, Endler NS. Substance abuse and panic-related anxiety: a critical review. Behav Res Ther 1990;28(5):385–93.

Cox BJ, Norton GR, Dorward J, Fergusson PA. The relationship between panic attacks and chemical dependencies. Addict Behav 1989;14(1):53–60.

Cox BJ, Swinson RP, Endler NS. A review of the psychopharmacology of panic disorder: Individual differences and non specific factors. Can J Psychiatry 1991;36(2):130–8.

Coyle PK, Sterman AB. Focal neurologic symptoms in panic attacks. Am J Psychiatry 1986 May;143(5):648–9.

Craske MG, Barlow DH. A review of the relationship between panic and avoidance. Clin Psychol Rev 1988;8(6):667–85.

Craske MG, Barlow DH. Nocturnal panic. J Nerv Ment Dis 1989 Mar;177(3):160–7.

Craske MG, Krueger MT. Prevalence of nocturnal panic in a college population. J Anxiety Disord 1990;4(2):125–39.

Craske MG, Miller PP, Rotunda R, Barlow DH. A descriptive report of features of initial unexpected panic attacks in minimal and extensive avoiders. Behav Res Ther 1990;28(5):395–400.

Craske MG, Rapee RM, Barlow DH. The significance of panic-expectancy for individual patterns of avoidance. Behav Ther 1988;19(4):577–592.

Dager SR, Comess KA, Saal AK, Sisk EJ, Beach KW, Dunner DL. Diagnostic reliability of M-mode echocardiography for detecting mitral valve prolapse in 50 consecutive panic patients. Compr Psychiatry 1989 Sep-Oct;30(5):369–75.

Dager SR, Khan A, Comess KA, Raisys V, Dunner DL. Mitral valve abnormalities and catecholamine activity in anxious patients. Psychiatry Res 1987 Jan;20(1):13–8.

Dajas F, Nin A, Barbeito L. Urinary norepinephrine excretion in panic and phobic disorders. J Neural Transm 1986;65(1):75–81.

de Ruiter C, Garssen B. Social anxiety and fear of bodily sensations in panic disorder and agoraphobia: A matched comparison. J Psychopathol Behav Assess 1989;11(2):175–184.

de Ruiter C, Garssen B, Rijken H, Kraaimaat F. The hyperventilation syndrome in panic disorder, agoraphobia and generalized anxiety disorder. Behav Res Ther 1989; 27(4):447–52.

de Ruiter C, Rijken H, Garssen B, Van Schaik A, Kraaimaat F. Comorbidity among the anxiety disorders. J Anxiety Disord 1989;3(2):57–68.

Deltito JA, Cassano GB. "Panic-attack disorders." Clinical and biological correlates. Encephale 1985 Jul-Aug;11(4):163–5.

Deltito JA, Perugi G, Maremmani I, Mignani V, Cassano GB. The importance of separation anxiety in the differentiation of panic disorder from agoraphobia. Psychiatr Dev 1986 Autumn;4(3):227–36.

DeMet E, Stein MK, Tran C, Chicz-DeMet A, Sangdahl C, Nelson J. Caffeine taste test for panic disorder: adenosine receptor supersensitivity. Psychiatry Res 1989 Dec;30(3):231–42.

Den Boer JA, Westenberg HG, Klompmakers AA, van Lint LE. Behavioral biochemical and neuroendocrine concomitants of lactate-induced panic anxiety. Biol Psychiatry 1989 Oct;26(6):612–22.

Dillon DJ, Gorman JM, Liebowitz MR, Fyer AJ, Klein DF. Measurement of lactate–induced panic and anxiety. Psychiatry Res 1987 Feb;20(2):97–105.

Donnell CD, McNally RJ. Anxiety sensitivity and history of panic as predictors of response to hyperventilation. Behav Res Ther 1989;27(4):325–32.

Dube S, Jones DA, Bell J, Davies A, Ross E, Sitaram N. Interface of panic and depression: clinical and sleep EEG correlates. Psychiatry Res 1986 Oct;19(2):119–33.

Dube S, Jones DA, Bell J, et al. Interface of panic and depression: Clinical and sleep EEG correlates. Psychiatry Res 1986;19(2):119–33.

Dunner DL. Anxiety and panic: relationship to depression and cardiac disorders. Psychosomatics 1985 Nov;26(11 Suppl):18–22.

Edlund MJ, McNamara ME, Millman RP. Sleep apnea and panic attacks. Compr Psychiatry 1991 Mar-Apr;32(2):130–2.

Edlund MJ, Swann AC, Clothier J. Patients with panic attacks and abnormal EEG results. Am J Psychiatry 1987 Apr;144(4):508–9.

Ehlers A, Margraf J, Roth WT, Taylor AU, Maddock RJ, Sheikh J, Kopell ML, McClenahan KL, Gossard D, Blowers GH, et al. Lactate infusions and panic attacks: do patients and controls respond differently? Psychiatry Res 1986 Apr;17(4):295–308.

Eriksson E, Westberg P, Alling C, Thuresson K, Modigh K. Cerebrospinal fluid levels of monoamine metabolites in panic disorder. Psychiatry Res 1991;36(3):243–51.

Evans L. Panic disorder. A new definition to anxiety. Curr Ther 1987;28(11):19–21.

Faludi G, Kasko M, Perenyi A, Arato M, Frecska E. The dexamethasone suppression test in panic disorder and major depressive episodes. Biol Psychiatry 1986 Sep;21(11):1008–14.

Faravelli C, Albanesi G. Agoraphobia with panic attacks: 1-year prospective follow up. Compr Psychiatry 1987;28(6):481–7.

Faravelli C, Pallanti S, Frassine R, Albanesi G, Guerrini Degl'Innocenti B. Panic attacks with and without agoraphobia: a comparison. Psychopathology 1988;21(1):51–6.

Fava GA, Grandi S, Canestrari R. Prodromal symptoms in panic disorder with agoraphobia. Am J Psychiatry 1988 Dec;145(12):1564–7.

Fava GA, Grandi S, Saviotti FM, Conti S. Hypochondriasis with panic attacks. Psychosomatics 1990 Summer;31(3):351–3.

Fava M, Anderson K, Rosenbaum JF. "Anger attacks": possible variants of panic and major depressive disorders. Am J Psychiatry 1990 Jul;147(7):867–70.

Fava M, Rosenbaum JF, MacLaughlin RA, Tesar GE, Pollack MH, Cohen LS, Hirsch M. Dehydroepiandrosterone-sulfate/cortisol ratio in panic disorder. Psychiatry Res 1989 Jun;28(3):345–50.

Fawcett J. Targeting treatment in patients with mixed symptoms of anxiety and depression. J Clin Psychiatry 1990 Nov;51 Suppl:40–3.

Fier M. Panic disorder and agoraphobia. N J Med 1990 Jun;87(6):475–6.

Fisher DC, Wutchiett RJ. MMPI profiles of persons having panic disorder with agoraphobia. Phobia Pract Res J 1990 Spring-Summer;3(1):19–25.

Fishman SM, Sheehan DV, Carr DB. Thyroid indices in panic disorder. J Clin Psychiatry 1985 Oct;46(10):432–3.

Fleming B, Faulk A. Discriminating factors in panic disorder with and without agoraphobia. J Anxiety Disord 1989;3(4):209–19.

Freedman RR, Ianni P, Ettedgui E, Puthezhath N. Ambulatory monitoring of panic disorder. Arch Gen Psychiatry 1985 Mar;42(3):244–8.

Freinhar JP, Alvarez WA. Organic claustrophobia: An association between panic and carbon dioxide? Int J Psychosom 1987;34(2):18–9.

Fried R, Golden WL. The role of psychophysiological hyperventilation assessment in cognitive behavior therapy. J Cogn Psychother Int Q 1989;3(1):5–14.

Friedman S, Paradis C. African–American patients with panic disorder and agoraphobia. J Anxiety Disord 1991;5(1):35–41.

Fyer MR, Uy J, Martinez J, Goetz R, Klein DF, Fyer A, Liebowitz MR, Gorman J. CO2 challenge of patients with panic disorder. Am J Psychiatry 1987 Aug;144(8):1080–2.

Gaffney FA, Fenton BJ, Lane LD, Lake CR. Hemodynamic, ventilatory, and biochemical responses of panic patients and normal controls with sodium lactate infusion and spontaneous panic attacks. Arch Gen Psychiatry 1988 Jan;45(1):53–60.

Ganellen RJ, Matuzas W, Uhlenhuth EH, Glass R, Easton CR. Panic disorder, agoraphobia, and anxiety-relevant cognitive style. J Affective Disord 1986 Nov-Dec;11(3):219–25.

Garland EJ, Smith DH. Panic disorder on a child psychiatric consultation service. J Am Acad Child Adolesc Psychiatry 1990 Sep;29(5):785–8.

Garvey M, Noyes R Jr, Cook B. Comparison of panic disordered patients with high versus low MHPG. J Affective Disord 1990 Sep;20(1):7–12.

Garvey M, Noyes R Jr, Cook B. Does situational panic disorder represent a specific panic disorder subtype? Compr Psychiatry 1987 Jul–Aug;28(4):329–33.

Garvey M, Noyes R Jr, Cook B, Tollefson G. The relationship of panic disorder and its treatment outcome to 24-hour urinary MHPG levels. Psychiatry Res 1989 Oct;30(1):53–61.

Garvey MJ, Cook B, Noyes R Jr. The occurrence of a prodrome of generalized anxiety in panic disorder. Compr Psychiatry 1988 Sep-Oct;29(5):445–9.

Garvey MJ, Tollefson GD, Orsulak PJ. Elevations of urinary MHPG in depressed patients with panic attacks. Psychiatry Res 1987 Mar;20(3):183–7.

Garvey MJ, Tollefson GD, Tuason VB. Comparison of major depressions with and without panic attacks. Compr Psychiatry 1987;28(1):65–7.

Gelder MG. Panic disorder: fact or fiction? Psychol Med 1989 May;19(2):277–83.

Gelder MG. The classification of anxiety disorders. Br J Psychiatry Suppl 1989 May;(4):28–32.

George DT, Anderson P, Nutt DJ, Linnoila M. Aggressive thoughts and behavior: another symptom of panic disorder? Acta Psychiatr Scand 1989 May;79(5):500–2.

George MS, Lydiard RB. Inability to walk as a symptom of panic disorder and social phobia. Neuropsychiatr Neuropsychol Behav Neurol 1989;2(3):219–23.

George DT, Nutt DJ, Dwyer BA, Linnoila M. Alcoholism and panic disorder: is the co-morbidity more than coincidence? Acta Psychiatr Scand 1990 Feb;81(2):97–107.

George DT, Nutt DJ, Waxman RP, Linnoila M. Panic response to lactate administration in alcoholic and nonalcoholic patients with panic disorder. Am J Psychiatry 1989 Sep;146(9):1161–5.

George DT, Zerby A, Noble S, Nutt DJ. Panic attacks and alcohol withdrawal: Can subjects differentiate the symptoms? Biol Psychiatry 1988;24(2):240–3.

Goetz RR, Gorman JM, Dillon DJ, Papp LA, Hollander E, Fyer AJ, Liebowitz MR, Klein DF. Do panic disorder patients indiscriminately endorse somatic complaints? Psychiatry Res 1989 Aug;29(2):207–13.

Gold DD Jr. Panic attacks: Diagnosis and management. Cardiovasc Rev Rep 1988;9(1):35–7, 40.

Goldberg R, Morris P, Christian F, Badger J, Chabot S, Edlund M. Panic disorder in cardiac outpatients. Psychosomatics 1990 Spring;31(2):168–73.

Goldberg RJ. Clinical presentations of panic–related disorders. J Anxiety Disord 1988;2(1):61–75.

Goldstein S, Halbreich U, Asnis G, Endicott J, Alvir J. The hypothalamic-pituitary-adrenal system in panic disorder. Am J Psychiatry 1987 Oct;144(10):1320–3.

Gorman JM. Panic disorders. Mod Probl Pharmacopsychiatry 1987;22:36–90.

Gorman JM, Battista D, Goetz RR, Dillon DJ, Liebowitz MR, Fyer AJ, Kahn JP, Sandberg D, Klein DF. A comparison of sodium bicarbonate and sodium lactate infusion in the induction of panic attacks. Arch Gen Psychiatry 1989 Feb;46(2):145–50.

Gorman JM, Cohen BS, Liebowitz MR, Fyer AJ, Ross D, Davies SO, Klein DF. Blood gas changes and hypophosphatemia in lactate-induced panic. Arch Gen Psychiatry 1986 Nov;43(11):1067–71.

Gorman JM, Davies M, Steinman R, Liebowitz MR, Fyer AJ, Coromilas J, Klein DF. An objective marker of lactate-induced panic. Psychiatry Res 1987 Dec;22(4):341–8.

Gorman JM, Goetz RR, Dillon D, Liebowitz MR, Fyer AJ, Davies S, Klein DF. Sodium D-lactate infusion of panic disorder patients. Neuropsychopharmacology 1990 Jun;3(3):181–9.

Gorman JM, Goetz RR, Uy J, Ross D, Martinez J, Fyer AJ, Liebowitz MR, Klein DF. Hyperventilation occurs during lactate-induced panic. J Anxiety Disord 1988;2(3):193–202.

Gorman JM, Liebowitz MR, Fyer AJ, Fyer MR, Klein DF. Possible respiratory abnormalities in panic disorder. Psychopharmacol Bull 1986;22(3):797–801.

Gorman JM, Papp LA, Martinez J, Goetz RR, Hollander E, Liebowitz MR, Jordan F. High-dose carbon dioxide challenge test in anxiety disorder patients. Biol Psychiatry 1990 Nov 1;28(9):743–57.

Gorman JM, Uy J. Respiratory physiology and pathological anxiety. Gen Hosp Psychiatry 1987 Nov;9(6):410–9.

Green MA, Curtis GC. Personality disorders in panic patients: Response to termination of antipanic medication. J Pers Disord 1988;2(4):303–14.

Griez E, de Loof C, Pols H, Zandbergen J, Lousberg H. Specific sensitivity of patients with panic attacks to carbon dioxide inhalation. Psychiatry Res 1990 Feb;31(2):193–9.

Griez E, Pols HJ, van den Hout MA. Acid-base balance in real life panic. J Affective Disord 1987 May-Jun;12(3):263–6.

Griez E, van den Hout MA, Verstappen F. Body fluids after CO_2 inhalation: insight into panic mechanisms? Eur Arch Psychiatry Neurol Sci 1987;236(6):369–71.

Griez E, Zandbergen J, Pols H, de Loof C. Response to 35% CO_2 as a marker of panic in severe anxiety. Am J Psychiatry 1990 Jun;147(6):796–7.

Griez EJ, Lousberg H, van den Hout MA, van der Molen GM. CO_2 vulnerability in panic disorder. Psychiatry Res 1987 Feb;20(2):87–95.

Griffin GC. From panic attacks to lethal arrhythmias. Postgrad Med 1990;88(6):19.

Grunhaus L. Clinical and psychobiological characteristics of simultaneous panic disorder and major depression. Am J Psychiatry 1988 Oct;145(10):1214–21.

Grunhaus L, Birmaher B. The clinical spectrum of panic attacks. J Clin Psychopharmacol 1985 Apr;5(2):93–9.

Grunhaus L, Flegel P, Haskett RF, Greden JF. Serial dexamethasone suppression tests in simultaneous panic and depressive disorders. Biol Psychiatry 1987 Mar;22(3):332–8.

Grunhaus L, Haskett RF, Pande AC. Catecholamine and cortisol response to yohimbine infusions in comorbidity of depression and panic attacks. Eur J Pharmacol 1990;183(5):1652–3.

Grunhaus L, King D, Greden JF, Flegel P. Depression and panic in patients with borderline personality disorder. Biol Psychiatry 1985 Jun;20(6):688–92.

Grunhaus L, Rabin D, Harel Y, Greden JF, Feinberg M, Hermann R. Simultaneous panic and depressive disorders: clinical and sleep EEG correlates. Psychiatry Res 1986 Apr;17(4):251–9.

Grunhaus L, Tiongco D, Haskett RF, Greden JF. The dexamethasone suppression test in inpatients with panic disorder or agoraphobia with panic attacks. Biol Psychiatry 1987 Apr;22(4):517–21.

Grunhaus LJ, Cameron O, Pande AC, Haskett RF, Hollingsworth PJ, Smith CB. Comorbidity of panic disorder and major depressive disorder: effects on platelet alpha 2 adrenergic receptors. Acta Psychiatr Scand 1990 Mar;81(3):216–9.

Gurguis GNM, Cameron OG, Ericson WA, Curtis GC. The daily distribution of panic attacks. Compr Psychiatry 1988;29(1):1–3.

Hauri PJ, Friedman M, Ravaris CL. Sleep in patients with spontaneous panic attacks. Sleep 1989 Aug;12(4):323–37.

Hayward C, Killen JD, Taylor CB. Panic attacks in young adolescents. Am J Psychiatry 1989 Aug;146(8):1061–2.

Hayward C, Taylor CB, Roth WT, King R, Agras WS. Plasma lipid levels in patients with panic disorder or agoraphobia. Am J Psychiatry 1989 Jul;146(7):917–9.

Hebenstreit M, Buller R, Maier W, Philipp M, Frommberger U. The personality sphere in patients with panic attacks. Pharmacopsychiatry 1988 Nov;21(6):463–4.

Hibbert G, Pilsbury D. Hyperventilation in panic attacks. Ambulant monitoring of transcutaneous carbon dioxide. Br J Psychiatry 1988 Jul;153:76–80.

Hoehn-Saric R, McLeod DR, Zimmerli WD. Psychophysiological response patterns in panic disorder. Acta Psychiatr Scand 1991 Jan;83(1):4–11.

Hoes MJ, Colla P, van Doorn P, Folgering H, de Swart J. Hyperventilation and panic attacks. J Clin Psychiatry 1987 Nov;48(11):435–7.

Hollander E, Liebowitz MR, Cohen B, Gorman JM, Fyer AJ, Papp LA, Klein DF. Prolactin and sodium lactate-induced panic. Psychiatry Res 1989 May;28(2):181–91.

Hollander E, Liebowitz MR, Gorman JM, Cohen B, Fyer A, Klein DF. Cortisol and sodium lactate-induced panic. Arch Gen Psychiatry 1989 Feb;46(2):135–40.

Hollifield M, Katon W, Spain D, Pule L. Anxiety and depression in a village in Lesotho, Africa: a comparison with the United States. Br J Psychiatry 1990 Mar;156:343–50.

Holmberg G. The nosologic specificity of panic disorder/agoraphobia. Proceedings of the World Psychiatric Association on the Psychopathology of Panic Disorders: Many faces of panic disorder (1988, Espoo, Finland). Psychiatr Fenn 1989;Suppl:53–7.

Holt PE, Andrews G. Hyperventilation and anxiety in panic disorder, social phobia, GAD and normal controls. Behav Res Ther 1989;27(4):453–60.

Hudson JI, Pope HG Jr. Affective spectrum disorder: does antidepressant response identify a family of disorders with a common pathophysiology? Am J Psychiatry 1990 May;147(5):552–64.

Innis RB, Charney DS, Heninger GR. Differential 3H-imipramine platelet binding in patients with panic disorder and depression. Psychiatry Res 1987 May;21(1):33–41.

Jacob RG. Panic disorder and the vestibular system. Psychiatr Clin North Am 1988 Jun;11(2):361–74.

Jacob RG, Lilienfeld SO, Furman JMR, Durrant JD, Turner SM. Panic disorder with vestibular dysfunction: Further clinical observations and description of space and motion phobic stimuli. J Anxiety Disord 1989;3(2):117–30.

Jacob RG, Muller MB, Turner SM, Wall C 3d. Otoneurological examination in panic disorder and agoraphobia with panic attacks: a pilot study. Am J Psychiatry 1985 Jun;142(6):715–20.

Jefferson JW. Anxiety and the aching heart. Stress Med 1987;3(1):33–9.

Johannessen DJ, Cowley DS, Walker RD, Jensen CF, Parker L. Prevalence, onset, and clinical recognition of panic states in hospitalized male alcoholics. Am J Psychiatry 1989 Sep;146(9):1201–3.

Johnson J, Weissman MM, Klerman GL. Panic disorder, comorbidity, and suicide attempts. Arch Gen Psychiatry 1990 Sep;47(9):805–8.

Johnston AL, File SE. Profiles of the antipanic compounds, triazolobenzodiazepines and phenelzine, in two animal tests of anxiety. Psychiatry Res 1988 Jul;25(1):81–90.

Judd FK, Norman TR, Burrows GD, McIntyre IM. The dexamethasone suppression test in panic disorder. Pharmacopsychiatry 1987 May;20(3):99–101.

Kahn JP, Drusin RE, Klein DF. Idiopathic cardiomyopathy and panic disorder: clinical association in cardiac transplant candidates. Am J Psychiatry 1987 Oct;144(10):1327–30.

Kahn RS, Wetzler S, Asnis GM, Kling MA, Suckow RF, Van Praag HM. Pituitary hormone responses to meta-chlorophenylpiperazine in panic disorder and healthy control subjects. Psychiatry Res 1991;37(1):25–34.

Kane FJ Jr, Wittels E, Harper RG. Chest pain and anxiety disorder. Tex Med 1990 Jul;86(7):104–10.

Kasdorf JA, Kasdorf JL, Janzen WB. Panic attacks: Are they spontaneous? Phobia Pract Res J 1988 Spring;1(1):32–47.

Katerndahl DA. Infrequent and limited-symptom panic attacks. J Nerv Ment Dis 1990 May;178(5):313–7.

Katerndahl DA. Panic is panic: homogeneity of the panic attack experience. Fam Pract Res J 1990 Spring-Summer;9(2):147–55.

Katerndahl DA. The sequence of panic symptoms. J Fam Pract 1988 Jan;26(1):49–52.

Katerndahl DA, Gabel LL, Monk JS. Comparative symptomatology of phobic and nonphobic panic attacks. Fam Pract Res J 1986 Winter;6(2):106–13.

Kathol RG, Noyes R, Lopez A. Similarities in hypothalamic-pituitary-adrenal axis activity between patients with panic disorder and those experiencing external stress. Psychiatr Clin North Am 1988 Jun;11(2):335–48.

Kathol RG, Noyes R Jr, Lopez AL, Reich JH. Relationship of urinary free cortisol levels in patients with panic disorder to symptoms of depression and agoraphobia. Psychiatry Res 1988 May;24(2):211–21.

Katon WJ. Chest pain, cardiac disease, and panic disorder. J Clin Psychiatry 1990 May;51 Suppl: 27-30; discussion 50–3.

Katon W, Roy-Byrne PP. Panic disorder in the medically ill. J Clin Psychiatry 1989 Aug;50(8):299–302.

Katon W, Vitaliano PP, Anderson K, et al. Panic disorder: Residual symptoms after the acute attacks abate. Compr Psychiatry 1987;28(2):151–8.

Katon W, Vitaliano PP, Russo J, Jones M, Anderson K. Panic disorder. Spectrum of severity and somatization. J Nerv Ment Dis 1987 Jan;175(1):12–9.

Kenardy J, Evans L, Oei TP. Attributional style and panic disorder. J Behav Ther Exp Psychiatry 1990 Mar;21(1):9–13.

Keyl PM, Eaton WW. Risk factors for the onset of panic disorder and other panic attacks in a prospective, population-based study. Am J Epidemiol 1990 Feb;131(2):301–11.

King LJ. Major depressive disorder and panic disorder in children of parenɩs with alcohol dependence. Ann Clin Psychiatry 1989;1(4):269–270.

King RJ, Bayon EP, Clark DB, Taylor CB. Tonic arousal and activity: relationships to personality and personality disorder traits in panic patients. Psychiatry Res 1988 Jul;25(1):65–72.

Klein DF, Klein HM. The status of panic disorder. Curr Opin Psychiatry 1988;1(2):177–83.

Klein DF, Klein HM. The utility of the panic disorder concept. Eur Arch Psychiatry Neurol Sci 1989;238(5-6):268–79.

Kleiner L. Agoraphobia or panic disorder? Behav Ther 1986 Jan;9(1):14–5.

Klerman GL, Freedman DX, Shader RI. The separation of panic and agoraphobia from other anxiety disorders: Introduction of the conference proceedings. J Psychiatr Res 1988;22 Suppl 1:3–5.

Knott VJ, Lapierre YD. Effects of lactate-induced panic attacks on brain stem auditory evoked potentials. Neuropsychobiology 1986;16(1):9–14.

Knott VJ, Lapierre YD. Neuropsychophysiological correlates of lactate-induced panic. Prog Neuropsychopharmacol Biol Psychiatry 1988;12(2-3):183–92.

Koehler K, Vartzopoulos D, Ebel H. The relationship of panic attacks to autonomically labile generalized anxiety. Compr Psychiatry 1988;29(2):91–7.

Koenigsberg HW, Pollak C, Sullivan T. The sleep lactate infusion: arousal and the panic mechanism. Biol Psychiatry 1987 Jun;22(6):789–91.

Kopp MS, Arato M, Magyar I, Buza K. Basal adrenocortical activity and DST in electrodermally differentiated subgroups of panic patients. Int J Psychophysiol 1989 Mar;7(1):77–83.

Krakowski AJ. Panic disorder associated with mitral valve prolapse: psychosomatic implications. Psychother Psychosom 1987;47(3-4):211–8.

Kushner MG, Beitman BD. Panic attacks without fear: an overview. Behav Res Ther 1990;28(6):469–79.

Kushner MG, Beitman BD, Beck NC. Factors predictive of panic disorder in cardiology patients with chest pain and no evidence of coronary artery disease: a cross-validation. J Psychosom Res 1989;33(2):207–15.

Kushner MG, Sher KJ, Beitman BD. The relation between alcohol problems and the anxiety disorders. Am J Psychiatry 1990 Jun;147(6):685–95.

Kwon S-M, Evans L, Oei TPS. Factor structure of the mobility inventory for agoraphobia: A validational study with Australian samples of agoraphobic patients. J Psychopathol Behav Assess 1990;12(4):365–74.

Lane JW, Pollard CA, Cox GL. Validity study of the Anxiety Symptoms Interview. J Clin Psychol 1990 Jan;46(1):52–7.

Lapierre YD. Clinical and biological correlates of panic states. Prog Neuropsychopharmacol Biol Psychiatry 1987;11(2-3):91–6.

Last CG, Strauss CC. Panic disorder in children and adolescents. J Anxiety Disord 1989;3(2):87–95.

Lee MA, Flegel P, Greden JF, Cameron OG. Anxiogenic effects of caffeine on panic and depressed patients. Am J Psychiatry 1988 May;145(5):632–5.

Lelliott P, Bass C. Symptom specificity in patients with panic. Br J Psychiatry 1990 Oct;157:593–7.

Lepine JP, Chignon JM, Teherani M. Onset of panic disorder and suicide attempts. Psychiatr Psychobiol 1990;5(6):339–42.

Lepola U. Recognition of panic disorder. Nord Psykiatr Tidsskr 1989;43(6):511–3.

Lepola U, Jolkkonen J, Pitkanen A, Riekkinen P, Rimon R. Cerebrospinal fluid monoamine metabolites and neuropeptides in patients with panic disorder. Ann Med 1990;22(4):237–9.

Lepola U, Nousiainen U, Puranen M, Riekkinen R, Rimon R. EEG and CT findings in patients with panic disorders. Biol Psychiatry 1990;28(8):721–7.

Lesser IM. The relationship between panic disorder and depression. J Anxiety Disord 1988;2(1):3–15.

Lesser IM, Rubin RT. Diagnostic considerations in panic disorders. J Clin Psychiatry 1986 Jun;47 Suppl:4–10.

Lesser IM, Rubin RT, Lydiard RB, Swinson R, Pecknold J. Past and current thyroid function in subjects with panic disorder. J Clin Psychiatry 1987 Dec;48(12):473–6.

Lesser IM, Rubin RT, Pecknold JC, Rifkin A, Swinson RP, Lydiard RB, Burrows GD, Noyes R Jr, DuPont RL Jr. Secondary depression in panic disorder and agoraphobia. I. Frequency, severity, and response to treatment. Arch Gen Psychiatry 1988 May;45(5):437–43.

Lesser IM, Rubin RT, Rifkin A, Swinson RP, Ballenger JC, Burrows GD, DuPont RL, Noyes R, Pecknold JC. Secondary depression in panic disorder and agoraphobia. II. Dimensions of depressive symptomatology and their response to treatment. J Affective Disord 1989 Jan-Feb;16(1):49–58.

Levin AP, Doran AR, Liebowitz MR, Fyer AJ, Gorman JM, Klein DF, Paul SM. Pituitary adrenocortical unresponsiveness in lactate-induced panic. Psychiatry Res 1987 May;21(1):23–32.

Levinson HN. A cerebellar-vestibular explanation for fears/phobias: hypothesis and study. Percept Mot Skills 1989 Feb;68(1):67–84.

Lewis RP, Wooley CF, Kolibash AJ, Boudoulas H. The mitral valve prolapse epidemic: fact or fiction. Trans Am Clin Climatol Assoc 1986;98:222–36.

Liberthson RR, King ME. "Mitral valve prolapse in a psychiatric setting: Diagnostic assessment, research, and clinical implications": Comment. Integr Psychiatry 1987 Mar;5(1):56–7.

Liebowitz MR, Ballenger J, Barlow DH, Davidson J, Foa EB, Fyer A. New perspectives on anxiety disorders in DSM-IV and ICD-10. Drug Ther 1990;20 Suppl:129–36.

Liebowitz MR, Fyer AJ, Gorman JM, Dillon D, Davies S, Stein JM, Cohen BS, Klein DF. Specificity of lactate infusions in social phobia versus panic disorders. Am J Psychiatry 1985 Aug;142(8):947–50.

Liebowitz MR, Gorman JM, Fyer AJ, Levitt M, Dillon D, Levy G, Appleby IL, Anderson S, Palij M, Davies SO, et al. Lactate provocation of panic attacks. II. Biochemical and physiological findings. Arch Gen Psychiatry 1985 Jul;42(7):709–19.

Linnoila MI. Anxiety and alcoholism. J Clin Psychiatry 1989 Nov;50 Suppl:26–9.

Lousberg H, Griez E, van den Hout MA. Carbon dioxide chemosensitivity in panic disorder. Acta Psychiatr Scand 1988 Feb;77(2):214–8.

Lucas JA, Telch MJ, Bigler ED. Memory functioning in panic disorder: A neuropsychological perspective. J Anxiety Disord 1991;5(1):1–20.

Luchins DJ, Rose RP. Late-life onset of panic disorder with agoraphobia in three patients. Am J Psychiatry 1989 Jul;146(7):920–1.

Lydiard RB, Laraia MT, Howell EF, Ballenger JC. Can panic disorder present as irritable bowel syndrome? J Clin Psychiatry 1986 Sep;47(9):470–3.

Lydiard RB, Zealberg J, Laraia MT, Fossey M, Prockow V, Gross J, Ballenger JC. Electroencephalography during sleep of patients with panic disorder. J Neuropsychiatry Clin Neurosci 1989;1(4):372–6.

Macaulay JL, Kleinknecht RA. Panic and panic attacks in adolescents. J Anxiety Disord 1989;3(4):221–41.

Maddock RJ, Blacker KH. Response to treatment in panic disorder with associated depression. Psychopathology 1991;24(1):1–6.

Maddock RJ, Mateo-Bermudez J. Elevated serum lactate following hyperventilation during glucose infusion in panic disorder. Biol Psychiatry 1990 Feb 15;27(4):411–8.

Maier W, Buller R, Frommberger U, Philipp M. One-year follow-up of cardiac anxiety syndromes. Outcome and predictors of course. Eur Arch Psychiatry Neurol Sci 1987;237(1):16–20.

Maier W, Buller R, Rieger H, Benkert O. The cardiac anxiety syndrome—a subtype of panic attacks. Eur Arch Psychiatry Neurol Sci 1985;235(3):146–52.

Maier W, Buller R, Sonntag A, Heuser I. Subtypes of panic attacks and ICD-9 classification. Eur Arch Psychiatry Neurol Sci 1986;235(6):361–6.

Maier W, Rosenberg R, Argyle N, Buller R, Roth M, Brandon S, Benkert O. Avoidance behaviour and major depression in panic disorder: a report from the Cross-National Collaborative Panic Study. Psychiatr Dev 1989 Summer;7(2):123–42.

Manu P, Matthews DA, Lane TJ. Panic disorder among patients with chronic fatigue. South Med J 1991 Apr;84(4):451–6.

Margraf J. Ambulatory psychophysiological monitoring of panic attacks. J Psychophysiol 1990;4(4):321–30.

Margraf J, Ehlers A, Roth WT. Mitral valve prolapse and panic disorder: a review of their relationship. Psychosom Med 1988 Mar-Apr;50(2):93–113.

Margraf J, Ehlers A, Roth WT. Panic attack associated with perceived heart rate acceleration: A case report. Behav Ther 1987;18(1):84–9.

Margraf J, Ehlers A, Roth WT. Sodium lactate infusions and panic attacks: a review and critique. Psychosom Med 1986 Jan-Feb;48(1-2):23–51.

Margraf J, Taylor B, Ehlers A, Roth WT, Agras WS. Panic attacks in the natural environment. J Nerv Ment Dis 1987 Sep;175(9):558–65.

Marks I. Agoraphobia, panic disorder and related conditions in the DSM-III-R and ICD-10. J Psychopharmacol 1987;1(1):6–12.

Marriott JA. The cord component in panic attack syndrome: Five case studies. Aust J Clin Hypnother Hypnosis 1989 Mar;10(1):17–24.

Marshall JR. Are some irritable bowel syndromes actually panic disorders? Postgrad Med 1988 May 1;83(6):206–9.

Marshall JR. Hyperventilation syndrome or panic disorder—what's in the name? Hosp Pract [Off] 1987 Oct 15;22(10):105-8, 111-2, 117–8.

Mathew RJ, Wilson WH. Behavioral and cerebrovascular effects of caffeine in patients with anxiety disorders. Acta Psychiatr Scand 1990 Jul;82(1):17–22.

Mathew RJ, Wilson WH, Tant S. Responses to hypercarbia induced by acetazolamide in panic disorder patients. Am J Psychiatry 1989 Aug;146(8):996–1000.

Mavissakalian M. The relationship between panic disorder/agoraphobia and personality disorders. Psychiatr Clin North Am 1990 Dec;13(4):661–84.

Mavissakalian M, Hamann MS. Correlates of DSM-III personality disorder in panic disorder and agoraphobia. Compr Psychiatry 1988 Nov-Dec;29(6):535–44.

Mavissakalian M, Hamann MS. DSM-III personality disorder in agoraphobia: II. Changes with treatment. Comp Psychiatry 1987 Jul-Aug;28(4):356–61.

Mavissakalian M, Hamann MS, Jones B. A comparison of DSM-III personality disorders in panic/agoraphobia and obsessive-compulsive disorder. Compr Psychiatry 1990 May-Jun;31(3):238–44.

McGrath PJ, Stewart JW, Liebowitz MR, Markowitz JM, Quitkin FM, Klein DF, Gorman JM. Lactate provocation of panic attacks in depressed outpatients. Psychiatry Res 1988 Jul;25(1):41–7.

McIntyre IM, Judd FK, Burrows GD, Armstrong SM, Norman TR. Plasma concentrations of melatonin in panic disorder. Am J Psychiatry 1990 Apr;147(4):462–4.

McIntyre IM, Norman TR, Marriott PF, Burrows GD. The pineal hormone melatonin in panic disorder. J Affective Disord 1987 May–Jun;12(3):203–6.

McNally RJ, Riemann BC, Kim E. Selective processing of threat cues in panic disorder. Behav Res Ther 1990;28(5):407–12.

Mellman TA, Uhde TW. Electroencephalographic sleep in panic disorder. A focus on sleep-related panic attacks. Arch Gen Psychiatry 1989 Feb;46(2):178–84.

Mellman TA, Uhde TW. Obsessive-compulsive symptoms in panic disorder. Am J Psychiatry 1987 Dec;144(12):1573–6.

Mellman TA, Uhde TW. Patients with frequent sleep panic: clinical findings and response to medication treatment. J Clin Psychiatry 1990 Dec;51(12):513–6.

Mellman TA, Uhde TW. Sleep panic attacks: new clinical findings and theoretical implications. Am J Psychiatry 1989 Sep;146(9):1204–7.

Metz A, Sichel DA, Goff DC. Postpartum panic disorder. J Clin Psychiatry 1988 Jul;49(7):278–9.

Middleton HC. Cardiovascular dystonia in recovered panic patients. J Affective Disord 1990 Aug;19(4):229–36.

Modestin J. Symptomatic panic disorder in borderline personality disorder. Eur J Psychiatry 1989 Jul-Sep;3(3):133–7.

Moreau DL, Weissman M, Warner V. Panic disorder in children at high risk for depression. Am J Psychiatry 1989 Aug;146(8):1059–60.

Mukerji V, Beitman BD, Alpert MA, Lamberti JW, DeRosear L, Basha IM. Panic disorder: a frequent occurrence in patients with chest pain and normal coronary arteries. Angiology 1987 Mar;38(3):236–40.

Munjack DJ, Brown RA, McDowell DE. Comparison of social anxiety in patients with social phobia and panic disorder. J Nerv Ment Dis 1987 Jan;175(1):49–51.

Munjack DJ, Palmer R. Thyroid hormones in panic disorder, panic disorder with agoraphobia, and generalized anxiety disorder. J Clin Psychiatry 1988 Jun;49(6):229–31.

Murphy DL, Pigott TA. A comparative examination of a role for serotonin in obsessive compulsive disorder, panic disorder, and anxiety. J Clin Psychiatry 1990 Apr;51 Suppl:53–8; discussion 59–60.

Murray JB. Psychopharmacological investigation of panic disorder by means of lactate infusion. J Gen Psychol 1987 Jul;114(3):297–311.

Neenan P, Felkner J, Reich J. Schizoid personality traits developing secondary to panic disorder. J Nerv Ment Dis 1986 Aug;174(8):483.

Nelles WB, Barlow DH. Do children panic? Clin Psychol Rev 1988;8(4):359–72.

Nesse RM, Cameron OG, Buda AJ, McCann DS, Curtis GC, Huber-Smith MJ. Urinary catecholamines and mitral valve prolapse in panic-anxiety patients. Psychiatry Res 1985 Jan;14(1):67–75.

Nordahl TE, Semple WE, Gross M, Mellman TA, Stein MB, Goyer P, King AC, Uhde TW, Cohen RM. Cerebral glucose metabolic differences in patients with panic disorder. Neuropsychopharmacology 1990 Aug;3(4):261–72.

Norton GR, Harrison B, Hauch J, Rhodes L. Characteristics of people with infrequent panic attacks. J Abnorm Psychol 1985;94(2):216–21.

Noyes R. Is panic disorder a disease for the medical model? Psychosomatics 1987 Nov;28 (11):582–4, 586.

Noyes R, Reich J, Clancy J, O'Gorman TW. Reduction in hypochondriasis with treatment of panic disorder [published erratum appears in Br J Psychiatry 1987 Feb;150:273]. Br J Psychiatry 1986 Nov;149:631–5.

Noyes R Jr. The comorbidity and mortality of panic disorder. Psychiatr Med 1990;8(2):41–66.

Noyes R Jr, Clancy J, Garvey MJ, Anderson DJ. Is agoraphobia a variant of panic disorder or a separate illness? J Anxiety Disord 1987;1(1):3–13.

Noyes R Jr, Cook B, Garvey M, Summers R. Reduction of gastrointestinal symptoms following treatment for panic disorder. Psychosomatics 1990 Winter;31(1):75–9.

Noyes R Jr, Crowe RR, Harris EL, Hamra BJ, McChesney CM, Chaudhry DR. Relationship between panic disorder and agoraphobia. A family study. Arch Gen Psychiatry 1986 Mar;43(3):227–32.

Noyes R Jr, Reich J, Christiansen J, Suelzer M, Pfohl B, Coryell WA. Outcome of panic disorder. Relationship to diagnostic subtypes and comorbidity. Arch Gen Psychiatry 1990 Sep;47(9):809–18.

Nutzinger DO, Zapotoczky HG. The influence of depression on the outcome of cardiac phobia (panic disorder). Psychopathology 1985;18(2-3):155–62.

Oei TP, Gross PR, Evans L. Phobic disorders and anxiety states: how do they differ? Aust N Z J Psychiatry 1989 Mar;23(1):81–8.

Oei TPS, Wanstall K, Evans L. Sex differences in panic disorder with agoraphobia. J Anxiety Disord 1990;4(4):317–24.

Ontiveros A, Fontaine R. Panic attacks and multiple sclerosis. Biol Psychiatry 1990 Mar;27(6):672–3.

Ontiveros A, Fontaine R, Breton G, Elie R, et al. Correlation of severity of panic disorder and neuroanatomical changes on magnetic resonance imaging. J Neuropsychiatry Clin Neurosci 1989 Fall;1(4):404–8.

Orenstein H, Peskind A, Raskind MA. Thyroid disorders in female psychiatric patients with panic disorder or agoraphobia. Am J Psychiatry 1988 Nov;145(11):1428–30.

Orsini A, Sciuto G, Smeraldi E. A familial validation of dissection between panic and generalized anxiety disorders. New Trends Exp Clin Psychiatry 1990;6(2):69–77.

Ottaviani R, Beck RT. Cognitive aspects of panic disorders. J Anxiety Disord 1987;1(1):15–28.

Overall JE, Sheehan DV. Multivariate analysis of changes in panic frequency counts. Clin Neuropharmacol 1986;9 Suppl 4:155–7.

Pain MC, Biddle N, Tiller JW. Panic disorder, the ventilatory response to carbon dioxide and respiratory variables. Psychosom Med 1988 Sep-Oct;50(5):541–8.

Papp LA, Goetz R, Cole R, Klein DF, Jordan F, Liebowitz MR, Fyer AJ, Hollander E, Gorman JM. Hypersensitivity to carbon dioxide in panic disorder. Am J Psychiatry 1989 Jun;146(6):779–81.

Papp LA, Martinez JM, Klein DF, Ross D, Liebowitz MR, Fyer AJ, Hollander E, Gorman JM. Arterial blood gas changes in panic disorder and lactate-induced panic. Psychiatry Res 1989 May;28(2):171–80.

Paulsen AS, Crowe RR, Noyes R, Pfohl B. Reliability of the telephone interview in diagnosing anxiety disorders. Arch Gen Psychiatry 1988 Jan;45(1):62–3.

Pecknold JC, Chang H, Fleury D, Koszychi D, Quirion R, Nair NP, Suranyi-Cadotte BE. Platelet imipramine binding in patients with panic disorder and major familial depression. J Psychiatr Res 1987;21(3):319–26.

Pecknold JC, Luthe L. Sleep studies and neurochemical correlates in panic disorder and agoraphobia. Prog Neuropsychopharmacol Biol Psychiatry 1990;14(5):753–8.

Pecknold JC, Suranyi-Cadotte B, Chang H, Nair NP. Serotonin uptake in panic disorder and agoraphobia. Neuropsychopharmacology 1988 May;1(2):173–6.

Perugi G, Deltito J, Soriani A, Musetti L, Petracca A, Nisita C, Maremmani I, Cassano GB. Relationships between panic disorder and separation anxiety with school phobia. Compr Psychiatry 1988 Mar–Apr;29(2):98–107.

Peters JC, Alpert M, Beitman BD, Kushner M, Webel R. Panic disorder associated with permanent pacemaker implantation. Psychosomatics 1990 Summer;31(3):345–7.

Pohl R, Yeragani VK, Balon R, Rainey JM, Lycaki H, Ortiz A, Berchou R, Weinberg P. Isoproterenol-induced panic attacks. Biol Psychiatry 1988 Dec;24(8):891–902.

Pollack MH, Otto MW, Rosenbaum JF, Sachs GS, O'Neil C, Asher R, Meltzer-Brody S. Longitudinal course of panic disorder: findings from the Massachusetts General Hospital Naturalistic Study. J Clin Psychiatry 1990 Dec;51 Suppl A:12–6.

Pollard CA, Cox GL. Social-evaluative anxiety in panic disorder and agoraphobia. Psychol Rep 1988 Feb;62(1):323–6.

Pollard CA, Detrick P, Flynn T, Frank M. Panic attacks and related disorders in alcohol-dependent, depressed, and nonclinical samples. J Nerv Ment Dis 1990 Mar;178(3):180–5.

Pollock C, Andrews G. Defense styles associated with specific anxiety disorders. Am J Psychiatry 1989 Nov;146(11):1500–2.

Rachman S, Levitt K. Panics and their consequences. Behav Res Ther 1985;23(5):585–600.

Rachman S, Levitt K, Lopatka C. A simple method for distinguishing between expected and unexpected panics. Behav Res Ther 1987;25(2):149–54.

Rachman S, Levitt K, Lopatka C. Experimental analyses of panic. III. Claustrophobic subjects. Behav Res Ther 1988;26(1):41–52.

Rachman S, Lopatka C, Levitt K. Experimental analyses of panic. II. Panic patients. Behav Res Ther 1988;26(1):33–40.

Raj A, Sheehan DV. Mitral valve prolapse and panic disorder. Bull Menninger Clin 1990 Spring;54(2):199–208.

Rapaport MH, Risch SC, Gillin JC, Golshan S, Janowsky DS. Blunted growth hormone response to peripheral infusion of human growth hormone-releasing factor in patients with panic disorder. Am J Psychiatry 1989 Jan;146(1):92–5.

Rapee R. Differential response to hyperventilation in panic disorder and generalized anxiety disorder. J Abnorm Psychol 1986;95(1):24–8.

Rapee RM. Distinctions between panic disorder and generalized anxiety disorder: clinical presentation. Aust N Z J Psychiatry 1985 Sep;19(3):227–32.

Rapee RM, Ancis JR, Barlow DH. Emotional reactions to physiological sensations: Panic disorder patients and non-clinical Ss. Behav Res Ther 1988;26(3):265–9.

Rapee RM, Craske MG, Barlow DH. Subject-described features of panic attacks using self-monitoring. J Anxiety Disord 1990;4(2):171–81.

Raymond C. Chest pain not always what it seems; panic disorder may be cause in some. JAMA 1989 Feb 24;261(8):1101–2.

Reich J. DSM-III personality disorders and family history of mental illness. J Nerv Ment Dis 1988 Jan;176(1):45–9.

Reich J, Chaudry D. Personality of panic disorder alcohol abusers. J Nerv Ment Dis 1987 Apr;175(4):224–8.

Reich J, Noyes R, Yates W. Anxiety symptoms distinguishing social phobia from panic and generalized anxiety disorders. J Nerv Ment Dis 1988 Aug;176(8):510–3.

Reich J, Noyes R Jr, Coryell W, O'Gorman TW. The effect of state anxiety on personality measurement. Am J Psychiatry 1986 Jun;143(6):760–3.

Reich J, Noyes R Jr, Hirschfeld R, Coryell W, O'Gorman T. State and personality in depressed and panic patients. Am J Psychiatry 1987 Feb;144(2):181–7.

Reich J, Noyes R Jr, Troughton E. Dependent personality disorder associated with phobic avoidance in patients with panic disorder. Am J Psychiatry 1987 Mar;144(3):323–6.

Reich J, Troughton E. Comparison of DSM-III personality disorders in recovered depressed and panic disorder patients. J Nerv Ment Dis 1988 May;176(5):300–4.

Reich J, Troughton E. Frequency of DSM-III personality disorders in patients with panic disorder: comparison with psychiatric and normal control subjects. Psychiatry Res 1988 Oct;26(1):89–100.

Reich JH. DSM-III personality disorders and the outcome of treated panic disorder. Am J Psychiatry 1988 Sep;145(9):1149–52.

Reich JH, Green AI. Effect of personality disorders on outcome of treatment. J Nerv Ment Dis 1991 Feb;179(2):74–82.

Reich P. Panic attacks and the risk of suicide [editorial]. N Engl J Med 1989 Nov 2;321(18):1260–1.

Reiman EM. The study of panic disorder using positron emission tomography. Psychiatr Dev 1987 Spring;5(1):63–78.

Reiman EM, Raichle ME, Robins E, Mintun MA, Fusselman MJ, Fox PT, Price JL, Hackman KA. Neuroanatomical correlates of a lactate-induced anxiety attack. Arch Gen Psychiatry 1989 Jun;46(6):493–500.

Rickels K, Schweizer E, Case WG. The uncontrolled case report: A double-edged sword. J Nerv Ment Dis 1988 Jan;176(1):50–2.

Rifkin A, Nakai BS. Difficulty walking as a symptom of panic disorder. Comp Psychiatry 1987 Sep-Oct;28(5):428–9.

Rosenbaum JF. Limited-symptom panic attacks. Psychosomatics 1987 Aug;28(8):407–12.

Rosenberg NK, Andersen R. Rorschach-profile in panic disorder. Scand J Psychol 1990;31(2):99–109.

Rosenberg R, Bech P, Plenge P, et al. MAO activity and ^{3}H-imipramine binding in platelets from patients with panic disorder. Nord Psykiatr Tidsskr 1986;40(6):440.

Rosenberg R, Bech P, Mellergard M, Ottosson J-O. Secondary depression in panic disorder: An indicator of severity with a weak effect on outcome in alprazolam and imipramine treatment. Acta Psychiatr Scand Suppl 1991;83(365):39–45.

Rosenberg R, Ottosson J-O, Bech P, Mellergard M, Rosenberg NK. Validation criteria for panic disorders as a nosological entity. Acta Psychiatr Scand Suppl 1991;83(365):7–17.

Rosenblat H. Panic attacks triggered by photic stimulation. Am J Psychiatry 1989 Jun;146(6):801–2.

Roth WT, Ehlers A, Taylor CB, Margraf J, Agras WS. Skin conductance habituation in panic disorder patients. Biol Psychiatry 1990 Jun 1;27(11):1231–43.

Roy-Byrne PP, Bierer LM, Uhde TW. The dexamethasone suppression test in panic disorder: Comparison with normal controls. Biol Psychiatry 1985;20(11):1237–40.

Roy-Byrne PP, Cowley DS, Greenblatt DJ, Shader RI, Hommer D. Reduced benzodiazepine sensitivity in panic disorder. Arch Gen Psychiatry 1990 Jun;47(6):534–8.

Roy-Byrne PP, Lewis N, Villacres E, Diem H, Greenblatt DJ, Shader RI, Veith R. Preliminary evidence of benzodiazepine subsensitivity in panic disorder. Biol Psychiatry 1989 Nov;26(7):744–8.

Roy-Byrne PP, Mellman TA, Uhde TW. Biologic findings in panic disorder: neuroendocrine and sleep-related abnormalities. J Anxiety Disord 1988;2(1):17–29.

Roy-Byrne PP, Schmidt P, Cannon RO, Diem H, Rubinow DR. Microvascular angina and panic disorder. Int J Psychiatry Med 1989;19(4):315–25.

Roy-Byrne PP, Uhde TW. Panic disorder and major depression: Biological relationships. Psychopharmacol Bull 1985;21(3):551–4.

Roy-Byrne PP, Uhde TW, Gold PW, Rubinow DR, Post RM. Neuroendocrine abnormalities in panic disorder. Psychopharmacol Bull 1985;21(3):546–50.

Roy-Byrne PP, Uhde TW, Post RM. Effects of one night's sleep deprivation on mood and behavior in panic disorder. Patients with panic disorder compared with depressed patients and normal controls. Arch Gen Psychiatry 1986 Sep;43(9):895–9.

Roy-Byrne PP, Uhde TW, Post RM, Gallucci W, Chrousos GP, Gold PW. The corticotropin-releasing hormone stimulation test in patients with panic disorder. Am J Psychiatry 1986 Jul;143(7):896–9.

Roy-Byrne P, Uhde TW, Post RM, King AC, Buchsbaum MS. Normal pain sensitivity in patients with panic disorder. Psychiatry Res 1985 Jan;14(1):77–84.

Roy-Byrne PP, Uhde TW, Rubinow DR, Post RM. Reduced TSH and prolactin responses to TRH in patients with panic disorder. Am J Psychiatry 1986 Apr;143(4):503–7.

Roy-Byrne PP, Uhde TW, Sack DA, Linnoila M, Post RM. Plasma HVA and anxiety in patients with panic disorder. Biol Psychiatry 1986 Jul;21(8–9):849–53.

Russell JL, Kushner MG, Beitman BD, Bartels KM. Nonfearful panic disorder in neurology patients validated by lactate challenge. Am J Psychiatry 1991 Mar;148(3):361–4.

Sabelli HC, Javaid JI, Fawcett J, Kravitz HM, Wynn P. Urinary phenylacetic acid in panic disorder with and without depression. Acta Psychiatr Scand 1990 Jul;82(1):14–6.

Salkovskis PM, Warwick HMC, Clark DM, Wessels DJ. A demonstration of acute hyperventilation during naturally occurring panic attacks. Behav Res Ther 1986;24(1):91–4.

Sanderson WC, Rapee RM, Barlow DH. Panic induction via inhalation of 5.5% CO_2 enriched air: a single subject analysis of psychological and physiological effects. Behav Res Ther 1988;26(4):333–5.

Sanderson WC, Wetzler S. Five percent carbon dioxide challenge: valid analogue and marker of panic disorder? Biol Psychiatry 1990 Apr 1;27(7):689–701.

Scharfman EL. "Relaxation–induced panic (RIP): When resting isn't peaceful": Commentary. Integr Psychiatry 1987 Jun;5(2):110–2.

Schittecatte M, Charles G, Depauw Y, Mesters P, Wilmotte J. Growth hormone response to clonidine in panic disorder patients. Psychiatry Res 1988 Feb;23(2):147–51.

Schneider LS, Munjack D, Severson JA, Palmer R. Platelet [3H]imipramine binding in generalized anxiety disorder, panic disorder, and agoraphobia with panic attacks. Biol Psychiatry 1987 Jan;22(1):59–66.

Schneier FR, Fyer AJ, Martin LY, Ross D, Mannuzza S, Liebowitz MR, Gorman JM, Klein DF. A comparison of phobic subtypes within panic disorder. J Anxiety Disord 1991;5(1):65–75.

Schweizer E, Winokur A, Rickels K. Insulin-induced hypoglycemia and panic attacks. Am J Psychiatry 1986 May;143(5):654–5.

Scrignar CB. Postpanic anxiety disorder: diagnosis and treatment. South Med J 1986 Apr;79(4):400–4.

Seibyl JP, Krystal JH, Charney DS. Marijuana (cannabis) use is anecdotally said to precipitate anxiety symptoms in patients with panic disorder. Is there any research evidence to support this? Also, can marijuana use precipitate or expose paranoia in patients with an underlying bipolar disorder? J Clin Psychopharmacol 1990 Feb;10(1):78.

Shear MK, Kligfield P, Harshfield G, Devereux RB, Polan JJ, Mann JJ, Pickering T, Frances AJ. Cardiac rate and rhythm in panic patients. Am J Psychiatry 1987 May;144(5):633–7.

Sheehan DV, Carr DB, Fishman SM, Walsh MM, Peltier-Saxe D. Lactate infusion in anxiety research: its evolution and practice. J Clin Psychiatry 1985 May;46(5):158–65.

Siegel L, Jones WC, Wilson JO. Economic and life consequences experienced by a group of individuals with panic disorder. J Anxiety Disord 1990;4(3):201–11.

Sietsema KE, Simon JI, Wasserman K. Pulmonary hypertension presenting as a panic disorder. Chest 1987 Jun;91(6):910–2.

Sklare DA, Stein MB, Pikus AM, Uhde TW. Disequilibrium and audiovestibular function in panic disorder: symptom profiles and test findings. Am J Otol 1990 Sep;11(5):338–41.

Spitz MC. Panic disorder in seizure patients: a diagnostic pitfall. Epilepsia 1991 Jan-Feb;32(1):33–8.

Starcevic V. Pathological fear of death, panic attacks, and hypochondriasis. Am J Psychoanal 1989 Dec;49(4):347–61.

Stein MB. Panic disorder and medical illness. Psychosomatics 1986;27(12):833–40.

Stein MB, Schmidt PJ, Rubinow DR, Uhde TW. Panic disorder and the menstrual cycle: panic disorder patients, healthy control subjects, and patients with premenstrual syndrome. Am J Psychiatry 1989 Oct;146(10):1299–303.

Stein MB, Shea CA, Uhde TW. Social phobic symptoms in patients with panic disorder: practical and theoretical implications. Am J Psychiatry 1989 Feb;146(2):235–8.

Stein MB, Tancer ME, Uhde TW. Major depression in patients with panic disorder: factors associated with course and recurrence. J Affective Disord 1990 Aug;19(4):287–96.

Stein MB, Uhde TW. Autoimmune thyroiditis and panic disorder. Am J Psychiatry 1989 Feb;146(2):259–60.

Stein MB, Uhde TW. Endocrine, cardiovascular, and behavioral effects of intravenous protirelin in patients with panic disorder. Arch Gen Psychiatry 1991 Feb;48(2):148–56.

Stein MB, Uhde TW. Panic disorder and major depression. A tale of two syndromes [published erratum appears in Psychiatr Clin North Am 1988 Dec;11(4):following vii]. Psychiatr Clin North Am 1988 Jun;11(2):441–61.

Stein MB, Uhde TW. Thyroid indices in panic disorder. Am J Psychiatry 1988 Jun;145(6):745–7.

Stewart RS, Devous MD Sr, Rush AJ, Lane L, Bonte FJ. Cerebral blood flow changes during sodium-lactate-induced panic attacks. Am J Psychiatry 1988 Apr;145(4):442–9.

Stewart WF, Linet MS, Celentano DD. Migraine headaches and panic attacks. Psychosom Med 1989 Sep-Oct;51(5):559–69.

Street LL, Craske MG, Barlow DH. Sensations, cognitions and the perception of cues associated with expected and unexpected panic attacks. Behav Res Ther 1989;27(2):189–98.

Szuster RR, Pontius EB, Campos PE. Marijuana sensitivity and panic anxiety. J Clin Psychiatry 1988 Nov;49(11):427–9.

Tancer ME, Stein MB, Moul DE, Uhde TW. Normal serum cholesterol in panic disorder. Biol Psychiatry 1990 Jan 1;27(1):99–101.

Tancer ME, Stein MB, Uhde TW. Effects of thyrotropin-releasing hormone on blood pressure and heart rate in phobic and panic patients: a pilot study. Biol Psychiatry 1990 Apr 1;27(7):781–3.

Tancer ME, Stein MB, Uhde TW. Paradoxical growth-hormone responses to thyrotropin-releasing hormone in panic disorder. Biol Psychiatry 1990 Jun 1;27(11):1227–30.

Targum SD. Differential responses to anxiogenic challenge studies in patients with major depressive disorder and panic disorder. Biol Psychiatry 1990 Jul 1;28(1):21–34.

Targum SD. Panic attack frequency and vulnerability to anxiogenic challenge studies. Psychiatry Res 1991 Jan;36(1):75–83.

Tavel ME. Hyperventilation syndrome—hiding behind pseudonyms? Chest 1990 Jun;97(6):1285–8.

Taylor CB, King R, Ehlers A, Margraf J, Clark D, Hayward C, Roth WT, Agras S. Treadmill exercise test and ambulatory measures in panic attacks. Am J Cardiol 1987 Dec 28;60(18):48J–52J.

Taylor CB, Sheikh J, Agras WS, Roth WT, Margraf J, Ehlers A, Maddock RJ, Gossard D. Ambulatory heart rate changes in patients with panic attacks. Am J Psychiatry 1986 Apr;143(4):478–82.

Telch MJ, Lucas JA, Nelson P. Nonclinical panic in college students: an investigation of prevalence and symptomatology. J Abnorm Psychol 1989 Aug;98(3):300–6.

Thompson AH, Bland RC, Orn HT. Relationship and chronology of depression, agoraphobia, and panic disorder in the general population. J Nerv Ment Dis 1989 Aug;177 (8):456–63.

Thyer BA, Himle J, Curtis GC, et al. A comparison of panic disorder and agoraphobia with panic attacks. Compr Psychiatry 1985;26(2):208–14.

Thyer BA, Parrish RT, Himle J, et al. Case histories and shorter communications. Alcohol abuse among clinically anxious patients. Behav Res Ther 1986;24(3):357–359.

Turner SM, McCann BS, Beidel DC, Mezzich JE. DSM-III classification of the anxiety disorders: a psychometric study. J Abnorm Psychol 1986 May;95(2):168–72.

Turner SM, Williams SL, Beidel DC, Mezzich JE. Panic disorder and agoraphobia with panic attacks: Covariation along the dimensions of panic and agoraphobic fear. J Abnorm Psychol 1986;95(4):384–8.

Tyrer P. Classification of anxiety disorders: A critique of DSM-III. J Affect Disord 1986 Sep-Oct;11(2):99–104.

Tyrer P, Seivewright N, Ferguson B, Murphy S, Darling C, Brothwell J, Kingdon D, Johnson AL. The Nottingham Study of Neurotic Disorder: relationship between personality status and symptoms. Psychol Med 1990 May;20(2):423–31.

Uhde TW, Berrettini WH, Roy-Byrne PP, Boulenger JP, Post RM. Platelet [3H]imipramine binding in patients with panic disorder. Biol Psychiatry 1987 Jan;22(1):52–8.

Uhde TW, Boulenger JP, Roy-Byrne PP, Geraci MF, Vittone BJ, Post RM. Longitudinal course of panic disorder: clinical and biological considerations. Prog Neuropsychopharmacol Biol Psychiatry 1985;9(1):39–51.

Uhde TW, Joffe RT, Jimerson DC, Post RM. Normal urinary free cortisol and plasma MHPG in panic disorder: clinical and theoretical implications. Biol Psychiatry 1988 Mar 15;23(6):575–85.

Uhde TW, Kellner CH. Cerebral ventricular size in panic disorder. J Affective Disord 1987 Mar-Apr;12(2):175–8.

Uhde TW, Mellman TA. "Relaxation-induced panic (RIP): When resting isn't peaceful": Commentary. Integr Psychiatry 1987 Jun;5(2):101–4.

van den Hout MA, De Jong P, Zandbergen J, Merckelbach H. Waning of panic sensations during prolonged hyperventilation. Behav Res Ther 1990;28(5):445–8.

van den Hout MA, Griez E, van der Molen GM, Lousberg H. Pulmonary carbon dioxide and panic-arousing sensations after 35% carbon dioxide inhalation: hypercapnia/hyperoxia versus hypercapnia/normoxia. J Behav Ther Exp Psychiatry 1987 Mar;18(1):19–23.

van den Hout MA, van der Molen GM, Griez E, Lousberg H. Specificity of interoceptive fear to panic disorders. J Psychopathol Behav Assess 1987;9(1):99–106.

Villacres EC, Hollifield M, Katon WJ, Wilkinson CW, Veith RC. Sympathetic nervous system activity in panic disorder. Psychiatry Res 1987 Aug;21(4):313–21.

Vitiello B, Behar D, Wolfson S, McLeer SV. Diagnosis of panic disorder in prepubertal children. J Am Acad Child Adolesc Psychiatry 1990 Sep;29(5):782–4.

von Bardeleben U, Holsboer F. Human corticotropin releasing hormone: clinical studies in patients with affective disorders, alcoholism, panic disorder and in normal controls. Prog Neuropsychopharmacol Biol Psychiatry 1988;12 Suppl:S165–87.

Weiler MA, Val ER, Gaviria M, Prasad RB, Lahmeyer HW, Rodgers P. Panic disorder is borderline personality disorder. Psychiatr J Univ Ott 1988 Sep;13(3):140–3.

Weiss KJ. Panic disorder: fear disguised as medical illness. J Med Soc N J 1985 Feb;82(2):141–2.

Weissman MM. Panic and generalized anxiety: are they separate disorders? J Psychiatr Res 1990;24 Suppl 2:157–62.

Weissman MM. Panic disorder: impact on quality of life. J Clin Psychiatry 1991 Feb;52 Suppl:6–8; discussion 9.

Weissman MM. The hidden patient: unrecognized panic disorder. J Clin Psychiatry 1990 Nov;51 Suppl:5–8.

Weissman MM, Klerman GL, Markowitz JS, Ouellette R. Suicidal ideation and suicide attempts in panic disorder and attacks. N Engl J Med 1989 Nov 2;321(18):1209–14.

Weissman MM, Markowitz JS, Ouellette R, Greenwald S, Kahn JP. Panic disorder and cardiovascular/ cerebrovascular problems: results from a community survey. Am J Psychiatry 1990 Nov;147(11):1504–8.

Weissman NJ, Shear MK, Kramer-Fox R, Devereux RB. Contrasting patterns of autonomic dysfunction in patients with mitral valve prolapse and panic attacks. Am J Med 1987 May;82(5):880–8.

Wetzler S, Kahn RS, Cahn W, van Praag HM, Asnis GM. Psychological test characteristics of depressed and panic patients. Psychiatry Res 1990 Feb;31(2):179–92.

White WB, Baker LH. Ambulatory blood pressure monitoring in patients with panic disorder. Arch Intern Med 1987 Nov;147(11):1973–5.

Whiteford HA, Evans L. Agoraphobia and the dexamethasone suppression test: Atypical depression? Aust N Z J Psychiatry 1984;18(4):374–7.

Woodruff BJ, Clum GA, Broyles SE. MMPI correlates of panic disorder and panic attacks. J Anxiety Disord 1989;3(2):107–15.

Woods SW, Charney DS. Applications of the pharmacologic challenge strategy in panic disorders research. J Anxiety Disord 1988;2(1):31–49.

Woods SW, Charney DS, Delgado PL, Heninger GR. The effect of long-term imipramine treatment on carbon dioxide-induced anxiety in panic disorder patients. J Clin Psychiatry 1990 Dec;51(12):505–7.

Woods SW, Charney DS, Goodman WK, Heninger GR. Carbon dioxide-induced anxiety. Behavioral, physiologic, and biochemical effects of carbon dioxide in patients with panic disorders and healthy subjects. Arch Gen Psychiatry 1988 Jan;45(1):43–52.

Yeragani V, Balon R, Pohl R. Lactate infusions in panic disorder patients and normal controls: autonomic measures and subjective anxiety. Acta Psychiatr Scand 1989 Jan;79 (1):32–40.

Yeragani VK, Balon R, Pohl R, Ortiz A, Weinberg P, Rainey JM. Do higher preinfusion heart rates predict laboratory-induced panic attacks? Biol Psychiatry 1987 May;22(5):554–8.

Yeragani VK, Balon R, Pohl R, Ramesh C, Glitz D, Weinberg P, Merlos B. Decreased R-R variance in panic disorder patients. Acta Psychiatr Scand 1990 Jun;81(6):554–9.

Yeragani VK, Balon R, Rainey JM, Ortiz A, Berchou R, Lycaki H, Pohl R. Effects of laboratory-induced panic-anxiety on subsequent provocative infusions. Psychiatry Res 1988 Feb;23(2):161–6.

Yeragani VK, Meiri PC, Pohl R, Balon R, Desai N, Golec S. Heart rate and blood pressure changes during postural change and isometric handgrip exercise in patients with panic disorder and normal controls. Acta Psychiatr Scand 1990 Jan;81(1):9–13.

Yeragani VK, Pohl R, Balon R, Ramesh C, Glitz D, Sherwood P. Risk factors for cardiovascular illness in panic disorder patients. Neuropsychobiology 1990-91;23(3):134–9.

Yeragani VK, Pohl R, Balon R, Weinberg P, Berchou R, Rainey JM. Preinfusion anxiety predicts lactate-induced panic attacks in normal controls. Psychosom Med 1987 Jul-Aug;49(4):383–9.

Yeragani VK, Pohl R, Rainey JM, Balon R, Ortiz A, Lycaki H, Gershon S. Pre-infusion heart rates and laboratory-induced panic anxiety. Acta Psychiatr Scand 1987 Jan;75(1):51–4.

Yeragani VK, Rainey JM Jr, Pohl R, Balon R, Berchou R, Jolly S, Lycaki H. Preinfusion anxiety and laboratory-induced panic attacks in panic disorder patients. J Clin Psychiatry 1988 Aug;49(8):302–6.

Zander JR, McNally RJ. Bio-informational processing in agoraphobia. Special Issue: A selection of papers to mark The Third World Congress of Behavior Therapy. Behav Res Ther 1988;26(5):421–9.

Zane MD. "Relaxation-induced panic (RIP): When resting isn't peaceful": Commentary. Integr Psychiatry 1987 Jun;5(2):106–8.

Zitrin CM. "Relaxation-induced panic (RIP): When resting isn't peaceful": Commentary. Integr Psychiatry 1987 Dec;5(4):294-5.

Epidemiology

Angst J, Dobler-Mikola A. The Zurich Study. V. Anxiety and phobia in young adults. Eur Arch Psychiatry Neurol Sci 1985;235(3):171–8.

Anthony JC, Tien AY, Petronis KR. Epidemiologic evidence on cocaine use and panic attacks. Am J Epidemiol 1989 Mar;129(3):543–9.

Faravelli C, Guerrini Degl'Innocenti B, Giardinelli L. Epidemiology of anxiety disorders in Florence. Acta Psychiatr Scand 1989 Apr;79(4):308–12.

Joyce PR, Bushnell JA, Oakley-Browne MA, Wells JE, Hornblow AR. The epidemiology of panic symptomatology and agoraphobic avoidance. Compr Psychiatry 1989 Jul-Aug;30(4):303–12.

Karno M, Golding JM, Burnam MA, Hough RL, Escobar JI, Wells KM, Boyer R. Anxiety disorders among Mexican Americans and non-Hispanic whites in Los Angeles. J Nerv Ment Dis 1989 Apr;177(4):202–9.

Karno M, Hough RL, Burnam MA, Escobar JI, Timbers DM, Santana F, Boyd JH. Lifetime prevalence of specific psychiatric disorders among Mexican Americans and non-Hispanic whites in Los Angeles. Arch Gen Psychiatry 1987 Aug;44(8):695–701.

Katon W, Vitaliano PP, Russo J, Cormier L, Anderson K, Jones M. Panic disorder: epidemiology in primary care. J Fam Pract 1986 Sep;23(3):233–9.

Klerman GL, Weissman MM, Ouellette R, Johnson J, Greenwald S. Panic attacks in the community. Social morbidity and health care utilization. JAMA 1991 Feb 13;265(6):742–6.

Lepine JP, Lellouch J, Lovell A, Teherani M, Ha C, Verdier-Taillefer MH, Rambourg N, Lemperiere T. Anxiety and depressive disorders in a French population: methodology and preliminary results. Psychiatr Psychobiol 1989;4(5):267–74.

Lepine JP, Pariente P, Boulenger JP, Hardy P, Zarifian E, Lemperiere T, Lellouch J. Anxiety disorders in a French general psychiatric outpatient sample. Comparison between DSM-III and DSM-III-R criteria. Soc Psychiatry Psychiatr Epidemiol 1989 Nov;24(6):301–8.

Maier W, Buller R. One-year follow-up of panic disorder. Outcome and prognostic factors. Eur Arch Psychiatry Neurol Sci 1988;238(2):105–9.

Markowitz JS, Weissman MM, Ouellette R, Lish JD, Klerman GL. Quality of life in panic disorder. Arch Gen Psychiatry 1989 Nov;46(11):984–92.

Otakpor AN. A prospective study of panic disorder in a Nigerian psychiatric out-patient population. Acta Psychiatr Scand 1987 Nov;76(5):541–4.

Regier DA, Narrow WE, Rae DS. The epidemiology of anxiety disorders: the Epidemiologic Catchment Area (ECA) experience. J Psychiatr Res 1990;24 Suppl 2:3–14.

Reich J. The epidemiology of anxiety. J Nerv Ment Dis 1986 Mar;174(3):129–36.

Salge RA, Beck JG, Logan AC. A community survey of panic. J Anxiety Disord 1988;2(2):157–67.

Stirton RF, Brandon S. Preliminary report of a community survey of panic attacks and panic disorder. J R Soc Med 1988 Jul;81(7):392–3.

Takahashi S, Nakamura M, Iida H, Iritani S, Fujii M, Yamashita Y, Yoichi I. Prevalence of panic disorder and other subtypes of anxiety disorder and their background. Jpn J Psychiatry Neurol 1987 Mar;41(1):9–18.

Thyer BA, Parrish RT, Curtis GC, Nesse RM, Cameron OG. Ages of onset of DSM-III anxiety disorders. Compr Psychiatry 1985 Mar-Apr;26(2):113–22.

Vollrath M, Angst J. Outcome of panic and depression in a seven-year follow-up: results of the Zurich study. Acta Psychiatr Scand 1989 Dec;80(6):591–6.

Vollrath M, Koch R, Angst J. The Zurich Study. IX. Panic disorder and sporadic panic: symptoms, diagnosis, prevalence, and overlap with depression. Eur Arch Psychiatry Neurol Sci 1990;239(4):221–30.

Von Korff MR, Eaton WW, Keyl PM. The epidemiology of panic attacks and panic disorder. Results of three community surveys. Am J Epidemiol 1985 Dec;122(6):970–81.

Weissman MM. Epidemiology of panic disorder and agoraphobia. Psychiatr Med 1990;8(2):3–13.

Weissman MM, Leaf PJ, Blazer DG, Boyd JH, Florio L. The relationship between panic disorder and agoraphobia: an epidemiologic perspective. Psychopharmacol Bull 1986;22(3):787–91.

Weissman MM, Leaf PJ, Holzer CE 3d, Merikangas KR. The epidemiology of anxiety disorders: a highlight of recent evidence. Psychopharmacol Bull 1985;21(3):538–41.

Weissman MM, Merikangas KR. The epidemiology of anxiety and panic disorders: an update. J Clin Psychiatry 1986 Jun;47 Suppl:11–7.

Zgourides GD, Warren R. Prevalence of panic in adolescents: a brief report. Psychol Rep 1988 Jun;62(3):935–7.

Etiology and Maintenance

Aronson TA, Logue CM. On the longitudinal course of panic disorder: development history and predictors of phobic complications. Compr Psychiatry 1987 Jul-Aug;28(4):344–55.

Aronson TA, Whitaker-Azmitia P, Caraseti I. Differential reactivity to lactate infusions: the relative role of biological, psychological, and conditioning variables. Biol Psychiatry 1989 Feb 15;25(4):469–81.

Ayuso JL, Alfonso S, Rivera A. Childhood separation anxiety and panic disorder: a comparative study. Prog Neuropsychopharmacol Biol Psychiatry 1989;13(5):665–71.

Ballenger JC. Toward an integrated model of panic disorder. Am J Orthopsychiatry 1989 Apr;59(2):284–93.

Balon R, Jordan M, Pohl R, Yeragani VK. Family history of anxiety disorders in control subjects with lactate-induced panic attacks. Am J Psychiatry 1989 Oct;146(10):1304–6.

Bass C, Gardner W. Emotional influences on breathing and breathlessness. J Psychosom Res 1985;29(6):599–609.

Baum M. An animal model for situational panic attacks. Behav Res Ther 1986;24(5):509–12.

Ben-Noun L. Mitral valve prolapse syndrome, panic disorder and agoraphobia. Practitioner 1989 Mar 22;233(1465):379–80.

Brown SL, Charney DS, Woods SW, Heninger GR, Tallman J. Lymphocyte beta-adrenergic receptor binding in panic disorder. Psychopharmacology (Berlin) 1988;94(1):24–8.

Burrows GD, Judd FK, Hopper JL. The biology of panic-genetic evidence. Int J Clin Pharmacol Res 1989;9(2):147–9.

Cameron OG, Nesse RM. Systemic hormonal and physiological abnormalities in anxiety disorders. Psychoneuroendocrinology 1988;13(4):287–307.

Cameron OG, Smith CB, Lee MA, Hollingsworth PJ, Hill EM, Curtis GC. Adrenergic status in anxiety disorders: platelet alpha 2-adrenergic receptor binding, blood pressure, pulse, and plasma catecholamines in panic and generalized anxiety disorder patients and in normal subjects. Biol Psychiatry 1990 Jul 1;28(1):3–20.

Carney RM, Freedland KE, Ludbrook PA, Saunders RD, Jaffe AS. Major depression, panic disorder, and mitral valve prolapse in patients who complain of chest pain. Am J Med 1990 Dec;89(6):757–60.

Charney DS, Heninger GR. Abnormal regulation of noradrenergic function in panic disorders. Effects of clonidine in healthy subjects and patients with agoraphobia and panic disorder. Arch Gen Psychiatry 1986 Nov;43(11):1042–54.

Charney DS, Heninger GR, Jatlow PI. Increased anxiogenic effects of caffeine in panic disorders. Arch Gen Psychiatry 1985 Mar;42(3):233–43.

Charney DS, Innis RB, Duman RS, Woods SW, Heninger GR. Platelet alpha-2-receptor binding and adenylate cyclase activity in panic disorder. Psychopharmacology (Berlin) 1989;98(1):102–7.

Charney DS, Woods SW, Goodman WK, Heninger GR. Neurobiological mechanisms of panic anxiety: biochemical and behavioral correlates of yohimbine-induced panic attacks. Am J Psychiatry 1987 Aug;144(8):1030–6.

Charney DS, Woods SW, Goodman WK, Heninger GR. Serotonin function in anxiety. II. Effects of the serotonin agonist MCPP in panic disorder patients and healthy subjects. Psychopharmacology (Berlin) 1987;92(1):14–24.

Charney DS, Woods SW, Nagy LM, Southwick SM, Krystal JH, Heninger GR. Noradrenergic function in panic disorder. J Clin Psychiatry 1990 Dec;51 Suppl A:5–11.

Coulehan JL. Mitral valve prolapse as metaphor. Perspect Biol Med 1988 Winter;31(2):252–9.

Cowley DS, Roy-Byrne PP. Psychosocial aspects. Psychiatr Ann 1988 Aug;18(8):464–7.

Craske MG, Barlow DH. Nocturnal panic: response to hyperventilation and carbon dioxide challenges. J Abnorm Psychol 1990 Aug;99(3):302–7.

Crowe RR. Mitral valve prolapse and panic disorder. Psychiatr Clin North Am 1985 Mar;8(1):63–71.

Crowe RR. Panic disorder: genetic considerations. J Psychiatr Res 1990;24 Suppl 2:129–34.

Crowe RR. The genetics of panic disorder and agoraphobia. Psychiatr Dev 1985 Summer;3(2):171–85.

Crowe RR, Noyes R Jr, Wilson AF, Elston RC, Ward LJ. A linkage study of panic disorder. Arch Gen Psychiatry 1987 Nov;44(11):933–7.

Crowe RR, Noyes R Jr, Samuelson S, Wesner R, Wilson R. Close linkage between panic disorder and alpha-haptoglobin excluded in 10 families. Arch Gen Psychiatry 1990 Apr;47(4):377–80.

Crowe RR, Noyes R Jr, Persico AM. Pro-opiomelanocortin (POMC) gene excluded as a cause of panic disorder in a large family. J Affective Disord 1987 Jan-Feb;12(1):23–7.

Dager SR, Saal AK, Comess KA, Dunner DL. Mitral valve prolapse and the anxiety disorders. Hosp Community Psychiatry 1988 May;39(5):517–27.

De Loof C, Zandbergen J, Lousberg H, Pols H, Griez E. The role of life events in the onset of panic disorder. Behav Res Ther 1989;27(4):461–3.

de Montigny C. Cholecystokinin tetrapeptide induces panic-like attacks in healthy volunteers. Preliminary findings. Arch Gen Psychiatry 1989 Jun;46(6):511–7.

Deltito JA, Argyle N, Buller R, Nutzinger D, Ottosson JO, Brandon S, Mellergard M, Shera D. The sequence of improvement of the symptoms encountered in patients with panic disorder. Compr Psychiatry 1991 Mar-Apr;32(2):120–9.

Den Boer JA, Westenberg HG. Behavioral, neuroendocrine, and biochemical effects of 5-hydroxytryptophan administration in panic disorder. Psychiatry Res 1990 Mar;31(3) :267–78.

Den Boer JA, Westenberg HG, Verhoeven WM. Biological aspects of panic anxiety. Psychiatric Ann 1990 Sep;20(9):494–500, 502.

Edlund MJ, Swann AC, Davis CM. Plasma MHPG in untreated panic disorder. Biol Psychiatry 1987 Dec;22(12):1491–5.

Ehlers A, Margraf J, Roth WT, Taylor CB, Birbaumer N. Anxiety induced by false heart rate feedback in patients with panic disorder. Behav Res Ther 1988;26(1):1–11.

Evans L. Some biological aspects of panic disorder. Int J Clin Pharmacol Res 1989;9(2):139–45.

Familial analysis of panic disorder and agoraphobia. Gruppo Italiano Disturbi d'Ansia. J Affective Disord 1989 Jul-Aug;17(1):1–8.

Faravelli C. Life events preceding the onset of panic disorder. J Affective Disord 1985 Jul;9(1):103–5.

Faravelli C, Pallanti S. Recent life events and panic disorder. Am J Psychiatry 1989 May;146(5):622–6.

Fontaine R, Breton G, Dery R, Fontaine S, Elie R. Temporal lobe abnormalities in panic disorder: an MRI study. Biol Psychiatry 1990 Feb 1;27(3):304–10.

Fontana DJ, Carbary TJ, Commissaris RL. Effects of acute and chronic anti-panic drug administration on conflict behavior in the rat. Psychopharmacology (Berlin) 1989;98(2):157–62.

Fontana DJ, Commissaris RL. Effects of acute and chronic imipramine administration on conflict behavior in the rat: a potential "animal model" for the study of panic disorder? Psychopharmacology (Berlin) 1988;95(2):147–50.

Friedman S, Sunderland GS, Rosenblum LA. A nonhuman primate model of panic disorder. Psychiatry Res 1988 Jan;23(1):65–75.

Fyer AJ, Liebowitz MR, Gorman JM, Davies SO, Klein DF. Lactate vulnerability of remitted panic patients. Psychiatry Res 1985 Feb;14(2):143–8.

Gelder MG. Panic attacks: new approaches to an old problem. Br J Psychiatry 1986 Sep;149:346–52.

Gentil V. Towards an integrated model for panic disorder. Stress Med 1988;4(3):131–4.

George DT, Adinoff B, Ravitz B, Nutt DJ, De Jong J, Berrettini W, Mefford IN, Costa E, Linnoila M. A cerebrospinal fluid study of the pathophysiology of panic disorder associated with alcoholism. Acta Psychiatr Scand 1990 Jul;82(1):1–7.

George DT, Nutt DJ, Walker WV, Porges SW, Adinoff B, Linnoila M. Lactate and hyperventilation substantially attenuate vagal tone in normal volunteers. A possible mechanism of panic provocation? Arch Gen Psychiatry 1989 Feb;46(2):153–6.

Gold PW, Pigott TA, Kling MA, Kalogeras K, Chrousos GP. Basic and clinical studies with corticotropin-releasing hormone. Implications for a possible role in panic disorder. Psychiatr Clin North Am 1988 Jun;11(2):327–34.

Gorman J, Liebowitz MR, Fyer AJ, Levitt M, Baron M, Davies S, Klein DF. Platelet mono-amine oxidase activity in patients with panic disorder. Biol Psychiatry 1985 Aug;20(8):852–7.

Gorman JM. "Relaxation-induced panic (RIP): When resting isn't peaceful": Commentary. Integr Psychiatry 1987 Jun;5(2):100–1.

Gorman JM, Fyer MR, Goetz R, Askanazi J, Liebowitz MR, Fyer AJ, Kinney J, Klein DF. Ventilatory physiology of patients with panic disorder [published erratum appears in Arch Gen Psychiatry 1991 Feb;48(2):181]. Arch Gen Psychiatry 1988 Jan;45(1):31–9.

Gorman JM, Goetz RR, Fyer M, King DL, Fyer AJ, Liebowitz MR, Klein DF. The mitral valve prolapse—panic disorder connection. Psychosom Med 1988 Mar-Apr;50(2):114–22.

Gorman JM, Liebowitz MR, Fyer AJ, Stein J. A neuroanatomical hypothesis for panic disorder. Am J Psychiatry 1989 Feb;146(2):148–61.

Gorman JM, Shear MK, Devereaux RB, King DL, Klein DF. Prevalence of mitral valve prolapse in panic disorder: effect of echocardiographic criteria. Psychosom Med 1986 Mar-Apr;48(3-4):167–71.

Gottlieb SH. Mitral valve prolapse: from syndrome to disease. Am J Cardiol 1987 Dec 28;60(18):53J–58J.

Griez E, Zandbergen J, Lousberg H, van den Hout M. Effects of low pulmonary CO2 on panic anxiety. Compr Psychiatry 1988 Sep-Oct;29(5):490–7.

Gurguis GN, Uhde TW. Effect of yohimbine on plasma homovanillic acid in panic disorder patients and normal controls. Biol Psychiatry 1990 Aug 15;28(4):292–6.

Gurguis GN, Uhde TW. Plasma 3-methoxy-4-hydroxyphenylethylene glycol (MHPG) and growth hormone responses to yohimbine in panic disorder patients and normal con-trols. Psychoneuroendocrinology 1990;15(3):217–24.

Heninger GR, Charney DS. Monoamine receptor systems and anxiety disorders. Psychiatr Clin North Am 1988 Jun;11(2):309–26.

Heninger GR, Charney DS, Price LH. Noradrenergic and serotonergic receptor system function in panic disorder and depression. Acta Psychiatr Scand Suppl 1988;341:138–50.

Hibbert G, Pilsbury D. Hyperventilation: is it a cause of panic attacks? Br J Psychiatry 1989 Dec;155: 805–9.

Hickie I, Silove D. A family panics. Aust N Z J Psychiatry 1989 Sep;23(3):418–21.

Holt PE, Andrews G. Provocation of panic: three elements of the panic reaction in four anxiety disorders. Behav Res Ther 1989;27(3):253–61.

Hopper JL, Judd FK, Derrick PL, Macaskill GT, Burrows GD. A family study of panic disorder: reanalysis using a regressive logistic model that incorporates a sibship environ-ment. Genet Epidemiol 1990;7(2):151–61.

Hopper JL, Judd FK, Derrick PL, Burrows GD. A family study of panic disorder. Genet Epidemiol 1987;4(1):33–41.

Humble M. Etiology and mechanisms of anxiety disorders. Acta Psychiatr Scand Suppl 1987;335:15–30.

Judd FK, Burrows GD, Hay DA. Genetic aspects of panic disorder. Aust N Z J Psychiatry 1987;21:197–210.

Judd FK, Burrows GD, Hay DA. Panic disorder: evidence for genetic vulnerability. Aust N Z J Psychiatry 1987 Jun;21(2):197–208.

Kagan BL. A molecular mechanism of panic attacks. Specul Sci Technol 1989;12(3):199–208.

Kahn JP, Gorman JM, King DL, Fyer AJ, Liebowitz MR, Klein DF. Cardiac left ventricular hypertrophy and chamber dilatation in panic disorder patients: implications for idiopathic dilated cardiomyopathy. Psychiatry Res 1990 Apr;32(1):55–61.

Kahn RS, Asnis GM, Wetzler S, van Praag HM. Neuroendocrine evidence for serotonin receptor hypersensitivity in panic disorder. Psychopharmacology (Berlin) 1988;96(3):360–4.

Kahn RS, Van Praag HM. A serotonin hypothesis of panic disorder. Hum Psychopharmacol 1988;3(4):285–8.

Kahn RS, Van Praag HM. Panic disorder: A presynaptic serotonin defect? Psychiatry Res 1990 Feb;31(2):209–10.

Kahn RS, Wetzler S, van Praag HM, Asnis GM, Strauman T. Behavioral indications for serotonin receptor hypersensitivity in panic disorder. Psychiatry Res 1988 Jul;25(1):101–4.

Katerndahl DA. Comparison of panic symptom sequences and pathophysiologic models. J Behav Ther Exp Psychiatry 1990 Jun;21(2):101–11.

Kenardy J, Evans L, Oei TPS. Cognitions and heart rate in panic disorders during everyday activity. J Anxiety Disord 1989;3(1):33–43.

Kenardy J, Oei Tian P, Ryan P, Evans L. Attribution of panic attacks: Patient perspective. J Anxiety Disord 1988;2(3):243–51.

Kenardy J, Oei TP, Evans L. Hyperventilation and panic attacks. Aust N Z J Psychiatry 1990 Jun;24(2):261–7.

Klein DF, Gorman JM. A model of panic and agoraphobic development. Acta Psychiatr Scand Suppl 1987;335:87–95.

Knott VJ. Neuroelectrical activity related to panic disorder. Prog Neuropsychopharmacol Biol Psychiatry 1990;14(5):697–707.

Leckman JF, Weissman MM, Merikangas KR, Pauls DL, Prusoff BA, Kidd KK. Major depression and panic disorder: a family study perspective. Psychopharmacol Bull 1985;21(3):543–5.

Lelliott P, Marks I, McNamee G, Tobena A. Onset of panic disorder with agoraphobia. Toward an integrated model. Arch Gen Psychiatry 1989 Nov;46(11):1000–4.

Leonard BE. Changes in biogenic amine neurotransmitters in panic disorder. Stress Med 1990;6(4):267–74.

Levinson HN. The cerebellar-vestibular predisposition to anxiety disorders. Percept Mot Skills 1989 Feb;68(1):323–38.

Ley R. Hyperventilation and lactate infusion in the production of panic attacks. Clin Psychol Rev 1988;8(1):1–18.

Ley R. Panic attacks during relaxation and relaxation-induced anxiety: a hyperventilation interpretation. J Behav Ther Exp Psychiatry 1988 Dec;19(4):253–9.

Ley R. Panic attacks during sleep: a hyperventilation-probability model. J Behav Ther Exp Psychiatry 1988 Sep;19(3):181–92.

Ley R. Panic disorder and agoraphobia: fear of fear or fear of the symptoms produced by hyperventilation? J Behav Ther Exp Psychiatry 1987 Dec;18(4):305–16.

Liberthson R, Sheehan DV, King ME, Weyman AE. The prevalence of mitral valve prolapse in patients with panic disorders. Am J Psychiatry 1986 Apr;143(4):511–5.

Liebowitz MR, Gorman JM, Fyer A, Dillon D, Levitt M, Klein DF. Possible mechanisms for lactate's induction of panic. Am J Psychiatry 1986 Apr;143(4):495–502.

Lilienfeld SO, Jacob RG, Furman JM. Vestibular dysfunction followed by panic disorder with agoraphobia. J Nerv Ment Dis 1989 Nov;177(11):700–1.

Lynch P, Bakal DA, Whitelaw W, Fung T. Chest muscle activity and panic anxiety: a preliminary investigation. Psychosom Med 1991 Jan-Feb;53(1):80–9.

Marazziti D, Michelini S, Martini C, Giannaccini G, Lucacchini A, Cassano GB. Further investigation on benzodiazepine binding inhibitory activity in patients with major depression or panic disorder and in healthy volunteers. Neuropsychobiology 1989;21(1):14–6.

Margraf J, Ehlers A, Roth WT. Biological models of panic disorder and agoraphobia—a review. Behav Res Ther 1986;24(5):553–67.

Martin NG, Jardine R, Andrews G, Heath AC. Anxiety disorders and neuroticism: are there genetic factors specific to panic? Acta Psychiatr Scand 1988 Jun;77(6):698–706.

Maser JD, Woods SW. The biological basis of panic: psychological interactions. Psychiatr Med 1990;8(3):121–47.

Matuzas W, Al-Sadir J, Uhlenhuth EH, Glass RM. Mitral valve prolapse and thyroid abnormalities in patients with panic attacks. Am J Psychiatry 1987 Apr;144(4):493–6.

Matuzas W, Al-Sadir J, Uhlenhuth EH, Glass RM, Easton C. Correlates of mitral valve prolapse among patients with panic disorder. Psychiatry Res 1989 May;28(2):161–70.

Mazza DL, Martin D, Spacavento L, Jacobsen J, Gibbs H. Prevalence of anxiety disorders in patients with mitral valve prolapse. Am J Psychiatry 1986 Mar;143(3):349–52.

McIntyre IM, Judd FK, Burrows GD, Norman TR. Serotonin in panic disorder: platelet uptake and concentration. Int Clin Psychopharmacol 1989 Jan;4(1):1–6.

Middleton HC. An enhanced hypotensive response to clonidine can still be found in panic patients despite psychological treatment. J Anxiety Disord 1990;4(3):213–9.

Mutchler K, Crowe RR, Noyes R Jr, Wesner RW. Exclusion of the tyrosine hydroxylase gene in 14 panic disorder pedigrees. Am J Psychiatry 1990 Oct;147(10):1367–9.

Norman TR, Acevedo A, McIntyre IM, Judd FK, Burrows GD. A kinetic analysis of platelet monoamine oxidase activity in patients with panic attacks. J Affective Disord 1988 Sep-Oct;15(2):127–30.

Norman TR, Burrows GD, Judd FK, McIntyre IM. Serotonin and panic disorders: a review of clinical studies. Int J Clin Pharmacol Res 1989;9(2):151–7.

Norman TR, Gregory MS, Judd FK, Burrows GD, McIntyre IM. Platelet serotonin uptake in panic disorder: comparison with normal controls and the effect of treatment. Aust N Z J Psychiatry 1988 Dec;22(4):390–5.

Norman TR, Judd FK, Burrows GD, McIntyre IM. Platelet serotonin uptake in panic disorder patients: a replication study. Psychiatry Res 1989 Oct;30(1):63–8.

Norman TR, Judd FK, Gregory M, James RH, Kimber NM, McIntyre IM, Burrows GD. Platelet serotonin uptake in panic disorder. J Affective Disord 1986 Jul-Aug;11(1):69–72.

Norman TR, Judd FK, Staikos V, Burrows GD, McIntyre IM. High-affinity platelet [3H]LSD binding is decreased in panic disorder. J Affective Disord 1990 Jun;19(2):119–23.

Norman TR, Sartor DM, Judd FK, Burrows GD, Gregory MS, McIntyre IM. Platelet serotonin uptake and 3H-imipramine binding in panic disorder. J Affective Disord 1989 Jul-Aug;17(1):77–81.

Nutt DJ. Altered central alpha 2-adrenoceptor sensitivity in panic disorder. Arch Gen Psychiatry 1989 Feb;46(2):165–9.

Nutt DJ. Endocrine response to syncope in panic disorder. Psychiatry Res 1989 Jun;28(3):351–3.

Nutt DJ. Increased central alpha 2-adrenoceptor sensitivity in panic disorder. Psychopharmacology (Berlin) 1986;90(2):268–9.

Nutt DJ. The pharmacology of human anxiety. Pharmacol Ther 1990;47(2):233–66.

Nutt DJ, Fraser S. Platelet binding studies in panic disorder. J Affective Disord 1987 Jan-Feb;12(1):7–11.

Nutt DJ, Glue P, Lawson C, Wilson S. Flumazenil provocation of panic attacks. Evidence for altered benzodiazepine receptor sensitivity in panic disorder. Arch Gen Psychiatry 1990 Oct;47(10):917–25.

Pauli P, Marquardt C, Hartl L, Nutzinger DO, Holzl R, Strian F. Anxiety induced by cardiac perceptions in patients with panic attacks: a field study. Behav Res Ther 1991;29(2):137–45.

Pohl R, Ettedgui E, Bridges M, Lycaki H, Jimerson D, Kopin I, Rainey JM. Plasma MHPG levels in lactate and isoproterenol anxiety states. Biol Psychiatry 1987 Sep;22(9):1127–36.

Pols H, Griez E. Serotonin in panic anxiety. Acta Psychiatr Belg 1988 Mar-Apr;88(2):162–72.

Price RA, Kidd KK, Weissman MM. Early onset (under age 30 years) and panic disorder as markers for etiologic homogeneity in major depression. Arch Gen Psychiatry 1987 May;44(5):434–40.

Rachman S, Levitt K, Lopatka C. Panic: the links between cognitions and bodily symptoms—I. Behav Res Ther 1987;25(5):411–23.

Rainey JM Jr, Nesse RM. Psychobiology of anxiety and anxiety disorders. Psychiatr Clin North Am 1985 Mar;8(1):133–44.

Rapaport MH, Risch SC, Golshan S, Gillin JC. Neuroendocrine effects of ovine corticotropin-releasing hormone in panic disorder patients. Biol Psychiatry 1989 Aug;26(4):344–8.

Rapee RM, Litwin EM, Barlow DH. Impact of life events on subjects with panic disorder and on comparison subjects. Am J Psychiatry 1990 May;147(5):640–4.

Rapee R, Mattick R, Murrell E. Cognitive mediation in the affective component of spontaneous panic attacks. J Behav Ther Exp Psychiatry 1986 Dec;17(4):245–53.

Reiman EM, Raichle ME, Robins E, Butler FK, Herscovitch P, Fox P, Perlmutter J. The application of positron emission tomography to the study of panic disorder. Am J Psychiatry 1986 Apr;143(4):469–77.

Reiss S. Expectancy model of fear, anxiety, and panic. Clin Psychol Rev 1991;11(2):141–53.

Rosenbaum JF. A psychopharmacologist's perspective on panic disorder. Bull Menninger Clin 1990 Spring;54(2):184–98.

Rosenbaum JF, Biederman J, Gersten M, Hirshfeld DR, Meminger SR, Herman JB, Kagan J, Reznick JS, Snidman N. Behavioral inhibition in children of parents with panic disorder and agoraphobia. A controlled study. Arch Gen Psychiatry 1988 May;45(5):463–70.

Rosenbaum JF, Biederman J, Hirshfeld DR, Bolduc EA, Faraone SV, Kagan J, Snidman N, Reznick JS. Further evidence of an association between behavioral inhibition and anxiety disorders: results from a family study of children from a nonclinical sample. J Psychiatr Res 1991;25(1–2):49–65.

Roth M. Some recent developments in relation to agoraphobia and related disorders and their bearing upon theories of their causation. First Gerald J. Sarwer-Foner Clinical Symposium: Current trends in psychiatry (1986, Ottawa, Canada). Psychiatr J Univ Ottawa 1987 Sep;12(3):150–5.

Roy-Byrne P, Geraci M, Uhde TW. Life events obtained via interview: the effect of time of recall on data obtained in controls and patients with panic disorder. J Affective Disord 1987 Jan-Feb;12(1):57–62.

Roy-Byrne PP, Geraci M, Uhde TW. Life events and course of illness in patients with panic disorder. Am J Psychiatry 1986 Aug;143(8):1033–5.

Roy-Byrne PP, Geraci M, Uhde TW. Life events and the onset of panic disorder. Am J Psychiatry 1986 Nov;143(11):1424–7.

Roy-Byrne PP, Uhde TW. Exogenous factors in panic disorder: clinical and research implications. J Clin Psychiatry 1988 Feb;49(2):56–61.

Salkovskis PM. The importance of behavior in the maintenance of anxiety and panic: A cognitive account. Behav Psychother 1991;19(1):6–19.

Salkovskis PM, Clark DM. Affective responses to hyperventilation: a test of the cognitive model of panic. Behav Res Ther 1990;28(1):51–61.

Sanderson WC, Beck AT. Classical conditioning model of panic disorder: response to Wolpe and Rowan. Behav Res Ther 1989;27(5):581–4.

Sanderson WC, Rapee RM, Barlow DH. The influence of an illusion of control on panic attacks induced via inhalation of 5.5% carbon dioxide-enriched air. Arch Gen Psychiatry 1989 Feb;46(2):157–62.

Sevin BH. Mitral valve prolapse, panic states, and anxiety. A dilemma in perspective. Psychiatr Clin North Am 1987 Mar;10(1):141–50.

Shean GD. Interpersonal aspects of agoraphobia: Therapeutic implications. 96th Annual Convention of the American Psychological Association: The Adopted Child Syndrome: What therapists should know (1988, Atlanta, Georgia). Psychother Priv Pract 1990;8(3):101–22.

Shear MK. Pathophysiology of panic: a review of pharmacologic provocative tests and naturalistic monitoring data. J Clin Psychiatry 1986 Jun;47 Suppl:18–26.

Silove D. Severe threat in the genesis of panic disorder. Aust N Z J Psychiatry 1987 Dec;21(4):591–600.

Smeraldi E, Orsini A, Gasperini M, Sciuto G, Battaglia M, Cassano GB, Perugi G, Migani W, Faravelli C, Pallanti S, Bressa G. Familial analysis of panic disorder and agoraphobia. J Affect Disord 1989;17(1):1–8.

Starkman MN, Cameron OG, Nesse RM, Zelnik T. Peripheral catecholamine levels and the symptoms of anxiety: studies in patients with and without pheochromocytoma. Psychosom Med 1990 Mar-Apr;52(2):129–42.

Stein MB, Uhde TW. Cortisol response to clonidine in panic disorder: comparison with depressed patients and normal controls. Biol Psychiatry 1988 Jul;24(3):322–30.

Stein MB, Uhde TW. Infrequent occurrence of EEG abnormalities in panic disorder. Am J Psychiatry 1989 Apr;146(4):517–20.

Targum SD, Marshall LE. Fenfluramine provocation of anxiety in patients with panic disorder. Psychiatry Res 1989 Jun;28(3):295–306.

Teicher MH. Biology of anxiety. Med Clin North Am 1988 Jul;72(4):791–814.

Telch MJ, Brouillard M, Telch CF, Agras WS, Taylor CB. Role of cognitive appraisal in panic-related avoidance. Behav Res Ther 1989;27(4):373–83.

Thyer BA, Himle J, Fischer D. Is parental death a selective precursor to either panic disorder or agoraphobia? A test of the separation anxiety hypothesis. J Anxiety Disord 1988;2(4):333–8.

Thyer BA, Nesse RM, Curtis GC, Cameron OG. Case histories and shorter communications. Panic disorder: A test of the separation anxiety hypothesis. Behav Res Ther 1986;24(2):209–11.

Torgersen S. Childhood and family characteristics in panic and generalized anxiety disorders. Am J Psychiatry 1986 May;143(5):630–2.

Torgersen S. Comorbidity of major depression and anxiety disorders in twin pairs. Am J Psychiatry 1990 Sep;147(9):1199–202.

Tweed JL, Schoenbach VJ, George LK, Blazer DG. The effects of childhood parental death and divorce on six-month history of anxiety disorders. Br J Psychiatry 1989 Jun;154:823–8.

van den Hout MA, van der Molen GM, Griez E, Lousberg H, Nansen A. Reduction of CO_2-induced anxiety in patients with panic attacks after repeated CO_2 exposure. Am J Psychiatry 1987 Jun;144(6):788–91.

van der Molen GM, van den Hout MA, van Dieren AC, Griez E. Childhood separation anxiety and adult-onset panic disorders. J Anxiety Disord 1989;3(2):97–106.

Vitaliano PP, Katon W, Russo J, Maiuro RD, Anderson K, Jones M. Coping as an index of illness behavior in panic disorder. J Nerv Ment Dis 1987 Feb;175(2):78–84.

Wall M, Tuchman M, Mielke D. Panic attacks and temporal lobe seizures associated with a right temporal lobe arteriovenous malformation: case report. J Clin Psychiatry 1985 Apr;46(4):143–5.

Warren R, Zgourides G, Englert M. Relationships between catastrophic cognitions and body sensations in anxiety disordered, mixed diagnosis, and normal subjects. Behav Res Ther 1990;28(4):355–7.

Warren R, Zgourides G, Jones A. Cognitive bias and irrational belief as predictors of avoidance. Behav Res Ther 1989;27(2):181–8.

Watkins PL, Clum GA, Borden JW, Broyles S, Hayes J. Imagery-induced arousal in individuals with panic disorder. Cogn Ther Res 1990;14(1):37–46.

Weilburg JB, Bear DM, Sachs G. Three patients with concomitant panic attacks and seizure disorder: possible clues to the neurology of anxiety. Am J Psychiatry 1987 Aug;144(8):1053–6.

Westenberg HG, den Boer JA. Serotonin function in panic disorder: effect of 1-5-hydroxytryptophan in patients and controls. Psychopharmacology (Berlin) 1989;98(2):283–5.

Wolpe J, Rowan VC. Classical conditioning and panic disorder: Reply to Sanderson and Beck. Behav Res Ther 1989;27(5):583–4.

Wolpe J, Rowan VC. Panic disorder: A product of classical conditioning. Behav Res Ther 1988;26(6):441–50.

Woods SW, Charney DS, Silver JM, Krystal JH, Heninger GR. Behavioral, biochemical, and cardiovascular responses to the benzodiazepine receptor antagonist flumazenil in panic disorder. Psychiatry Res 1991 Feb;36(2):115–27.

Yeragani VK, Meiri PC, Balon R, Patel H, Pohl R. History of separation anxiety in patients with panic disorder and depression and normal controls. Acta Psychiatr Scand 1989 Jun;79(6):550–6.

Yeragani VK, Rainey JM, Pohl R, Ortiz A, Weinberg P, Gershon S. Thyroid hormone levels in panic disorder. Can J Psychiatry 1987 Aug;32(6):467–9.

Zandbergen J, Lousberg HH, Pols H, de Loof C, Griez EJ. Hypercarbia versus hypocarbia in panic disorder. J Affective Disord 1990 Feb;18(2):75–81.

Zandbergen J, Pols H, De Loof C, Lousberg H, Griez E. Effect of hypercapnia and other disturbances in the acid-base-balance on panic disorder. Hillside J Clin Psychiatry 1989;11(2):185–97.

Zeanah CH. Atypical panic attacks and lack of resolution of mourning. Gen Hosp Psychiatry 1988 Sep;10(5):373–7.

Zucker D, Taylor CB, Brouillard M, Ehlers A, Margraf J, Telch M, Roth WT, Agras WS. Cognitive aspects of panic attacks. Content, course and relationship to laboratory stressors. Br J Psychiatry 1989 Jul;155:86–91.

Primary Care, Family Practice, and Services

Anixter WL. Panic disorder and agoraphobia. An update for primary care physicians. N C Med J 1988 Oct;49(10):507–11.

Aronson TA, Craig TJ, Thomason S, Logue C. Health care utilization patterns in panic disorder and agoraphobia: A naturalistic study in secondary prevention. J Anxiety Disord 1987;1(4):283–93.

Ballenger JC. Unrecognized prevalence of panic disorder in primary care, internal medicine and cardiology. Am J Cardiol 1987 Dec 28;60(18):39J–47J.

Bernstein JA, Sheridan E, Patterson R. Asthmatic patients with panic disorders: report of three cases with management and outcome. Ann Allergy 1991 Apr;66(4):311–4.

Boyd JH. Use of mental health services for the treatment of panic disorder. Am J Psychiatry 1986 Dec;143(12):1569–74.

Braverman BG. Calming a patient with panic disorder. Nursing 1990 Jan;20(1):32C, 32F.

Drug treatment of panic disorder: Discussion III. Hosp Pract 1990;25 Suppl 2:40–2.

Edlund MJ, Swann AC. The economic and social costs of panic disorder. Hosp Community Psychiatry 1987 Dec;38(12):1277–9, 1288.

Enright MF, Blue BA. Collaborative treatment of panic disorders by psychologists and family physicians. Psychother Priv Pract 1989;7(2):85–90.

Ferentz KS. Panic disorder and agoraphobia. Nondrug treatment options for primary care physicians. Postgrad Med 1990 Aug;88(2):185–92.

Giesecke ME. Panic disorder in university students: A review. J Am Coll Health 1987;36(3):149–57.

Hudson CJ. Anxiety disorders and substance abuse. Special Issue: Managing the dually diagnosed patient: Current issues and clinical approaches. J Chem Depend Treat 1990;3(2):119–38.

Katerndahl DA. Factors associated with persons with panic attacks seeking medical care. Fam Med 1990 Nov-Dec;22(6):462–6.

Katerndahl DA. Panic disorder in primary care settings: research agenda for the '90s [editorial]. Fam Pract Res J 1991 Mar;11(1):3–7.

Katerndahl DA. Patients' willingness to discuss phobic avoidance symptoms. Fam Pract Res J 1991 Mar;11(1):91–7.

Linnoila MI. Approaches to the treatment of alcoholism and anxiety. Drug Ther 1990;20 Suppl:27–34.

Marshall JR. Diagnosis and management of panic disorder in the emergency department. Emerg Care Q 1991;7(1):1–8.

Muskin PR. Panics, prolapse, and PVCs. Gen Hosp Psychiatry 1985 Jul;7(3):219–23.

Pollard CA, Lewis LM. Managing panic attacks in emergency patients. J Emerg Med 1989 Sep-Oct;7(5):547–52.

Pollard CA, Obermeier HJ, Cox GL. Inpatient treatment of complicated agoraphobia and panic disorder. Hosp Community Psychiatry 1987 Sep;38(9):951–8.

Raj A, Sheehan DV. Medical evaluation of panic attacks. J Clin Psychiatry 1987 Aug;48(8):309–13.

Rifkin A. Solving panic disorder problems. When your patients' fears thwart their lives. Postgrad Med 1990 Nov 1;88(6):133–8.

Rosenbaum JF. Drug treatment of panic disorder. Hosp Pract [Off] 1990 Jun;25 Suppl 2:31-9; discussion 40–2.

Ross CA, Walker JR, Norton GR, Neufeld K. Management of anxiety and panic attacks in immediate care facilities. Gen Hosp Psychiatry 1988 Mar;10(2):129–31.

Roundtable discussion: "Panic disorder: Epidemiology, diagnosis, and treatment in primary care." Symposium: New directions in biological psychiatry (1986, Coronado, California). J Clin Psychiatry 1986 Oct;47 Suppl:28–30.

Schatzberg AF, Ballenger JC. Decisions for the clinician in the treatment of panic disorder: when to treat, which treatment to use, and how long to treat. J Clin Psychiatry 1991 Feb;52 Suppl:26–31; discussion 32.

Shear MK, Frances AJ. Clinical presentation and evaluation. Psychiatr Ann 1988 Aug;18(8):448–56.

Shelton RC. Diagnosis and management of panic disorder. Compr Ther 1990 Dec;16(12):11–7.

Tobe EH. Pitfalls in the management of panic disorder. J Am Osteopath Assoc 1988;88(4):507–9.

Wood WG. The diagnosis and management of panic disorder. Psychiatr Med 1990;8(3):197–209.

Wulsin LR, Hillard JR, Geier P, Hissa D, Rouan GW. Screening emergency room patients with atypical chest pain for depression and panic disorder. Int J Psychiatry Med 1988;18(4):315–23.

Treatments

Pharmacological

Tricyclic Antidepressants

Albus M, Lecrubier Y, Maier W, Buller R, Rosenberg R, Hippius H. Drug treatment of panic disorder: early response to treatment as a predictor of final outcome. Acta Psychiatr Scand 1990 Nov;82(5):359–65.

Albus M, Maier W, Shera D, Bech P. Consistencies and discrepancies in self- and observer-rated anxiety scales. A comparison between the self- and observer-rated Marks-Sheehan scales. Eur Arch Psychiatry Clin Neurosci 1990;240(2):96–102.

Andersch S, Rosenberg NK, Kullingsjo H, Ottosson J-O, Bech P, Bruun-Hansen J, Hanson L, Lorentzen K, Mellergard M, Rasmussen S, Rosenberg R. Efficacy and safety of alprazolam, imipramine and placebo in treating panic disorder. A Scandinavian multicenter study. Acta Psychiatr Scand Suppl 1991;83(365):18–27.

Aronson TA. A naturalistic study of imipramine in panic disorder and agoraphobia. Am J Psychiatry 1987 Aug;144(8):1014–9.

Aronson TA. Treatment-emergent depression with antidepressants in panic disorder. Compr Psychiatry 1989 May-Jun;30(3):267–71.

Austin LS, Lydiard RB, Fossey MD, Zealberg JJ, Laraia MT, Ballenger JC. Panic and phobic disorders in patients with obsessive compulsive disorder. J Clin Psychiatry 1990 Nov;51(11):456–8.

Balestrieri M, Ruggeri M, Bellantuono C. Drug treatment of panic disorder—a critical review of controlled clinical trials. Psychiatr Dev 1989 Winter;7(4):337–50.

Ballenger JC. Pharmacotherapy of the panic disorders. J Clin Psychiatry 1986 Jun;47 Suppl:27–32.

Beardslee SL, Papadakis E, Fontana DJ, Commissaris RL. Antipanic drug treatments: failure to exhibit anxiolytic-like effects on defensive burying behavior. Pharmacol Biochem Behav 1990 Feb;35(2):451–5.

Brady KT, Zarzar M, Lydiard RB. Fluoxetine in panic disorder patients with imipramine-associated weight gain. J Clin Psychopharmacol 1989 Feb;9(1):66–7.

Buller R, Maier W, Goldenberg IM, Lavori PW, Benkert O. Chronology of panic and avoidance, age of onset in panic disorder, and prediction of treatment response. A report from the Cross-National Collaborative Panic Study. Eur Arch Psychiatry Clin Neurosci 1991;240(3):163–8.

Burrows GD. Managing long-term therapy for panic disorder. J Clin Psychiatry 1990 Nov;51 Suppl: 9–12.

Cassano GB, Petracca A, Perugi G, Nisita C, Musetti L, Mengali F, McNair DM. Clomipramine for panic disorder: I. The first 10 weeks of a long-term comparison with imipramine. J Affective Disord 1988 Mar-Apr;14(2):123–7.

Charney DS, Heninger GR. Noradrenergic function and the mechanism of action of anti-anxiety treatment. II. The effect of long-term imipramine treatment. Arch Gen Psychiatry 1985 May;42(5):473–81.

Charney DS, Woods SW, Goodman WK, Rifkin B, Kinch M, Aiken B, Quadrino LM, Heninger GR. Drug treatment of panic disorder: the comparative efficacy of imipramine, alprazolam, and trazodone. J Clin Psychiatry 1986 Dec;47(12):580–6.

Clark DB, Taylor CB, Roth WT, Hayward C, Ehlers A, Margraf J, Agras WS. Surreptitious drug use by patients in a panic disorder study. Am J Psychiatry 1990 Apr;147(4):507–9.

Cox BJ, Swinson RP, Endler NS. A review of the psychopharmacology of panic disorder: Individual differences and non specific factors. Can J Psychiatry 1991;36(2):130–8.

Crowe RR, Noyes R Jr. Panic disorder and agoraphobia. Dis Mon 1986 Jul;32(7):389–444.

Davis DM. Update on the treatment of panic attacks. J Med Assoc Ga 1988 Nov;77(11):831–2.

Deltito JA, Argyle N, Klerman GL. Patients with panic disorder unaccompanied by depression improve with alprazolam and imipramine treatment. J Clin Psychiatry 1991 Mar;52(3):121–7.

Deltito JA, Argyle N, Buller R, Nutzinger D, Ottosson JO, Brandon S, Mellergard M, Shera D. The sequence of improvement of the symptoms encountered in patients with panic disorder. Compr Psychiatry 1991 Mar-Apr;32(2):120–9.

Den Boer JA, Westenberg HG. Effect of a serotonin and noradrenaline uptake inhibitor in panic disorder; a double-blind comparative study with fluvoxamine and maprotiline. Int Clin Psychopharmacol 1988 Jan;3(1):59–74.

Den Boer JA, Westenberg HG, Kamerbeek WD, Verhoeven WM, Kahn RS. Effect of serotonin uptake inhibitors in anxiety disorders; a double-blind comparison of clomipramine and fluvoxamine. Int Clin Psychopharmacol 1987 Jan;2(1):21–32.

Dilsaver SC. Panic disorder. Am Fam Physician 1989 Jun;39(6):167–72.

Eriksson E, Westberg P, Alling C, Thuresson K, Modigh K. Cerebrospinal fluid levels of monoamine metabolites in panic disorder. Psychiatry Res 1991;36(3):243–51.

Eriksson E, Westberg P, Thuresson K, Modigh K, Ekman R, Widerlov E. Increased cerebrospinal fluid levels of endorphin immunoreactivity in panic disorder. Neuropsychopharmacology 1989 Sep;2(3):225–8.

Faludi G, Kecskemety P. Melipramine treatment of panic disease. Ther Hung 1987;35(3):129–35.

Fava GA, Grandi S, Saviotti FM, Conti S. Hypochondriasis with panic attacks. Psychosomatics 1990 Summer;31(3):351–3.

Fava M, Anderson K, Rosenbaum JF. "Anger attacks": possible variants of panic and major depressive disorders. Am J Psychiatry 1990 Jul;147(7):867–70.

Fishman SM, Sheehan DV, Carr DB. Thyroid indices in panic disorder. J Clin Psychiatry 1985 Oct;46(10):432–3.

Fontana DJ, Carbary TJ, Commissaris RL. Effects of acute and chronic anti-panic drug administration on conflict behavior in the rat. Psychopharmacology (Berlin) 1989;98(2):157–62.

Fontana DJ, Commissaris RL. Effects of acute and chronic imipramine administration on conflict behavior in the rat: a potential "animal model" for the study of panic disorder? Psychopharmacology (Berlin) 1988;95(2):147–50.

Friedman S, Sunderland GS, Rosenblum LA. A nonhuman primate model of panic disorder. Psychiatry Res 1988 Jan;23(1):65–75.

Fyer AJ. Agoraphobia. Mod Probl Pharmacopsychiatry 1987;22:91–126.

Fyer AJ, Liebowitz MR, Gorman JM, Davies SO, Klein DF. Lactate vulnerability of remitted panic patients. Psychiatry Res 1985 Feb;14(2):143–8.

George DT, Anderson P, Nutt DJ, Linnoila M. Aggressive thoughts and behavior: another symptom of panic disorder? Acta Psychiatr Scand 1989 May;79(5):500–2.

Giesecke ME. Panic disorder in university students: A review. J Am Coll Health 1987;36(3):149–57.

Gold DD Jr. Management of panic disorder: Case reports support a potential role for amoxapine. Hosp Formul 1990;25(11):1178–79, 1182–4.

Gold DD Jr. Panic attacks: Diagnosis and management. Cardiovasc Rev Rep 1988;9(1):35–7, 40.

Goodman WK, Charney DS. Therapeutic applications and mechanisms of action of monoamine oxidase inhibitor and heterocyclic antidepressant drugs. J Clin Psychiatry 1985 Oct;46(10 Pt 2):6–24.

Gorman JM, Liebowitz MR, Dillon D, Fyer AJ, Cohen BS, Klein DF. Antipanic drug effects during lactate infusion in lactate-refractory panic patients. Psychiatry Res 1987 Jul;21(3):205–12.

Green MA, Curtis GC. Personality disorders in panic patients: Response to termination of antipanic medication. J Pers Disord 1988;2(4):303–14.

Grunhaus L, Harel Y, Krugler T, Pande AC, Haskett RF. Major depressive disorder and panic disorder. Effects of comorbidity on treatment outcome with antidepressant medications. Clin Neuropharmacol 1988 Oct;11(5):454–61.

Grunhaus L, Rabin D, Greden JF. Simultaneous panic and depressive disorder: response to antidepressant treatments. J Clin Psychiatry 1986 Jan;47(1):4–7.

Heninger GR, Charney DS, Price LH. Noradrenergic and serotonergic receptor system function in panic disorder and depression. Acta Psychiatr Scand Suppl 1988;341:138–50.

Hudson JI, Pope HG Jr. Affective spectrum disorder: does antidepressant response identify a family of disorders with a common pathophysiology? Am J Psychiatry 1990 May;147(5):552–64.

Jann MW, Kurtz NM. Treatment of panic and phobic disorders. Clin Pharm 1987 Dec;6(12):947–62.

Judd FK, Burrows GD, Marriott PF, Farnbach P, Blair-West S, Normal TR. A short-term open trial of clomipramine in the treatment of patients with panic attacks. Hum Psychopharmacol 1991;6(1):53–60.

Judd FK, Norman TR, Burrows GD. Pharmacological treatment of panic disorder. Int Clin Psychopharmacol 1986 Jan;1(1):3–16.

Judd FK, Norman TR, Burrows GD. Pharmacotherapy of panic disorder. Int Rev Psychiatry 1990;2(3-4):399–409.

Kalus O, Asnis GM, Rubinson E, Kahn R, Harkavy Friedman JM, Iqbal N, Grosz D, Van Praag H, Cahn W. Desipramine treatment in panic disorder. J Affect Disord 1991;21(4):239–44.

Katon W. Panic disorder: epidemiology, diagnosis, and treatment in primary care. J Clin Psychiatry 1986 Oct;47 Suppl:21–30.

Katon W, Vitaliano PP, Russo J, Cormier L, Anderson K, Jones M. Panic disorder: epidemiology in primary care. J Fam Pract 1986 Sep;23(3):233–9.

King D, Nicolini H, de la Fuente JR. Abuse and withdrawal of panic treatment drugs. Psychiatr Ann 1990 Sep;20(9):525–8.

Klein DF. Psychopharmacologic treatment of panic disorder. Psychosomatics 1984;25(10 Suppl):32–6.

Klein DF, Gorman JM. A model of panic and agoraphobic development. Acta Psychiatr Scand Suppl 1987;335:87–95.

Klein DF, Klein HM. The status of panic disorder. Curr Opin Psychiatry 1988;1(2):177–83.

Klerman GL. Depression and panic anxiety: the effect of depressive co-morbidity on response to drug treatment of patients with panic disorder and agoraphobia. J Psychiatr Res 1990;24 Suppl 2: 27–41.

Klerman GL. Overview of the Cross-National Collaborative Panic Study. Arch Gen Psychiatry 1988 May;45(5):407–12.

Kupfer DJ. Lessons to be learned from long-term treatment of affective disorders: potential utility in panic disorder. J Clin Psychiatry 1991 Feb;52 Suppl:12–6; discussion 17.

Lepola U. Recognition of panic disorder. Nord Psykiatr Tidsskr 1989;43(6):511–3.

Lepola U, Heikkinen H, Rimon R, Riekkinen P. Clinical evaluation of alprazolam in patients with panic disorder: A double-blind comparison with imipramine. Hum Psychopharmacol 1990;5(2):159–63.

Lepola U, Jolkkonen J, Rim:on R, Riekkinen P. Long-term effects of alprazolam and im-ipramine on cerebrospinal fluid monoamine metabolites and neuropeptides in panic disorder. Neuropsychobiology 1989;21(4):182–6.

Liebowitz MR. Antidepressants in panic disorders. Br J Psychiatry Suppl 1989 Oct;(6):46–52.

Liebowitz MR. Imipramine in the treatment of panic disorder and its complications. Psy-chiatr Clin North Am 1985 Mar;8(1):37–47.

Liebowitz MR. Tricyclic antidepressants and monoamine oxidase inhibitors in the treat-ment of panic disorder: brief review. Psychopharmacol Bull 1989;25(1):17–20.

Liebowitz MR, Fyer AJ, Gorman JM, Campeas RB, Sandberg DP, Hollander E, Papp LA, Klein DF. Tricyclic therapy of the DSM-III anxiety disorders: a review with implications for further research. J Psychiatr Res 1988;22 Suppl 1:7–31.

Lingjaerde O. Lactate-induced panic attacks: possible involvement of serotonin reuptake stimulation. Acta Psychiatr Scand 1985 Aug;72(2):206–8.

Linnoila MI. Anxiety and alcoholism. J Clin Psychiatry 1989 Nov;50 Suppl:26–9.

Lydiard RB. Preliminary results of an open, fixed-dose study of desipramine in panic disorder. Psychopharmacol Bull 1987;23(1):139–40.

Lydiard RB, Ballenger JC. Antidepressants in panic disorder and agoraphobia. J Affective Disord 1987 Sep-Oct;13(2):153–68.

Lydiard RB, Ballenger JC. Panic-related disorders: Evidence for efficacy of the antidepres-sants. Special Issue: Perspectives on panic-related disorders. J Anxiety Disord 1988; 2(1):77–94.

Lydiard RB, Laraia MT, Ballenger JC, Howell EF. Emergence of depressive symptoms in patients receiving alprazolam for panic disorder. Am J Psychiatry 1987 May;144(5):664–5.

Lydiard RB, Roy-Byrne PP, Ballenger JC. Recent advances in the psychopharmacological treatment of anxiety disorders. Hosp Community Psychiatry 1988 Nov;39(11):1157–65.

Margraf J, Ehlers A, Roth WT, Clark DB, Sheikh J, Agras WS, Taylor CB. How "blind" are double-blind studies? J Consult Clin Psychol 1991 Feb;59(1):184–7.

Mattick RP, Andrews G, Hadzi-Pavlovic D, Christensen H. Treatment of panic and agora-phobia. An integrative review. J Nerv Ment Dis 1990 Sep;178(9):567–76.

Mavissakalian M. Differential effects of imipramine and behavior therapy on panic disorder with agoraphobia. Psychopharmacol Bull 1989;25(1):27–9.

Mavissakalian M. Sequential combination of imipramine and self-directed exposure in the treatment of panic disorder with agoraphobia. J Clin Psychiatry 1990 May;51(5):184–8.

Mavissakalian MR, Perel JM. Imipramine dose-response relationship in panic disorder with agoraphobia. Preliminary findings. Arch Gen Psychiatry 1989 Feb;46(2):127–31.

McTavish D, Benfield P. Clomipramine. An overview of its pharmacological properties and a review of its therapeutic use in obsessive compulsive disorder and panic disorder. Drugs 1990 Jan;39(1):136–53.

Mellergard M, Lorentzen K, Bech P, Ottosson J-O, Rosenberg R. A trend analysis of changes during treatment of panic disorder with alprazolam and imipramine. Acta Psychiatr Scand Suppl 1991;83(365):28–32.

Mellergard M, Rosenberg NK. Patterns of response during placebo treatment of panic disorder. Acta Psychiatr Scand 1990 Apr;81(4):340–4.

Mellman TA, Uhde TW. Patients with frequent sleep panic: clinical findings and response to medication treatment. J Clin Psychiatry 1990 Dec;51(12):513–6.

Middleton HC, Nutt DJ. Heart rate response to standing as an index of adaptation to imipramine during treatment of panic disorder. Hum Psychopharmacol 1988;3(3):191–4.

Modigh K. Antidepressant drugs in anxiety disorders. Acta Psychiatr Scand Suppl 1987;335:57–74.

Modigh K, Eriksson Elias, Lisjo P, Westburg P. Follow-up study of chlorimipramine in the treatment of panic disorder. Proceedings of the World Psychiatric Association on the Psychopathology of Panic Disorders: Many faces of panic disorder (1988, Espoo, Finland). Psychiatr Fenn 1989;Suppl:145–53.

Munjack DJ, Rebal R, Shaner R, et al. Imipramine versus propranolol for the treatment of panic attacks: A pilot study. Compr Psychiatry 1985;26(1):80–9.

Munjack DJ, Usigli R, Zulueta A, Crocker B, Adatia N, Buckwalter JG, Baltazar P, Kurvink W, Inglove H, Kelly R, et al. Nortriptyline in the treatment of panic disorder and agoraphobia with panic attacks. J Clin Psychopharmacol 1988 Jun;8(3):204–7.

Murphy DL, Pigott TA. A comparative examination of a role for serotonin in obsessive compulsive disorder, panic disorder, and anxiety. J Clin Psychiatry 1990 Apr;51 Suppl:53–8; discussion 59–60.

Murphy DL, Siever LJ, Insel TR. Therapeutic responses to tricyclic antidepressants and related drugs in non-affective disorder patient populations. Prog Neuropsychopharmacol Biol Psychiatry 1985;9(1):3–13.

Muskin PR. Panics, prolapse, and PVCs. Gen Hosp Psychiatry 1985 Jul;7(3):219–23.

Noyes R Jr, Garvey MJ, Cook BL. Follow-up study of patients with panic disorder and agoraphobia with panic attacks treated with tricyclic antidepressants. J Affective Disord 1989 Mar-Jun;16(2-3):249–57.

Noyes R Jr, Garvey MJ, Cook BL, Samuelson L. Problems with tricyclic antidepressant use in patients with panic disorder or agoraphobia: results of a naturalistic follow-up study. J Clin Psychiatry 1989 May;50(5):163–9.

Noyes R Jr, Perry P. Maintenance treatment with antidepressants in panic disorder. J Clin Psychiatry 1990 Dec;51 Suppl A:24–30.

Nutt DJ, Glue P. Imipramine in panic disorder. 1. Clinical response and pharmacological changes. J Psychopharmacol 1991;5(1):56–64.

Nutt DJ, Glue P. Irritability in panic disorder: Effects of imipramine treatment. Hum Psychopharmacol 1991;6(1):49–52.

O'Boyle M. Panic disorder: diagnosis and treatment. Tex Med 1989 Aug;85(8):46–9.

Otakpor AN. A prospective study of panic disorder in a Nigerian psychiatric out-patient population. Acta Psychiatr Scand 1987 Nov;76(5):541–4.

Overall JE, Sheehan DV. Multivariate analysis of changes in panic frequency counts. Clin Neuropharmacol 1986;9 Suppl 4:155–7.

Pecknold JC. Behavioral and combined therapy in panic states. Prog Neuropsychopharmacol Biol Psychiatry 1987;11(2-3):97–104.

Philipp M, Maier W, Buller R. Pharmacotherapy of panic attacks. Pharmacopsychiatry 1988 Nov;21(6):281–2.

Pohl R, Balon R, Yeragani VK, Gershon S. Serotonergic anxiolytics in the treatment of panic disorder: a controlled study with buspirone. Psychopathology 1989;22 Suppl 1:60–7.

Pohl R, Yeragani VK, Balon R. Effects of isoproterenol in panic disorder patients after antidepressant treatment. Biol Psychiatry 1990 Aug 1;28(3):203–14.

Pohl R, Yeragani VK, Balon R, Lycaki H. The jitteriness syndrome in panic disorder patients treated with antidepressants. J Clin Psychiatry 1988 Mar;49(3):100–4.

Pohl R, Yeragani VK, Ortiz A, Rainey JM Jr, Gershon S. Response of tricyclic–induced jitteriness to a phenothiazine in two patients. J Clin Psychiatry 1986 Aug;47(8):427.

Rickels K. Antianxiety therapy: potential value of long-term treatment. J Clin Psychiatry 1987 Dec;48 Suppl:7–11.

Rickels K, Case WG, Downing RW, Fridman R. One-year follow-up of anxious patients treated with diazepam. J Clin Psychopharmacol 1986;6(1):32–6.

Rifkin A, Siris SG. Panic disorder: response to sodium lactate and treatment with antidepressants. Prog Neuropsychopharmacol Biol Psychiatry 1985;9(1):33–8.

Rizley R, Kahn RJ, McNair DM, Frankenthaler LM. A comparison of alprazolam and imipramine in the treatment of agoraphobia and panic disorder. Psychopharmacol Bull 1986;22(1):167–72.

Rosenberg R, Bech P, Mellergard M, Ottosson J-O. Alprazolam, imipramine and placebo treatment of panic disorder: Predicting therapeutic response. Acta Psychiatr Scand Suppl 1991;83(365):46–52.

Rosenberg R, Bech P, Mellergard M, Ottosson J-O. Secondary depression in panic disorder: An indicator of severity with a weak effect on outcome in alprazolam and imipramine treatment. Acta Psychiatr Scand Suppl 1991;83(365):39–45.

Rosenberg NK, Mellergard M, Rosenberg R, Beck P, Ottosson J-O. Characteristics of panic disorder patients responding to placebo. Acta Psychiatr Scand Suppl 1991;83(365):33–8.

Sargent M. Panic disorder. Hosp Community Psychiatry 1990 Jun;41(6):621–3.

Schatzberg AF, Ballenger JC. Decisions for the clinician in the treatment of panic disorder: when to treat, which treatment to use, and how long to treat. J Clin Psychiatry 1991 Feb;52 Suppl:26–31; discussion 32.

Schifano F, Magni G. Panic attacks and major depression after discontinuation of long-term diazepam abuse. DICP 1989 Dec;23(12):989–90.

Schittecatte M, Charles G, Depauw Y, Mesters P, Wilmotte J. Growth hormone response to clonidine in panic disorder patients. Psychiatry Res 1988 Feb;23(2):147–51.

Schneier FR, Liebowitz MR, Davies SO, Fairbanks J, Hollander E, Campeas R, Klein DF. Fluoxetine in panic disorder. J Clin Psychopharmacol 1990 Apr;10(2):119–21.

Scrignar CB. Postpanic anxiety disorder: diagnosis and treatment. South Med J 1986 Apr;79(4):400–4.

Sheehan DV. Tricyclic antidepressants in the treatment of panic and anxiety disorders. 139th Annual Meeting of the American Psychiatric Association: Beyond depression: New uses of antidepressants (1986, Washington, DC). Psychosomatics 1986 Nov;27(11 Suppl):10–6.

Sheehan DV, Raj AB, Sheehan KH, Soto S. Is buspirone effective for panic disorder? J Clin Psychopharmacol 1990 Feb;10(1):3–11.

Sheehan DV, Raj AB, Sheehan KH, Soto S. The relative efficacy of buspirone, imipramine and placebo in panic disorder: a preliminary report. Pharmacol Biochem Behav 1988 Apr;29(4):815–7.

Sheehan DV, Sheehan KH. Pharmacological treatment of panic and anxiety disorders. ISI Atlas Sci Pharmacol 1987;1(3):254–6.

Sheehan DV, Soto S. Recent developments in the treatment of panic disorder. Acta Psychiatr Scand Suppl 1987;335:75–85.

Stein MB, Uhde TW. Triiodothyronine potentiation of tricyclic antidepressant treatment in patients with panic disorder. Biol Psychiatry 1990 Dec 15;28(12):1061–4.

Stewart RS. Pharmacologic treatment of panic disorder and agoraphobia. Hosp Formul 1990;25(4):416–22.

Sunderland G, Friedman S, Rosenblum LA. Imipramine and alprazolam treatment of lactate-induced acute endogenous distress in nonhuman primates. Am J Psychiatry 1989 Aug;146(8):1044–7.

Svebak S, Cameron A, Levander S. Clonazepam and imipramine in the treatment of panic attacks: a double-blind comparison of efficacy and side effects. J Clin Psychiatry 1990 May;51 Suppl:14–7; discussion 50–3.

Sverd J. Imipramine treatment of panic disorder in a boy with Tourette's syndrome. J Clin Psychiatry 1988 Jan;49(1):31–2.

Swinson RP. The acute treatment of anxiety and depression. Psychiatr J Univ Ott 1989 Jun;14(2):375–8; discussion 379–80.

Swinson RP, Pecknold JC, Kuch K. Psychopharmacological treatment of panic disorder and related states: a placebo controlled study of alprazolam. Prog Neuropsychopharmacol Biol Psychiatry 1987;11(2–3):105–13.

Taylor CB, Hayward C, King R, Ehlers A, Margraf J, Maddock R, Clark D, Roth WT, Agras WS. Cardiovascular and symptomatic reduction effects of alprazolam and imipramine in patients with panic disorder: results of a double-blind, placebo-controlled trial. J Clin Psychopharmacol 1990 Apr;10(2):112–8.

Taylor CB, King R, Margraf J, Ehlers A, Telch M, Roth WT, Agras WS. Use of medication and in vivo exposure in volunteers for panic disorder research. Am J Psychiatry 1989 Nov;146(11):1423–6.

Tesar GE, Rosenbaum JF. Successful use of clonazepam in patients with treatment-resistant panic disorder. J Nerv Ment Dis 1986 Aug;174(8):477–82.

Tobe EH. Pitfalls in the management of panic disorder. J Am Osteopath Assoc 1988;88(4):507–9.

Treatment outlines for the management of anxiety states. Aust N Z J Psychiatry 1985;19(2):138–51.

Tyrer P, Seivewright N, Ferguson B, Murphy S, Darling C, Brothwell J, Kingdon D, Johnson AL. The Nottingham Study of Neurotic Disorder: relationship between personality status and symptoms. Psychol Med 1990 May;20(2):423–31.

Tyrer P, Seivewright N, Murphy S, Ferguson B, Kingdon D, Barczak P, Brothwell J, Darling C, Gregory S, Johnson AL. The Nottingham study of neurotic disorder: comparison of drug and psychological treatments. Lancet 1988 Jul 30;2(8605):235–40.

Tyrer P, Shawcross C. Monoamine oxidase inhibitors in anxiety disorders. J Psychiatr Res 1988;22 Suppl 1:87–98.

Uhlenhuth EH, Matuzas W, Glass RM, Easton C. Response of panic disorder to fixed doses of alprazolam or imipramine. J Affective Disord 1989 Nov-Dec;17(3):261–70.

Wall M, Tuchman M, Mielke D. Panic attacks and temporal lobe seizures associated with a right temporal lobe arteriovenous malformation: case report. J Clin Psychiatry 1985 Apr;46(4):143–5.

Ware MR, DeVane CL. Imipramine treatment of panic disorder during pregnancy. J Clin Psychiatry 1990 Nov;51(11):482–4.

Westenberg HG, den Boer JA. Serotonin-influencing drugs in the treatment of panic disorder. Psychopathology 1989;22 Suppl 1:68–77.

Whiteford HA, Evans L. Agoraphobia and the dexamethasone suppression test: Atypical depression? Aust N Z J Psychiatry 1984;18(4):374–7.

Wood WG. The diagnosis and management of panic disorder. Psychiatr Med 1990; 8(3):197–209.

Woods SW, Charney DS, Delgado PL, Heninger GR. The effect of long-term imipramine treatment on carbon dioxide-induced anxiety in panic disorder patients. J Clin Psychiatry 1990 Dec;51(12):505–7.

Yeragani VK, Balon R, Pohl R. Schizophrenia, panic attacks, and antidepressants. Am J Psychiatry 1989 Feb;146(2):279.

Yeragani VK, Meiri P, Balon R, Pohl R, Golec S. Effect of imipramine treatment on changes in heart rate and blood pressure during postural and isometric handgrip tests. Eur J Clin Pharmacol 1990;38(2):139–44.

Yeragani VK, Pohl R, Balon R, Rainey JM, Berchou R, Ortiz A. Sodium lactate infusions after treatment with tricyclic antidepressants: behavioral and physiological findings. Biol Psychiatry 1988 Nov;24(7):767–74.

Yeragani VK, Rainey JM, Balon R, Berchou R, Lycaki H, Pohl R. The effect of tricyclic antidepressants on stress-induced heart rate changes in panic disorder patients. Acta Psychiatr Scand 1987 Sep;76(3):324–7.

Alprazolam

Albus M, Lecrubier Y, Maier W, Buller R, Rosenberg R, Hippius H. Drug treatment of panic disorder: early response to treatment as a predictor of final outcome. Acta Psychiatr Scand 1990 Nov;82(5):359–65.

Albus M, Maier W, Shera D, Bech P. Consistencies and discrepancies in self- and observer-rated anxiety scales. A comparison between the self- and observer-rated Marks-Sheehan scales. Eur Arch Psychiatry Clin Neurosci 1990;240(2):96–102.

Alexander PE, Alexander DD. Alprazolam treatment for panic disorders. J Clin Psychiatry 1986 Jun;47(6):301–4.

Andersch S, Rosenberg NK, Kullingsjo H, Ottosson J-O, Bech P, Bruun-Hansen J, Hanson L, Lorentzen K, Mellergard M, Rasmussen S, Rosenberg R. Efficacy and safety of alprazolam, imipramine and placebo in treating panic disorder. A Scandinavian multicenter study. Acta Psychiatr Scand Suppl 1991;83(365):18–27.

Ballenger JC. Efficacy of benzodiazepines in panic disorder and agoraphobia. J Psychiatr Res 1990;24 Suppl 2:15–25.

Ballenger JC, Burrows GD, DuPont RL Jr, Lesser IM, Noyes R Jr, Pecknold JC, Rifkin A, Swinson RP. Alprazolam in panic disorder and agoraphobia: results from a multicenter trial. I. Efficacy in short-term treatment. Arch Gen Psychiatry 1988 May;45(5):413–22.

Beitman BD, Basha IM, Trombka LH, Jayaratna MA, Russell B, Flaker G, Anderson S. Pharmacotherapeutic treatment of panic disorder in patients presenting with chest pain. J Fam Pract 1989 Feb;28(2):177–80.

Beitman BD, Basha IM, Trombka LH, Jayaratna MA, Russell BD, Tarr SK. Alprazolam in the treatment of cardiology patients with atypical chest pain and panic disorder. J Clin Psychopharmacol 1988 Apr;8(2):127–30.

Buller R, Maier W, Goldenberg IM, Lavori PW, Benkert O. Chronology of panic and avoidance, age of onset in panic disorder, and prediction of treatment response. A report from the Cross-National Collaborative Panic Study. Eur Arch Psychiatry Clin Neurosci 1991;240(3):163–8.

Burrows GD. Managing long-term therapy for panic disorder. J Clin Psychiatry 1990 Nov;51 Suppl: 9–12.

Burrows GD, Norman TR, Judd FK, Marriott PF. Short-acting versus long-acting benzodiazepines: discontinuation effects in panic disorders. J Psychiatr Res 1990;24 Suppl 2:65–72.

Carr DB, Fishman SM, Kasting NW, Sheehan DV. Vasopressin response to lactate infusion in normals and patients with panic disorder. Funct Neurol 1986 Apr-Jun;1(2):123–7.

Carr DB, Sheehan DV, Surman OS, Coleman JH, Greenblatt DJ, Heninger GR, Jones KJ, Levine PH, Watkins WD. Neuroendocrine correlates of lactate-induced anxiety and their response to chronic alprazolam therapy. Am J Psychiatry 1986 Apr;143(4):483–94.

Charney DS, Heninger GR. Noradrenergic function and the mechanism of action of antianxiety treatment. I. The effect of long-term alprazolam treatment. Arch Gen Psychiatry 1985 May;42(5):458–67.

Charney DS, Heninger GR. Serotonin function in panic disorders. The effect of intravenous tryptophan in healthy subjects and patients with panic disorder before and during alprazolam treatment. Arch Gen Psychiatry 1986 Nov;43(11):1059–65.

Charney DS, Woods SW. Benzodiazepine treatment of panic disorder: a comparison of alprazolam and lorazepam. J Clin Psychiatry 1989 Nov;50(11):418–23.

Charney DS, Woods SW, Goodman WK, Rifkin B, Kinch M, Aiken B, Quadrino LM, Heninger GR. Drug treatment of panic disorder: the comparative efficacy of imipramine, alprazolam, and trazodone. J Clin Psychiatry 1986 Dec;47(12):580–6.

Ciraulo DA, Antal EJ, Smith RB, Olson DR, Goldberg DA, Rand EH, Raskin RB, Phillips JP, Shader RI, Greenblatt DJ. The relationship of alprazolam dose to steady-state plasma concentrations. J Clin Psychopharmacol 1990 Feb;10(1):27–32.

Ciraulo DA, Barnhill JG, Boxenbaum HG, Greenblatt DJ, Smith RB. Pharmacokinetics and clinical effects of alprazolam following single and multiple oral doses in patients with panic disorder. J Clin Pharmacol 1986 Apr;26(4):292–8.

Clark DB, Taylor CB, Roth WT, Hayward C, Ehlers A, Margraf J, Agras WS. Surreptitious drug use by patients in a panic disorder study. Am J Psychiatry 1990 Apr;147(4):507–9.

Coryell W, Noyes R Jr, Clancy J, Crowe R, Chaudhry D. Abnormal escape from dexamethasone suppression in agoraphobia with panic attacks. Psychiatry Res 1985 Aug;15 (4):301–11.

Coryell W, Noyes R. HPA axis disturbance and treatment outcome in panic disorder. Biol Psychiatry 1988 Nov;24(7):762–6.

Coryell W, Noyes R. Placebo response in panic disorder. Am J Psychiatry 1988 Sep;145(9):1138–40.

Coryell W, Noyes R Jr, Schlechte J. The significance of HPA axis disturbance in panic disorder. Biol Psychiatry 1989 Apr 15;25(8):989–1002.

Cox BJ, Swinson RP, Endler NS. A review of the psychopharmacology of panic disorder: Individual differences and non specific factors. Can J Psychiatry 1991;36(2):130–8.

Dager SR, Khan A, Cowley D, Avery DH, Elder J, Roy-Byrne P, Dunner DL. Characteristics of placebo response during long-term treatment of panic disorder. Psychopharmacol Bull 1990;26(3):273–8.

Davidson JR. Continuation treatment of panic disorder with high-potency benzodiazepines. J Clin Psychiatry 1990 Dec;51 Suppl A:31–7.

Deltito JA, Argyle N, Buller R, Nutzinger D, Ottosson JO, Brandon S, Mellergard M, Shera D. The sequence of improvement of the symptoms encountered in patients with panic disorder. Compr Psychiatry 1991 Mar-Apr;32(2):120–9.

Deltito JA, Argyle N, Klerman GL. Patients with panic disorder unaccompanied by depression improve with alprazolam and imipramine treatment. J Clin Psychiatry 1991 Mar;52(3):121–7.

Dilsaver SC. Panic disorder. Am Fam Physician 1989 Jun;39(6):167–72.

Drug treatment of panic disorder: Discussion III. Hosp Pract 1990;25 Suppl 2:40–2.

Dunner DL, Ishiki D, Avery DH, Wilson LG, Hyde TS. Effect of alprazolam and diazepam on anxiety and panic attacks in panic disorder: a controlled study. J Clin Psychiatry 1986 Sep;47(9):458–60.

Edlund MJ, Swann AC. Low MHPG and continuing treatment in panic disorder. Prog Neuropsychopharmacol Biol Psychiatry 1989;13(5):701–7.

Edlund MJ, Swann AC, Clothier J. Patients with panic attacks and abnormal EEG results. Am J Psychiatry 1987 Apr;144(4):508–9.

Eriksson E. Brain neurotransmission in panic disorder. Acta Psychiatr Scand Suppl 1987;335:31–7.

Eriksson E, Carlsson M, Nilsson C, Soderpalm B. Does alprazolam, in contrast to diazepam, activate alpha 2-adrenoceptors involved in the regulation of rat growth hormone secretion? Life Sci 1986 Apr 21;38(16):1491–8.

Fava GA. Fading of therapeutic effects of alprazolam in agoraphobia. Case reports. Prog Neuropsychopharmacol Biol Psychiatry 1988;12(1):109–12.

Fava GA, Grandi S, Saviotti FM, Conti S. Hypochondriasis with panic attacks. Psychosomatics 1990 Summer;31(3):351–3.

Fava M, Rosenbaum JF, MacLaughlin RA, Tesar GE, Pollack MH, Cohen LS, Hirsch M. Dehydroepiandrosterone-sulfate/cortisol ratio in panic disorder. Psychiatry Res 1989 Jun;28(3):345–50.

Fishman SM, Sheehan DV, Carr DB. Thyroid indices in panic disorder. J Clin Psychiatry 1985 Oct;46(10):432–3.

Fyer AJ, Liebowitz MR, Gorman JM, Campeas R, Levin A, Davies SO, Goetz D, Klein DF. Discontinuation of alprazolam treatment in panic patients. Am J Psychiatry 1987 Mar;144(3):303–8.

Fyer AJ, Liebowitz MR, Gorman JM, Campeas R, Levin A, Sandberg D, Fyer M, Hollander E, Papp L, Goetz D, et al. Effects of clonidine on alprazolam discontinuation in panic patients: a pilot study. J Clin Psychopharmacol 1988 Aug;8(4):270–4.

Garvey M, Noyes R Jr, Cook B, Tollefson G. The relationship of panic disorder and its treatment outcome to 24-hour urinary MHPG levels. Psychiatry Res 1989 Oct;30(1):53–61.

Gastfriend DR, Rosenbaum JF. Adjunctive buspirone in benzodiazepine treatment of four patients with panic disorder. Am J Psychiatry 1989 Jul;146(7):914–6.

Giesecke ME. Panic disorder in university students: A review. J Am Coll Health 1987;36(3):149–57.

Gorman JM, Liebowitz MR, Dillon D, Fyer AJ, Cohen BS, Klein DF. Antipanic drug effects during lactate infusion in lactate-refractory panic patients. Psychiatry Res 1987 Jul;21(3):205–12.

Green MA, Curtis GC. Personality disorders in panic patients: Response to termination of antipanic medication. J Pers Disord 1988;2(4):303–14.

Hauri PJ, Friedman M, Ravaris CL. Sleep in patients with spontaneous panic attacks. Sleep 1989 Aug;12(4):323–37.

Herman JB, Brotman AW, Rosenbaum JF. Rebound anxiety in panic disorder patients treated with shorter-acting benzodiazepines. J Clin Psychiatry 1987 Oct;48 Suppl:22–8.

Herman JB, Rosenbaum JF, Brotman AW. The alprazolam to clonazepam switch for the treatment of panic disorder. J Clin Psychopharmacol 1987 Jun;7(3):175–8.

Huybrechts I. The pharmacology of alprazolam: a review. Clin Ther 1991 Jan-Feb;13(1):100–17.

Jann MW, Kurtz NM. Treatment of panic and phobic disorders. Clin Pharm 1987 Dec;6(12):947–62.

Johnston AL, File SE. Profiles of the antipanic compounds, triazolobenzodiazepines and phenelzine, in two animal tests of anxiety. Psychiatry Res 1988 Jul;25(1):81–90.

Katon W. Panic disorder: epidemiology, diagnosis, and treatment in primary care. J Clin Psychiatry 1986 Oct;47 Suppl:21–30.

Katon W, Vitaliano PP, Russo J, Cormier L, Anderson K, Jones M. Panic disorder: epidemiology in primary care. J Fam Pract 1986 Sep;23(3):233–9.

King D, Nicolini H, de la Fuente JR. Abuse and withdrawal of panic treatment drugs. Psychiatr Ann 1990 Sep;20(9):525–8.

Klein DF. Psychopharmacologic treatment of panic disorder. Psychosomatics 1984;25(10 Suppl):32–6.

Klerman GL. Depression and panic anxiety: the effect of depressive co-morbidity on response to drug treatment of patients with panic disorder and agoraphobia. J Psychiatr Res 1990;24 Suppl 2: 27–41.

Klerman GL. Overview of the Cross-National Collaborative Panic Study. Arch Gen Psychiatry 1988 May;45(5):407–12.

Klerman GL. Panic disorder: strategies for long-term treatment. J Clin Psychiatry 1991 Feb;52 Suppl:3–5.

Klerman GL, Ballenger JC, Burrows GD, DuPont RL, et al. "The 'efficacy' of alprazolam in panic disorder and agoraphobia: A critique of recent reports": Reply. Arch Gen Psychiatry 1989 Jul;46(7):670–2.

Klerman GL, Freedman DX, Shader RI. The separation of panic and agoraphobia from other anxiety disorders: Introduction of the conference proceedings. J Psychiatr Res 1988;22 Suppl 1:3–5.

Klosko JS, Barlow DH, Tassinari R, Cerny JA. A comparison of alprazolam and behavior therapy in treatment of panic disorder. J Consult Clin Psychol 1990 Feb;58(1):77–84.

Lepola U. Recognition of panic disorder. Nord Psykiatr Tidsskr 1989;43(6):511–3.

Lepola U, Heikkinen H, Rimon R, Riekkinen P. Clinical evaluation of alprazolam in patients with panic disorder: A double-blind comparison with imipramine. Hum Psychopharmacol 1990;5(2):159–63.

Lepola U, Jolkkonen J, Rim:on R, Riekkinen P. Long-term effects of alprazolam and imipramine on cerebrospinal fluid monoamine metabolites and neuropeptides in panic disorder. Neuropsychobiology 1989;21(4):182–6.

Lesser IM, Rubin RT, Pecknold JC, Rifkin A, Swinson RP, Lydiard RB, Burrows GD, Noyes R Jr, DuPont RL Jr. Secondary depression in panic disorder and agoraphobia. I. Frequency, severity, and response to treatment. Arch Gen Psychiatry 1988 May;45(5):437–43.

Lesser IM, Rubin RT, Rifkin A, Swinson RP, Ballenger JC, Burrows GD, DuPont RL, Noyes R, Pecknold JC. Secondary depression in panic disorder and agoraphobia. II. Dimensions of depressive symptomatology and their response to treatment. J Affective Disord 1989 Jan-Feb;16(1):49–58.

Liebowitz MR, Fyer AJ, Gorman JM, Campeas R, Levin A, Davies SR, Goetz D, Klein DF. Alprazolam in the treatment of panic disorders. J Clin Psychopharmacol 1986 Feb;6(1):13–20.

Linnoila MI. Anxiety and alcoholism. J Clin Psychiatry 1989 Nov;50 Suppl:26–9.

Lopez AL, Kathol RG, Noyes R Jr. Reduction in urinary free cortisol during benzodiazepine treatment of panic disorder. Psychoneuroendocrinology 1990;15(1):23–8.

Lydiard RB, Laraia MT, Ballenger JC, Howell EF. Emergence of depressive symptoms in patients receiving alprazolam for panic disorder. Am J Psychiatry 1987 May;144(5):664–5.

Lydiard RB, Roy-Byrne PP, Ballenger JC. Recent advances in the psychopharmacological treatment of anxiety disorders. Hosp Community Psychiatry 1988 Nov;39(11):1157–65.

Margraf J, Ehlers A, Roth WT, Clark DB, Sheikh J, Agras WS, Taylor CB. How "blind" are double-blind studies? J Consult Clin Psychol 1991 Feb;59(1):184–7.

Marks IM, de Albuquerque A, Cottraux J, Gentil V, et al. The "efficacy" of alprazolam in panic disorder and agoraphobia: A critique of recent reports. Arch Gen Psychiatry 1989 Jul;46(7):668–72.

Marshall JR. Diagnosis and management of panic disorder in the emergency department. Emerg Care Q 1991;7(1):1–8.

Mattick RP, Andrews G, Hadzi-Pavlovic D, Christensen H. Treatment of panic and agoraphobia. An integrative review. J Nerv Ment Dis 1990 Sep;178(9):567–76.

McIntyre IM, Judd FK, Burrows GD, Armstrong SM, Norman TR. Plasma concentrations of melatonin in panic disorder. Am J Psychiatry 1990 Apr;147(4):462–4.

Meco G, Capriani C, Bonifati U, Ecari U. Etizolam: A new therapeutic possibility in the treatment of panic disorder. Adv Ther 1989;6(4):196–206.

Mellergard M, Lorentzen K, Bech P, Ottosson J-O, Rosenberg R. A trend analysis of changes during treatment of panic disorder with alprazolam and imipramine. Acta Psychiatr Scand Suppl 1991;83(365):28–32.

Mellergard M, Rosenberg NK. Patterns of response during placebo treatment of panic disorder. Acta Psychiatr Scand 1990 Apr;81(4):340–4.

Mohns EB. Discontinuation and withdrawal problems of alprazolam. West J Med 1989;151(3):312.

Munjack DJ, Crocker B, Cabe D, Brown R, Usigli R, Zulueta A, McManus M, McDowell D, Palmer R, Leonard M. Alprazolam, propranolol, and placebo in the treatment of panic disorder and agoraphobia with panic attacks. J Clin Psychopharmacol 1989 Feb;9(1):22–7.

Nagy LM, Krystal JH, Woods SW, Charney DS. Clinical and medication outcome after short-term alprazolam and behavioral group treatment in panic disorder. 2.5 year naturalistic follow-up study. Arch Gen Psychiatry 1989 Nov;46(11):993–9.

Noyes R, Reich J, Clancy J, O'Gorman TW. Reduction in hypochondriasis with treatment of panic disorder [published erratum appears in Br J Psychiatry 1987 Feb;150:273]. Br J Psychiatry 1986 Nov;149:631–5.

Noyes R Jr, Cook B, Garvey M, Summers R. Reduction of gastrointestinal symptoms following treatment for panic disorder. Psychosomatics 1990 Winter;31(1):75–9.

Noyes R Jr, DuPont RL Jr, Pecknold JC, Rifkin A, Rubin RT, Swinson RP, Ballenger JC, Burrows GD. Alprazolam in panic disorder and agoraphobia: results from a multicenter trial. II. Patient acceptance, side effects, and safety. Arch Gen Psychiatry 1988 May;45(5):423–8.

Noyes R Jr, Garvey MJ, Cook B, Suelzer M. Controlled discontinuation of benzodiazepine treatment for patients with panic disorder. Am J Psychiatry 1991 Apr;148(4):517–23.

Noyes R Jr, Perry PJ, Crowe RR, Coryell WH, Clancy J, Yamada T, Gabel J. Seizures following the withdrawal of alprazolam. J Nerv Ment Dis 1986 Jan;174(1):50–2.

O'Boyle M. Panic disorder: diagnosis and treatment. Tex Med 1989 Aug;85(8):46–9.

Overall JE, Sheehan DV. Multivariate analysis of changes in panic frequency counts. Clin Neuropharmacol 1986;9 Suppl 4:155–7.

Pecknold JC. Behavioral and combined therapy in panic states. Prog Neuropsychopharmacol Biol Psychiatry 1987;11(2-3):97–104.

Pecknold JC, Fleury D. Alprazolam-induced manic episode in two patients with panic disorder. Am J Psychiatry 1986 May;143(5):652–3.

Pecknold JC, Swinson RP, Kuch K, Lewis CP. Alprazolam in panic disorder and agoraphobia: results from a multicenter trial. III. Discontinuation effects. Arch Gen Psychiatry 1988 May;45(5):429–36.

Pecknold JC, Swinson RP. Taper withdrawal studies with alprazolam in patients with panic disorder and agoraphobia. Psychopharmacol Bull 1986;22(1):173–6.

Pollack MH. Long-term management of panic disorder. J Clin Psychiatry 1990 May;51 Suppl:11–3; discussion 50–3.

Pollack MH, Otto MW, Rosenbaum JF, Sachs GS, O'Neil C, Asher R, Meltzer-Brody S. Longitudinal course of panic disorder: findings from the Massachusetts General Hospital Naturalistic Study. J Clin Psychiatry 1990 Dec;51 Suppl A:12–6.

Pollack MH, Rosenbaum JF. Benzodiazepines in panic-related disorders. Special Issue: Perspectives on panic-related disorders. J Anxiety Disord 1988;2(1):95–107.

Pollack MH, Rosenbaum JF, Tesar GE, Herman JB, Sachs GS. Clonazepam in the treatment of panic disorder and agoraphobia. Psychopharmacol Bull 1987;23(1):141–4.

Pyke RE, Greenberg HS. Double-blind comparison of alprazolam and adinazolam for panic and phobic disorders. J Clin Psychopharmacol 1989 Feb;9(1):15–21.

Pyke RE, Kraus M. Alprazolam in the treatment of panic attack patients with and without major depression. J Clin Psychiatry 1988 Feb;49(2):66–8.

Raj A, Sheehan DV. Panic anxiety: diagnosis, etiology, and treatment. Compr Ther 1986 Oct;12(10):7–15.

Rickels K, Case WG, Schweizer E. The drug treatment of anxiety and panic disorder. Stress Med 1988;4(4):231–9.

Rizley R, Kahn RJ, McNair DM, Frankenthaler LM. A comparison of alprazolam and imipramine in the treatment of agoraphobia and panic disorder. Psychopharmacol Bull 1986;22(1):167–72.

Rosenberg NK, Mellergard M, Rosenberg R, Beck P, Ottosson J-O. Characteristics of panic disorder patients responding to placebo. Acta Psychiatr Scand Suppl 1991;83(365):33–8.

Rosenberg R, Bech P, Mellergard M, Ottosson J-O. Alprazolam, imipramine and placebo treatment of panic disorder: Predicting therapeutic response. Acta Psychiatr Scand Suppl 1991;83(365):46–52.

Rosenberg R, Bech P, Mellergard M, Ottosson J-O. Secondary depression in panic disorder: An indicator of severity with a weak effect on outcome in alprazolam and imipramine treatment. Acta Psychiatr Scand Suppl 1991;83(365):39–45.

Roy-Byrne PP, Dager SR, Cowley DS, Vitaliano P, Dunner DL. Relapse and rebound following discontinuation of benzodiazepine treatment of panic attacks: alprazolam versus diazepam. Am J Psychiatry 1989 Jul;146(7):860–5.

Schweizer E, Fox I, Case G, Rickels K. Lorazepam vs. alprazolam in the treatment of panic disorder. Psychopharmacol Bull 1988;24(2):224–7.

Schweizer E, Pohl R, Balon R, Fox I, Rickels K, Yeragani VK. Lorazepam vs. alprazolam in the treatment of panic disorder. Pharmacopsychiatry 1990 Mar;23(2):90–3.

Scrignar CB. Postpanic anxiety disorder: diagnosis and treatment. South Med J 1986 Apr;79(4):400–4.

Sheehan DV. Benzodiazepines in panic disorder and agoraphobia. J Affective Disord 1987 Sep-Oct;13(2):169–81.

Sheehan DV. Monoamine oxidase inhibitors and alprazolam in the treatment of panic disorder and agoraphobia. Psychiatr Clin North Am 1985 Mar; 8(1):49–62.

Sheehan DV, Sheehan KH. Pharmacological treatment of panic and anxiety disorders. ISI Atlas Sci Pharmacol 1987;1(3):254–6.

Sheehan DV, Soto S. Recent developments in the treatment of panic disorder. Acta Psychiatr Scand Suppl 1987;335:75–85.

Smith GR, O'Rourke DF, Parker PE, Ford CV, et al. Panic and nausea instead of grief in an adolescent. J Am Acad Child Adolesc Psychiatry 1988 Jul;27(4):509–13.

Stewart RS. Pharmacologic treatment of panic disorder and agoraphobia. Hosp Formul 1990;25(4):416–22.

Sunderland G, Friedman S, Rosenblum LA. Imipramine and alprazolam treatment of lactate-induced acute endogenous distress in nonhuman primates. Am J Psychiatry 1989 Aug;146(8):1044–7.

Swinson RP, Pecknold JC, Kuch K. Psychopharmacological treatment of panic disorder and related states: a placebo controlled study of alprazolam. Prog Neuropsychopharmacol Biol Psychiatry 1987;11(2–3):105–13.

Taylor CB, Hayward C, King R, Ehlers A, Margraf J, Maddock R, Clark D, Roth WT, Agras WS. Cardiovascular and symptomatic reduction effects of alprazolam and imipramine in patients with panic disorder: results of a double-blind, placebo-controlled trial. J Clin Psychopharmacol 1990 Apr;10(2):112–8.

Tesar GE. High-potency benzodiazepines for short-term management of panic disorder: the U.S. experience. J Clin Psychiatry 1990 May;51 Suppl: 4–10; discussion 50–3.

Tesar GE, Rosenbaum JF, Pollack MH, Herman JB, Sachs GS, Mahoney EM, Cohen LS, McNamara M, Goldstein S. Clonazepam versus alprazolam in the treatment of panic disorder: interim analysis of data from a prospective, double-blind, placebo-controlled trial. J Clin Psychiatry 1987 Oct;48 Suppl:16–21.

Tesar GE, Rosenbaum JF, Pollack MH, Otto MW, Sachs GS, Herman JB, Cohen LS, Spier SA. Double-blind, placebo-controlled comparison of clonazepam and alprazolam for panic disorder. J Clin Psychiatry 1991 Feb;52(2):69–76.

Tiller JW. The new and newer antianxiety agents. Med J Aust 1989 Dec 4-18;151(11-12):697–701.

Tobe EH. Pitfalls in the management of panic disorder. J Am Osteopath Assoc 1988;88(4):507–9.

Tobena A, Sanchez R, Pose R, Masana J, et al. Brief treatment with alprazolam and behavioral guidance in panic disorder. Anxiety Res 1990 Nov;3(3):163–74.

Uhlenhuth EH, Matuzas W, Glass RM, Easton C. Response of panic disorder to fixed doses of alprazolam or imipramine. J Affective Disord 1989 Nov-Dec;17(3):261–70.

Warner MD, Peabody CA, Boutros NN, Whiteford HA. Alprazolam and withdrawal seizures. J Nerv Ment Dis 1990;178(3):208–9.

Wincor MZ, Munjack DJ, Palmer R. Alprazolam levels and response in panic disorder: preliminary results. J Clin Psychopharmacol 1991 Feb;11(1):48–51.

Wood WG. The diagnosis and management of panic disorder. Psychiatr Med 1990; 8(3):197–209.

Other Benzodiazepines

Andersch S, Rosenberg NK, Kullingsjo H, Ottosson J-O, Bech P, Bruun-Hansen J, Hanson L, Lorentzen K, Mellergard M, Rasmussen S, Rosenberg R. Efficacy and safety of alprazolam, imipramine and placebo in treating panic disorder. A Scandinavian multicenter study. Acta Psychiatr Scand Suppl 1991;83(365):18–27.

Aronson TA. Treatment-emergent depression with antidepressants in panic disorder. Compr Psychiatry 1989 May-Jun;30(3):267–71.

Aronson TA, Carasiti I, McBane D, Whitaker–Azmitia P. Biological correlates of lactate sensitivity in panic disorder. Biol Psychiatry 1989 Sep;26(5):463–77.

Balestrieri M, Ruggeri M, Bellantuono C. Drug treatment of panic disorder—a critical review of controlled clinical trials. Psychiatr Dev 1989 Winter;7(4):337–50.

Ballenger JC. Efficacy of benzodiazepines in panic disorder and agoraphobia. J Psychiatr Res 1990;24 Suppl 2:15–25.

Ballenger JC. Long-term pharmacologic treatment of panic disorder. J Clin Psychiatry 1991 Feb;52 Suppl:18–23; discussion 24–5.

Ballenger JC. Pharmacotherapy of the panic disorders. J Clin Psychiatry 1986 Jun;47 Suppl:27–32.

Beardslee SL, Papadakis E, Fontana DJ, Commissaris RL. Antipanic drug treatments: failure to exhibit anxiolytic-like effects on defensive burying behavior. Pharmacol Biochem Behav 1990 Feb;35(2):451–5.

Beaudry P, Fontaine R, Chouinard G, Annable L. An open clinical trial of clonazepam in the treatment of patients with recurrent panic attacks. Prog Neuropsychopharmacol Biol Psychiatry 1985;9(5–6):589–92.

Beaudry P, Fontaine R, Chouinard G, Annable L. Clonazepam in the treatment of patients with recurrent panic attacks. J Clin Psychiatry 1986 Feb;47(2):83–5.

Beckett A, Fishman SM, Rosenbaum JF. Clonazepam blockade of spontaneous and CO2 inhalation-provoked panic in a patient with panic disorder. J Clin Psychiatry 1986 Sep;47(9):475–6.

Bogdonoff MD. Benzodiazepine sensitivity in panic disorder. Drug Ther 1990;20(9):33.

Breier A, Charney DS, Heninger GR. The diagnostic validity of anxiety disorders and their relationship to depressive illness. Am J Psychiatry 1985 Jul;142(7):787–97.

Burrows GD. Managing long-term therapy for panic disorder. J Clin Psychiatry 1990 Nov;51 Suppl: 9–12.

Burrows GD, Norman TR, Judd FK, Marriott PF. Short-acting versus long-acting benzodiazepines: discontinuation effects in panic disorders. J Psychiatr Res 1990;24 Suppl 2:65–72.

Charney DS, Woods SW. Benzodiazepine treatment of panic disorder: a comparison of alprazolam and lorazepam. J Clin Psychiatry 1989 Nov;50(11):418–23.

Coryell W, Noyes R. Placebo response in panic disorder. Am J Psychiatry 1988 Sep;145(9):1138–40.

Coryell W, Noyes R Jr, Reich J. The prognostic significance of HPA-axis disturbance in panic disorder: a three-year follow-up. Biol Psychiatry 1991 Jan 15;29(2):96–102.

Coryell W, Noyes R Jr, Schlechte J. The significance of HPA axis disturbance in panic disorder. Biol Psychiatry 1989 Apr 15;25(8):989–1002.

Cowley DS, Roy-Byrne PP. Hyperventilation and panic disorder. Am J Med 1987 Nov;83(5):929–37.

Crowe RR, Noyes R Jr. Panic disorder and agoraphobia. Dis Mon 1986 Jul;32(7):389–444.

Dajas F, Nin A, Barbeito L. Urinary norepinephrine excretion in panic and phobic disorders. J Neural Transm 1986;65(1):75–81.

Davidson JR. Continuation treatment of panic disorder with high-potency benzodiazepines. J Clin Psychiatry 1990 Dec;51 Suppl A:31–7.

de Montigny C. Cholecystokinin tetrapeptide induces panic-like attacks in healthy volunteers. Preliminary findings. Arch Gen Psychiatry 1989 Jun;46(6):511–7.

Drug treatment of panic disorder: Discussion III. Hosp Pract 1990;25 Suppl 2:40–2.

Dunner DL, Ishiki D, Avery DH, Wilson LG, Hyde TS. Effect of alprazolam and diazepam on anxiety and panic attacks in panic disorder: a controlled study. J Clin Psychiatry 1986 Sep;47(9):458–60.

DuPont RL. Thinking about stopping treatment for panic disorder. J Clin Psychiatry 1990 Dec;51 Suppl A:38–45.

Eriksson E, Carlsson M, Nilsson C, Soderpalm B. Does alprazolam, in contrast to diazepam, activate alpha 2-adrenoceptors involved in the regulation of rat growth hormone secretion? Life Sci 1986 Apr 21;38(16):1491–8.

Evans L. Panic disorder. A new definition to anxiety. Curr Ther 1987;28(11):19–21.

Fava M, Anderson K, Rosenbaum JF. "Anger attacks": possible variants of panic and major depressive disorders. Am J Psychiatry 1990 Jul;147(7):867–70.

Fava M, Rosenbaum JF, MacLaughlin RA, Tesar GE, Pollack MH, Cohen LS, Hirsch M. Dehydroepiandrosterone-sulfate/cortisol ratio in panic disorder. Psychiatry Res 1989 Jun;28(3):345–50.

Fontaine R. Clonazepam for panic disorders and agitation. Psychosomatics 1985 Dec;26(12 Suppl):13–8.

Freedman DX. Benzodiazepines: therapeutic, biological and psychosocial issues. Symposium summary. J Psychiatr Res 1990;24 Suppl 2:169–74.

Garvey M, Noyes R Jr, Cook B, Tollefson G. The relationship of panic disorder and its treatment outcome to 24-hour urinary MHPG levels. Psychiatry Res 1989 Oct;30(1):53–61.

Gastfriend DR, Rosenbaum JF. Adjunctive buspirone in benzodiazepine treatment of four patients with panic disorder. Am J Psychiatry 1989 Jul;146(7):914–6.

Giesecke ME. Panic disorder in university students: A review. J Am Coll Health 1987;36(3):149–57.

Gold DD Jr. Panic attacks: Diagnosis and management. Cardiovasc Rev Rep 1988;9(1):35–7, 40.

Goodman WK, Charney DS, Price LH, Woods SW, Heninger GR. Ineffectiveness of clonidine in the treatment of the benzodiazepine withdrawal syndrome: report of three cases. Am J Psychiatry 1986 Jul;143(7):900–3.

Hayes PE, Schulz SC. Beta-blockers in anxiety disorders. J Affective Disord 1987 Sep-Oct;13(2):119–30.

Herman JB, Brotman AW, Rosenbaum JF. Rebound anxiety in panic disorder patients treated with shorter-acting benzodiazepines. J Clin Psychiatry 1987 Oct;48 Suppl:22–8.

Herman JB, Rosenbaum JF, Brotman AW. The alprazolam to clonazepam switch for the treatment of panic disorder. J Clin Psychopharmacol 1987 Jun;7(3):175–8.

Hollister LE. Anxiety: drug treatments for biologically determined disorders. Ration Drug Ther 1986 Apr;20(4):1–6.

Jann MW, Kurtz NM. Treatment of panic and phobic disorders. Clin Pharm 1987 Dec;6(12):947–62.

Johnston AL, File SE. Profiles of the antipanic compounds, triazolobenzodiazepines and phenelzine, in two animal tests of anxiety. Psychiatry Res 1988 Jul;25(1):81–90.

Judd FK, Burrows GD, Marriott PF, Norman TR. A short term open clinical trial of clobazam in the treatment of patients with panic attacks. Int Clin Psychopharmacol 1989 Oct;4(4):285–93.

Judd FK, Norman TR, Burrows GD. Pharmacological treatment of panic disorder. Int Clin Psychopharmacol 1986 Jan;1(1):3–16.

Judd FK, Norman TR, Burrows GD. Pharmacotherapy of panic disorder. Int Rev Psychiatry 1990;2(3–4):399–409.

Klein DF. Psychopharmacologic treatment of panic disorder. Psychosomatics 1984;25(10 Suppl):32–6.

Klerman GL. Panic disorder: strategies for long-term treatment. J Clin Psychiatry 1991 Feb;52 Suppl:3–5.

Klerman GL, Coleman JH, Purpura RP. The design and conduct of the Upjohn Cross-National Collaborative Panic Study. Psychopharmacol Bull 1986;22(1):59–64.

Kutcher SP, MacKenzie S. Successful clonazepam treatment of adolescents with panic disorder. J Clin Psychopharmacol 1988 Aug;8(4):299–301.

Lilienfeld SO, Jacob RG, Furman JM. Vestibular dysfunction followed by panic disorder with agoraphobia. J Nerv Ment Dis 1989 Nov;177(11):700–1.

Linnoila MI. Approaches to the treatment of alcoholism and anxiety. Drug Ther 1990;20 Suppl: 27–34.

Lopez AL, Kathol RG, Noyes R Jr. Reduction in urinary free cortisol during benzodiazepine treatment of panic disorder. Psychoneuroendocrinology 1990;15(1):23–8.

Lydiard RB. Pharmacological treatment. Psychiatr Ann 1988 Aug;18(8):468–72.

Lydiard RB, Howell EF, Laraia MT, Fossey MD, et al. Depression in patients receiving lorazepam for panic. Am J Psychiatry 1989 Sep;146(9):1230–1.

Lydiard RB, Laraia MT, Howell EF, Ballenger JC. Can panic disorder present as irritable bowel syndrome? J Clin Psychiatry 1986 Sep;47(9):470–3.

Lydiard RB, Laraia MT, Howell EF, Fossey MD, Reynolds RD, Ballenger JC. Phenelzine treatment of panic disorder: lack of effect on pyridoxal phosphate levels. J Clin Psychopharmacol 1989 Dec;9(6):428–31.

Lydiard RB, Roy-Byrne PP, Ballenger JC. Recent advances in the psychopharmacological treatment of anxiety disorders. Hosp Community Psychiatry 1988 Nov;39(11):1157–65.

Marks I. Behavioral and drug treatments of phobic and obsessive-compulsive disorders. Psychother Psychosom 1986;46(1-2):35–44.

Marshall JR. Diagnosis and management of panic disorder in the emergency department. Emerg Care Q 1991;7(1):1–8.

Mattick RP, Andrews G, Hadzi-Pavlovic D, Christensen H. Treatment of panic and agoraphobia. An integrative review. J Nerv Ment Dis 1990 Sep;178(9):567–76.

Meco G, Capriani C, Bonifati U, Ecari U. Etizolam: A new therapeutic possibility in the treatment of panic disorder. Adv Ther 1989;6(4):196–206.

Murray JB. Psychopharmacological investigation of panic disorder by means of lactate infusion. J Gen Psychol 1987 Jul;114(3):297–311.

Muskin PR. Panics, prolapse, and PVCs. Gen Hosp Psychiatry 1985 Jul;7(3):219–23.

Nasdahl CS, Johnston JA, Coleman JH, May CN, Druff JH. Protocols for the use of psychoactive drugs—Part IV: Protocol for the treatment of anxiety disorders. J Clin Psychiatry 1985 Apr;46(4):128–32.

Norman TR, Gregory MS, Judd FK, Burrows GD, McIntyre IM. Platelet serotonin uptake in panic disorder: comparison with normal controls and the effect of treatment. Aust N Z J Psychiatry 1988 Dec;22(4):390–5.

Noyes R Jr, Cook B, Garvey M, Summers R. Reduction of gastrointestinal symptoms following treatment for panic disorder. Psychosomatics 1990 Winter;31(1):75–9.

Noyes R Jr, Garvey MJ, Cook B, Suelzer M. Controlled discontinuation of benzodiazepine treatment for patients with panic disorder. Am J Psychiatry 1991 Apr;148(4):517–23.

Nutt DJ, Glue P, Lawson C, Wilson S. Flumazenil provocation of panic attacks. Evidence for altered benzodiazepine receptor sensitivity in panic disorder. Arch Gen Psychiatry 1990 Oct;47(10):917–25.

Ontiveros A, Fontaine R. Panic attacks and multiple sclerosis. Biol Psychiatry 1990 Mar;27(6):672–3.

Pollack MH. Clonazepam: a review of open clinical trials. J Clin Psychiatry 1987 Oct;48 Suppl:12–5.

Pollack MH. Long-term management of panic disorder. J Clin Psychiatry 1990 May;51 Suppl:11–3; discussion 50–3.

Pollack MH, Otto MW, Rosenbaum JF, Sachs GS, O'Neil C, Asher R, Meltzer-Brody S. Longitudinal course of panic disorder: findings from the Massachusetts General Hospital Naturalistic Study. J Clin Psychiatry 1990 Dec;51 Suppl A:12–6.

Pollack MH, Rosenbaum JF. Benzodiazepines in panic-related disorders. Special Issue: Perspectives on panic-related disorders. J Anxiety Disord 1988;2(1):95–107.

Pollack MH, Rosenbaum JF, Tesar GE, Herman JB, Sachs GS. Clonazepam in the treatment of panic disorder and agoraphobia. Psychopharmacol Bull 1987;23(1):141–4.

Pollack MH, Tesar GE, Rosenbaum JF, Spier SA. Clonazepam in the treatment of panic disorder and agoraphobia: a one-year follow-up. J Clin Psychopharmacol 1986 Oct;6(5):302–4.

Pyke RE, Greenberg HS. Double-blind comparison of alprazolam and adinazolam for panic and phobic disorders. J Clin Psychopharmacol 1989 Feb;9(1):15–21.

Reich JH. DSM-III personality disorders and the outcome of treated panic disorder. Am J Psychiatry 1988 Sep;145(9):1149–52.

Rickels K. Antianxiety therapy: potential value of long-term treatment. J Clin Psychiatry 1987 Dec;48 Suppl:7–11.

Rickels K. Clinical studies of "specific" anxiolytics as therapeutic agents. Psychopharmacol Ser 1987;3: 88–95.

Rickels K, Case WG, Downing RW, Fridman R. One-year follow-up of anxious patients treated with diazepam. J Clin Psychopharmacol 1986;6(1):32–6.

Rickels K, Case WG, Schweizer E. The drug treatment of anxiety and panic disorder. Stress Med 1988;4(4):231–9.

Rickels K, Schweizer EE. Benzodiazepines for treatment of panic attacks: a new look. Psychopharmacol Bull 1986;22(1):93–9.

Rickels K, Schweizer E, Case WG, Greenblatt DJ. Long-term therapeutic use of benzodiazepines. I. Effects of abrupt discontinuation [published erratum appears in Arch Gen Psychiatry 1991 Jan;48(1):51]. Arch Gen Psychiatry 1990 Oct;47(10):899–907.

Rifkin A. Benzodiazepines for anxiety disorders. Are the concerns justified? Postgrad Med 1990 Jan;87(1):209-11, 215–6, 219.

Rosenbaum JF. A psychopharmacologist's perspective on panic disorder. Bull Menninger Clin 1990 Spring;54(2):184–98.

Rosenbaum JF. Drug treatment of panic disorder. Hosp Pract [Off] 1990 Jun;25 Suppl 2:31–9; discussion 40–2.

Rosenbaum JF. Panic disorder: Diathesis and treatment issues. J Clin Psychiatry 1990;51(12 Suppl A):3–4.

Rosenblat H. Panic attacks triggered by photic stimulation. Am J Psychiatry 1989 Jun;146(6):801–2.

Roy-Byrne PP, Dager SR, Cowley DS, Vitaliano P, Dunner DL. Relapse and rebound following discontinuation of benzodiazepine treatment of panic attacks: alprazolam versus diazepam. Am J Psychiatry 1989 Jul;146(7):860–5.

Roy-Byrne PP, Lewis N, Villacres E, Diem H, Greenblatt DJ, Shader RI, Veith R. Preliminary evidence of benzodiazepine subsensitivity in panic disorder. Biol Psychiatry 1989 Nov;26(7):744–8.

Sargent M. Panic disorder. Hosp Community Psychiatry 1990 Jun;41(6):621–3.

Savoldi F, Somenzini G, Ecari U. Etizolam versus placebo in the treatment of panic disorder with agoraphobia: a double-blind study. Curr Med Res Opin 1990;12(3):185–90.

Schatzberg AF, Ballenger JC. Decisions for the clinician in the treatment of panic disorder: when to treat, which treatment to use, and how long to treat. J Clin Psychiatry 1991 Feb;52 Suppl:26–31; discussion 32.

Schifano F, Magni G. Panic attacks and major depression after discontinuation of long-term diazepam abuse. DICP 1989 Dec;23(12):989–90.

Schweizer E, Fox I, Case G, Rickels K. Lorazepam vs. alprazolam in the treatment of panic disorder. Psychopharmacol Bull 1988;24(2):224–7.

Schweizer E, Pohl R, Balon R, Fox I, Rickels K, Yeragani VK. Lorazepam vs. alprazolam in the treatment of panic disorder. Pharmacopsychiatry 1990 Mar;23(2):90–3.

Schweizer E, Rickels K. Buspirone in the treatment of panic disorder: A controlled pilot comparison with clorazepate. J Clin Psychopharmacol 1988 Aug;8(4):303.

Sheehan DV. Benzodiazepines in panic disorder and agoraphobia. J Affective Disord 1987 Sep-Oct;13(2):169–81.

Sheehan DV, Raj AB, Harnett-Sheehan K, Soto S, et al. Adinazolam sustained release formulation in the treatment of panic disorder: A pilot study. Ir J Psychol Med 1990 Sep;7(2):124–8.

Sheehan DV, Sheehan KH. Pharmacological treatment of panic and anxiety disorders. ISI Atlas Sci Pharmacol 1987;1(3):254–6.

Shelton RC. Diagnosis and management of panic disorder. Compr Ther 1990 Dec;16(12):11–7.

Spier SA, Tesar GE, Rosenbaum JF, Woods SW. Treatment of panic disorder and agoraphobia with clonazepam. J Clin Psychiatry 1986 May;47(5):238–42.

Stewart RS. Pharmacologic treatment of panic disorder and agoraphobia. Hosp Formul 1990;25(4):416–22.

Svebak S, Cameron A, Levander S. Clonazepam and imipramine in the treatment of panic attacks: a double-blind comparison of efficacy and side effects. J Clin Psychiatry 1990 May;51 Suppl:14–7; discussion 50–3.

Swartz M, Landerman R, George LK, Melville ML, Blazer D, Smith K. Benzodiazepine anti-anxiety agents: prevalence and correlates of use in a southern community. Am J Public Health 1991 May;81(5):592–6.

Swinson RP. The acute treatment of anxiety and depression. Psychiatr J Univ Ott 1989 Jun;14(2):375–8; discussion 379–80.

Taylor DP. Serotonin agents in anxiety. Ann New York Acad Sci 1990;600:545–57.

Taylor CB, Hayward C. Cardiovascular considerations in selection of anti-panic pharmacotherapy. J Psychiatr Res 1990;24 Suppl 2:43–9.

Taylor CB, King R, Margraf J, Ehlers A, Telch M, Roth WT, Agras WS. Use of medication and in vivo exposure in volunteers for panic disorder research. Am J Psychiatry 1989 Nov;146(11):1423–6.

Tesar GE. High-potency benzodiazepines for short-term management of panic disorder: the U.S. experience. J Clin Psychiatry 1990 May;51 Suppl:4–10; discussion 50–3.

Tesar GE, Rosenbaum JF. Successful use of clonazepam in patients with treatment-resistant panic disorder. J Nerv Ment Dis 1986 Aug;174(8):477–82.

Tesar GE, Rosenbaum JF, Pollack MH, Herman JB, Sachs GS, Mahoney EM, Cohen LS, McNamara M, Goldstein S. Clonazepam versus alprazolam in the treatment of panic disorder: interim analysis of data from a prospective, double-blind, placebo-controlled trial. J Clin Psychiatry 1987 Oct;48 Suppl:16–21.

Tesar GE, Rosenbaum JF, Pollack MH, Otto MW, Sachs GS, Herman JB, Cohen LS, Spier SA. Double-blind, placebo-controlled comparison of clonazepam and alprazolam for panic disorder. J Clin Psychiatry 1991 Feb;52(2):69–76.

Tiller JW. The new and newer antianxiety agents. Med J Aust 1989 Dec 4-18;151(11–12):697–701.

Treatment of syndromes or of symptoms in psychiatry? Lancet 1988;2(8607):373–4.

Treatment outlines for the management of anxiety states. Aust N Z J Psychiatry 1985;19(2):138–51.

Tyrer P, Seivewright N, Ferguson B, Murphy S, Darling C, Brothwell J, Kingdon D, Johnson AL. The Nottingham Study of Neurotic Disorder: relationship between personality status and symptoms. Psychol Med 1990 May;20(2):423–31.

Tyrer P, Seivewright N, Murphy S, Ferguson B, Kingdon D, Barczak P, Brothwell J, Darling C, Gregory S, Johnson AL. The Nottingham study of neurotic disorder: comparison of drug and psychological treatments. Lancet 1988 Jul 30;2(8605):235–40.

Uhde TW, Kellner CH. Cerebral ventricular size in panic disorder. J Affective Disord 1987 Mar-Apr;12(2):175–8.

Warneke LB. Benzodiazepines: abuse and new use. Can J Psychiatry 1991 Apr;36(3):194–205.

Williams RB Jr. Do benzodiazepines have a role in the prevention or treatment of coronary heart disease and other major medical disorders? J Psychiatr Res 1990;24 Suppl 2:51–6.

Wood WG. The diagnosis and management of panic disorder. Psychiatr Med 1990;8(3):197–209.

Woods SW, Charney DS, Silver JM, Krystal JH, Heninger GR. Behavioral, biochemical, and cardiovascular responses to the benzodiazepine receptor antagonist flumazenil in panic disorder. Psychiatry Res 1991 Feb;36(2):115–27.

Monoamine Oxidase Inhibitors

Balestrieri M, Ruggeri M, Bellantuono C. Drug treatment of panic disorder—a critical review of controlled clinical trials. Psychiatr Dev 1989 Winter;7(4):337–50.

Ballenger JC. Long-term pharmacologic treatment of panic disorder. J Clin Psychiatry 1991 Feb;52 Suppl:18–23; discussion 24–5.

Ballenger JC. Pharmacotherapy of the panic disorders. J Clin Psychiatry 1986 Jun;47 Suppl:27–32.

Beardslee SL, Papadakis E, Fontana DJ, Commissaris RL. Antipanic drug treatments: failure to exhibit anxiolytic-like effects on defensive burying behavior. Pharmacol Biochem Behav 1990 Feb;35(2):451–5.

Buigues J, Vallejo J. Therapeutic response to phenelzine in patients with panic disorder and agoraphobia with panic attacks. J Clin Psychiatry 1987 Feb;48(2):55–9.

Davis DM. Update on the treatment of panic attacks. J Med Assoc Ga 1988 Nov;77(11):831–2.

Dilsaver SC. Panic disorder. Am Fam Physician 1989 Jun;39(6):167–72.

Fishman SM, Sheehan DV, Carr DB. Thyroid indices in panic disorder. J Clin Psychiatry 1985 Oct;46(10):432–3.

Fontana DJ, Carbary TJ, Commissaris RL. Effects of acute and chronic anti-panic drug administration on conflict behavior in the rat. Psychopharmacology (Berlin) 1989;98(2):157–62.

Giesecke ME. Panic disorder in university students: A review. J Am Coll Health 1987;36(3):149–57.

Gold DD Jr. Management of panic disorder: Case reports support a potential role for amoxapine. Hosp Formul 1990;25(11):1178–79, 1182–4.

Gold DD Jr. Panic attacks: Diagnosis and management. Cardiovasc Rev Rep 1988;9(1):35–7, 40.

Goodman WK, Charney DS. Therapeutic applications and mechanisms of action of monoamine oxidase inhibitor and heterocyclic antidepressant drugs. J Clin Psychiatry 1985 Oct;46(10 Pt 2):6–24.

Gorman JM. Panic disorders. Mod Probl Pharmacopsychiatry 1987;22:36–90.

Hudson JI, Pope HG Jr. Affective spectrum disorder: does antidepressant response identify a family of disorders with a common pathophysiology? Am J Psychiatry 1990 May; 147(5):552–64.

Jann MW, Kurtz NM. Treatment of panic and phobic disorders. Clin Pharm 1987 Dec;6(12):947–62.

Johnston AL, File SE. Profiles of the antipanic compounds, triazolobenzodiazepines and phenelzine, in two animal tests of anxiety. Psychiatry Res 1988 Jul;25(1):81–90.

Judd FK, Norman TR, Burrows GD. Pharmacological treatment of panic disorder. Int Clin Psychopharmacol 1986 Jan;1(1):3–16.

Judd FK, Norman TR, Burrows GD. Pharmacotherapy of panic disorder. Int Rev Psychiatry 1990;2(3–4):399–409.

Katon W. Panic disorder: epidemiology, diagnosis, and treatment in primary care. J Clin Psychiatry 1986 Oct;47 Suppl:21–30.

Katon W, Vitaliano PP, Russo J, Cormier L, Anderson K, Jones M. Panic disorder: epidemiology in primary care. J Fam Pract 1986 Sep;23(3):233–9.

King D, Nicolini H, de la Fuente JR. Abuse and withdrawal of panic treatment drugs. Psychiatr Ann 1990 Sep;20(9):525–8.

Klein DF. Psychopharmacologic treatment of panic disorder. Psychosomatics 1984;25(10 Suppl):32–6.

Klein DF, Klein HM. The utility of the panic disorder concept. Eur Arch Psychiatry Neurol Sci 1989;238(5–6):268–79.

Liebowitz MR. Antidepressants in panic disorders. Br J Psychiatry Suppl 1989 Oct;(6):46–52.

Liebowitz MR. Tricyclic antidepressants and monoamine oxidase inhibitors in the treatment of panic disorder: brief review. Psychopharmacol Bull 1989;25(1):17–20.

Liebowitz MR, Ballenger J, Barlow DH, Davidson J, Foa EB, Fyer A. New perspectives on anxiety disorders in DSM-IV and ICD-10. Drug Ther 1990;20 Suppl:129–36.

Linnoila MI. Anxiety and alcoholism. J Clin Psychiatry 1989 Nov;50 Suppl:26–9.

Lydiard RB. Pharmacological treatment. Psychiatr Ann 1988 Aug;18(8):468–72.

Lydiard RB, Ballenger JC. Antidepressants in panic disorder and agoraphobia. J Affective Disord 1987 Sep-Oct;13(2):153–68.

Lydiard RB, Laraia MT, Howell EF, Ballenger JC. Can panic disorder present as irritable bowel syndrome? J Clin Psychiatry 1986 Sep;47(9):470–3.

Lydiard RB, Laraia MT, Howell EF, Fossey MD, Reynolds RD, Ballenger JC. Phenelzine treatment of panic disorder: lack of effect on pyridoxal phosphate levels. J Clin Psychopharmacol 1989 Dec;9(6):428–31.

Mattick RP, Andrews G, Hadzi-Pavlovic D, Christensen H. Treatment of panic and agoraphobia. An integrative review. J Nerv Ment Dis 1990 Sep;178(9):567–76.

Modigh K. Antidepressant drugs in anxiety disorders. Acta Psychiatr Scand Suppl 1987;335:57–74.

Murphy DL, Siever LJ, Insel TR. Therapeutic responses to tricyclic antidepressants and related drugs in non-affective disorder patient populations. Prog Neuropsychopharmacol Biol Psychiatry 1985;9(1):3–13.

Muskin PR. Panics, prolapse, and PVCs. Gen Hosp Psychiatry 1985 Jul;7(3):219–23.

Norman TR, Burrows GD. Monoamine oxidase, monoamine oxidase inhibitors, and panic disorder. J Neural Transm Suppl 1989;28:53–63.

Noyes R Jr, Perry P. Maintenance treatment with antidepressants in panic disorder. J Clin Psychiatry 1990 Dec;51 Suppl A:24–30.

O'Boyle M. Panic disorder: diagnosis and treatment. Tex Med 1989 Aug;85(8):46–9.

Overall JE, Sheehan DV. Multivariate analysis of changes in panic frequency counts. Clin Neuropharmacol 1986;9 Suppl 4:155–7.

Ozdaglar A, Wiedemann K, Lauer CJ, Krieg JC. Brofaromine (CGP 11305 A) in the treatment of panic disorders. Pharmacopsychiatry 1989;22(5):211–2.

Pecknold JC. Behavioral and combined therapy in panic states. Prog Neuropsychopharmacol Biol Psychiatry 1987;11(2–3):97–104.

Raj A, Sheehan DV. Panic anxiety: diagnosis, etiology, and treatment. Compr Ther 1986 Oct;12(10):7–15.

Rickels K. Antianxiety therapy: potential value of long-term treatment. J Clin Psychiatry 1987 Dec;48 Suppl:7–11.

Sargent M. Panic disorder. Hosp Community Psychiatry 1990 Jun;41(6):621–3.

Schatzberg AF, Ballenger JC. Decisions for the clinician in the treatment of panic disorder: when to treat, which treatment to use, and how long to treat. J Clin Psychiatry 1991 Feb;52 Suppl:26–31; discussion 32.

Scrignar CB. Postpanic anxiety disorder: diagnosis and treatment. South Med J 1986 Apr;79(4):400–4.

Sheehan DV. Monoamine oxidase inhibitors and alprazolam in the treatment of panic disorder and agoraphobia. Psychiatr Clin North Am 1985 Mar;8(1):49–62.

Sheehan DV, Sheehan KH. Pharmacological treatment of panic and anxiety disorders. ISI Atlas Sci Pharmacol 1987;1(3):254–6.

Sheehan DV, Soto S. Recent developments in the treatment of panic disorder. Acta Psychiatr Scand Suppl 1987;335:75–85.

Shelton RC. Diagnosis and management of panic disorder. Compr Ther 1990 Dec;16(12):11–7.

Stewart RS. Pharmacologic treatment of panic disorder and agoraphobia. Hosp Formul 1990;25(4):416–22.

Swinson RP, Pecknold JC, Kuch K. Psychopharmacological treatment of panic disorder and related states: a placebo controlled study of alprazolam. Prog Neuropsychopharmacol Biol Psychiatry 1987;11(2–3):105–13.

Taylor CB, Hayward C. Cardiovascular considerations in selection of anti-panic pharmacotherapy. J Psychiatr Res 1990;24 Suppl 2:43–9.

Tesar GE, Rosenbaum JF. Successful use of clonazepam in patients with treatment-resistant panic disorder. J Nerv Ment Dis 1986 Aug;174(8):477–82.

Treatment outlines for the management of anxiety states. Aust N Z J Psychiatry 1985;19(2):138–51.

Tyrer P, Shawcross C. Monoamine oxidase inhibitors in anxiety disorders. J Psychiatr Res 1988;22 Suppl 1:87–98.

Wesner RB, Noyes R Jr. Tolerance to the therapeutic effect of phenelzine in patients with panic disorder. J Clin Psychiatry 1988 Nov;49(11):450–1.

Westenberg HG, den Boer JA. Selective monoamine uptake inhibitors and a serotonin antagonist in the treatment of panic disorder. Psychopharmacol Bull 1989;25(1):119–23.

Westenberg HG, den Boer JA. Selective monoamine uptake inhibitors and a serotonin antagonist in the treatment of panic disorder. Psychopharmacol Bull 1989;25(1):124–7.

Whiteford HA, Evans L. Agoraphobia and the dexamethasone suppression test: Atypical depression? Aust N Z J Psychiatry 1984;18(4):374–7.

Wood WG. The diagnosis and management of panic disorder. Psychiatr Med 1990;8(3):197–209.

Other Pharmacological Treatments

Brady KT, Zarzar M, Lydiard RB. Fluoxetine in panic disorder patients with imipramine-associated weight gain. J Clin Psychopharmacol 1989 Feb;9(1):66–7.

Breier A, Charney DS, Heninger GR. The diagnostic validity of anxiety disorders and their relationship to depressive illness. Am J Psychiatry 1985 Jul;142(7):787–97.

Charney DS, Woods SW, Goodman WK, Rifkin B, Kinch M, Aiken B, Quadrino LM, Heninger GR. Drug treatment of panic disorder: the comparative efficacy of imipramine, alprazolam, and trazodone. J Clin Psychiatry 1986 Dec;47(12):580–6.

Clark DB, Taylor CB, Roth WT, Hayward C, Ehlers A, Margraf J, Agras WS. Surreptitious drug use by patients in a panic disorder study. Am J Psychiatry 1990 Apr;147(4):507–9.

Coryell W, Noyes R. Placebo response in panic disorder. Am J Psychiatry 1988 Sep;145(9):1138–40.

Dager SR, Khan A, Cowley D, Avery DH, Elder J, Roy-Byrne P, Dunner DL. Characteristics of placebo response during long-term treatment of panic disorder. Psychopharmacol Bull 1990;26(3):273–8.

Den Boer JA, Westenberg HG. Effect of a serotonin and noradrenaline uptake inhibitor in panic disorder; a double-blind comparative study with fluvoxamine and maprotiline. Int Clin Psychopharmacol 1988 Jan;3(1):59–74.

Den Boer JA, Westenberg HG, Kamerbeek WD, Verhoeven WM, Kahn RS. Effect of serotonin uptake inhibitors in anxiety disorders; a double-blind comparison of clomipramine and fluvoxamine. Int Clin Psychopharmacol 1987 Jan;2(1):21–32.

Den Boer JA, Westenberg HG, Mastenbroek B, van Ree JM. The ACTH (4-9) analog ORG 2766 in panic disorder: a preliminary study. Psychopharmacol Bull 1989;25(2):204–8.

Eriksson E, Carlsson M, Nilsson C, Soderpalm B. Does alprazolam, in contrast to diazepam, activate alpha 2-adrenoceptors involved in the regulation of rat growth hormone secretion? Life Sci 1986 Apr 21;38(16):1491–8.

Fyer AJ, Liebowitz MR, Gorman JM, Campeas R, Levin A, Sandberg D, Fyer M, Hollander E, Papp L, Goetz D, et al. Effects of clonidine on alprazolam discontinuation in panic patients: a pilot study. J Clin Psychopharmacol 1988 Aug;8(4):270–4.

Gastfriend DR, Rosenbaum JF. Adjunctive buspirone in benzodiazepine treatment of four patients with panic disorder. Am J Psychiatry 1989 Jul;146(7):914–6.

Gold DD Jr. Management of panic disorder: Case reports support a potential role for amoxapine. Hosp Formul 1990;25(11):1178-79, 1182–4.

Gold DD Jr. Panic attacks: Diagnosis and management. Cardiovasc Rev Rep 1988;9(1):35–7, 40.

Goodman WK, Charney DS, Price LH, Woods SW, Heninger GR. Ineffectiveness of clonidine in the treatment of the benzodiazepine withdrawal syndrome: report of three cases. Am J Psychiatry 1986 Jul;143(7):900–3.

Gorman JM, Liebowitz MR, Dillon D, Fyer AJ, Cohen BS, Klein DF. Antipanic drug effects during lactate infusion in lactate-refractory panic patients. Psychiatry Res 1987 Jul;21(3):205–12.

Gorman JM, Liebowitz MR, Fyer AJ, Goetz D, Campeas RB, Fyer MR, Davies SO, Klein DF. An open trial of fluoxetine in the treatment of panic attacks [published erratum appears in J Clin Psychopharmacol 1988 Feb;8(1):13]. J Clin Psychopharmacol 1987 Oct;7(5):329–32.

Griez E, Pols H, Lousberg H. Serotonin antagonism in panic disorder: an open trial with ritanserin. Acta Psychiatr Belg 1988;88(5–6):372–7.

Griez E, van den Hout MA. CO2 inhalation in the treatment of panic attacks. Behav Res Ther 1986;24(2):145–50.

Grunhaus LJ, Cameron O, Pande AC, Haskett RF, Hollingsworth PJ, Smith CB. Comorbidity of panic disorder and major depressive disorder: effects on platelet alpha 2 adrenergic receptors. Acta Psychiatr Scand 1990 Mar;81(3):216–9.

Hayes PE, Schulz SC. Beta-blockers in anxiety disorders. J Affective Disord 1987 Sep-Oct;13(2):119–30.

Heninger GR. Recent research on the neurobiology of panic. Curr Opin Psychiatry 1989;2(1):112–6.

Heninger GR, Charney DS, Price LH. Noradrenergic and serotonergic receptor system function in panic disorder and depression. Acta Psychiatr Scand Suppl 1988;341:138–50.

Jann MW, Kurtz NM. Treatment of panic and phobic disorders. Clin Pharm 1987 Dec;6(12):947–62.

Judd FK, Norman TR, Burrows GD. Pharmacotherapy of panic disorder. Int Rev Psychiatry 1990;2(3-4):399–409.

Klein E, Uhde TW. Controlled study of verapamil for treatment of panic disorder. Am J Psychiatry 1988 Apr;145(4):431–4.

Klerman GL. Panic disorder: strategies for long-term treatment. J Clin Psychiatry 1991 Feb;52 Suppl:3–5.

Levinson DF, Acquaviva J. Exacerbation of panic disorder during propranolol therapy. J Clin Psychopharmacol 1988 Jun;8(3):193–5.

Liegghio NE, Yeragani VK, Moore NC. Buspirone-induced jitteriness in three patients with panic disorder and one patient with generalized anxiety disorder. J Clin Psychiatry 1988 Apr;49(4):165–6.

Marconi PL, Gismondi R, Valigi R, Pancheri P. ALFA Project: An expert system on pharmacological treatment of panic attack disorder. New Trends Exp Clin Psychiatry 1988 Jan-Mar;4(1):25–36.

Mavissakalian M, Perel J, Bowler K, Dealy R. Trazodone in the treatment of panic disorder and agoraphobia with panic attacks. Am J Psychiatry 1987 Jun;144(6):785–7.

McNamara ME, Fogel BS. Anticonvulsant-responsive panic attacks with temporal lobe EEG abnormalities. J Neuropsychiatr Clin Neurosci 1990 Spring;2(2):193–6.

Mellergard M, Rosenberg NK. Patterns of response during placebo treatment of panic disorder. Acta Psychiatr Scand 1990 Apr;81(4):340–4.

Middleton HC. An enhanced hypotensive response to clonidine can still be found in panic patients despite psychological treatment. J Anxiety Disord 1990;4(3):213–9.

Munjack DJ, Crocker B, Cabe D, Brown R, Usigli R, Zulueta A, McManus M, McDowell D, Palmer R, Leonard M. Alprazolam, propranolol, and placebo in the treatment of panic disorder and agoraphobia with panic attacks. J Clin Psychopharmacol 1989 Feb;9(1):22–7.

Munjack DJ, Rebal R, Shaner R, et al. Imipramine versus propranolol for the treatment of panic attacks: A pilot study. Compr Psychiatry 1985;26(1):80–9.

Murphy DL, Pigott TA. A comparative examination of a role for serotonin in obsessive compulsive disorder, panic disorder, and anxiety. J Clin Psychiatry 1990 Apr;51 Suppl:53–8; discussion 59–60.

Nutt DJ. Altered central alpha 2-adrenoceptor sensitivity in panic disorder. Arch Gen Psychiatry 1989 Feb;46(2):165–9.

Nutt DJ. Increased central alpha 2-adrenoceptor sensitivity in panic disorder. Psychopharmacology (Berlin) 1986;90(2):268–9.

Ozdaglar A, Wiedemann K, Lauer CJ, Krieg JC. Brofaromine (CGP 11305 A) in the treatment of panic disorders. Pharmacopsychiatry 1989;22(5):211–2.

Pohl R, Balon R, Yeragani VK, Gershon S. Serotonergic anxiolytics in the treatment of panic disorder: a controlled study with buspirone. Psychopathology 1989;22 Suppl 1:60–7.

Pohl R, Yeragani VK, Balon R. Effects of isoproterenol in panic disorder patients after antidepressant treatment. Biol Psychiatry 1990 Aug 1;28(3):203–14.

Pohl R, Yeragani VK, Ortiz A, Rainey JM Jr, Gershon S. Response of tricyclic–induced jitteriness to a phenothiazine in two patients. J Clin Psychiatry 1986 Aug;47(8):427.

Primeau F, Fontaine R. GABAergic agents and panic disorder. Biol Psychiatry 1988 Dec;24(8):942–3.

Primeau F, Fontaine R, Beauclair L. Valproic acid and panic disorder. Can J Psychiatry 1990 Apr;35(3):248–50.

Rapaport MH, Risch SC, Gillin JC, Golshan S, Janowsky DS. Blunted growth hormone response to peripheral infusion of human growth hormone-releasing factor in patients with panic disorder. Am J Psychiatry 1989 Jan;146(1):92–5.

Reich J. The effect of personality on placebo response in panic patients. J Nerv Ment Dis 1990 Nov;178(11):699–702.

Reid TL, Raj BA, Sheehan DR. Ictal panic/epileptogenic activity: treatment with primidone. Psychosomatics 1988;29(4):431–3.

Rickels K, Case WG, Schweizer E. The drug treatment of anxiety and panic disorder. Stress Med 1988;4(4):231–9.

Robinson DS, Shrotriya RC, Alms DR, Messina M, Andary J. Treatment of panic disorder: nonbenzodiazepine anxiolytics, including buspirone. Psychopharmacol Bull 1989;25(1):21–6.

Rosenberg NK, Mellergard M, Rosenberg R, Beck P, Ottosson J-O. Characteristics of panic disorder patients responding to placebo. Acta Psychiatr Scand Suppl 1991;83(365):33–8.

Roy–Byrne PP, Uhde TW. Panic disorder and major depression: Biological relationships. Psychopharmacol Bull 1985;21(3):551–4.

Schittecatte M, Charles G, Depauw Y, Mesters P, Wilmotte J. Growth hormone response to clonidine in panic disorder patients. Psychiatry Res 1988 Feb;23(2):147–51.

Schneier FR, Liebowitz MR, Davies SO, Fairbanks J, Hollander E, Campeas R, Klein DF. Fluoxetine in panic disorder. J Clin Psychopharmacol 1990 Apr;10(2):119–21.

Schweizer E, Rickels K. Buspirone in the treatment of panic disorder: A controlled pilot comparison with clorazepate. J Clin Psychopharmacol 1988 Aug;8(4):303.

Sheehan DV, Raj AB, Sheehan KH, Soto S. Is buspirone effective for panic disorder? J Clin Psychopharmacol 1990 Feb;10(1):3–11.

Sheehan DV, Raj AB, Sheehan KH, Soto S. The relative efficacy of buspirone, imipramine and placebo in panic disorder: a preliminary report. Pharmacol Biochem Behav 1988 Apr;29(4):815–7.

Sheehan DV, Zak JP, Miller JA Jr, Fanous BS. Panic disorder: the potential role of serotonin reuptake inhibitors. J Clin Psychiatry 1988 Aug;49 Suppl: 30–6.

Stein MB, Uhde TW. Cortisol response to clonidine in panic disorder: comparison with depressed patients and normal controls [see comments]. Biol Psychiatry 1988 Jul;24(3):322–30.

Stewart RS. Pharmacologic treatment of panic disorder and agoraphobia. Hosp Formul 1990;25(4):416–22.

Stoudemire A, Ninan PT, Wooten V. Hypnogenic paroxysmal dystonia with panic attacks responsive to drug therapy. Psychosomatics 1987 May;28(5):280–1.

Taylor DP. Serotonin agents in anxiety. Ann New York Acad Sci 1990;600:545–57.

Tondo L, Burrai C, Scamonatti L, Toccafondi F, et al. Carbamazepine in panic disorder. Am J Psychiatry 1989 Apr;146(4):558–9.

Tundo A, Minnai G. Agoraphobic-panic disorder and carbamazepine. Med Sci Res 1989 Oct;17(19):801–2.

Uhde TW, Stein MB, Vittone BJ, Siever LJ, Boulenger JP, Klein E, Mellman TA. Behavioral and physiologic effects of short-term and long-term administration of clonidine in panic disorder. Arch Gen Psychiatry 1989 Feb;46(2):170–7.

Uhde TW, Stein MB, Post RM. Lack of efficacy of carbamazepine in the treatment of panic disorder. Am J Psychiatry 1988 Sep;145(9):1104–9.

Uhde TW, Vittone BJ, Siever LJ, Kaye WH, Post RM. Blunted growth hormone response to clonidine in panic disorder patients. Biol Psychiatry 1986 Sep;21(11):1081–5.

Westenberg HG, den Boer JA. Selective monoamine uptake inhibitors and a serotonin antagonist in the treatment of panic disorder. Psychopharmacol Bull 1989;25(1):119–23.

Westenberg HG, den Boer JA. Selective monoamine uptake inhibitors and a serotonin antagonist in the treatment of panic disorder. Psychopharmacol Bull 1989;25(1):124–7.

Westenberg HG, den Boer JA. Serotonin-influencing drugs in the treatment of panic disorder. Psychopathology 1989;22 Suppl 1:68–77.

Yeragani VK, Balon R, Pohl R. Schizophrenia, panic attacks, and antidepressants. Am J Psychiatry 1989 Feb;146(2):279.

Yeragani VK, Pohl R, Balon R. Lactate-induced panic and beta-adrenergic blockade. Psychiatry Res 1990 Apr;32(1):93–4.

Reviews

Balestrieri M, Ruggeri M, Bellantuono C. Drug treatment of panic disorder—a critical review of controlled clinical trials. Psychiatr Dev 1989 Winter;7(4):337–50.

Ballenger JC. Long-term pharmacologic treatment of panic disorder. J Clin Psychiatry 1991 Feb;52 Suppl:18–23; discussion 24–5.

Ballenger JC. Pharmacotherapy of the panic disorders. J Clin Psychiatry 1986 Jun;47 Suppl:27–32.

Burrows GD, Norman TR, Judd FK. Panic disorder: a treatment update. J Clin Psychiatry 1991 Jul;52 (7 Suppl):24–6.

Cassano GB, Perugi G, McNair DM. Panic disorder: review of the empirical and rational basis of pharmacological treatment. Pharmacopsychiatry 1988 Jul;21(4):157–65.

Davis DM. Update on the treatment of panic attacks. J Med Assoc Ga 1988 Nov;77(11):831–2.

Judd FK, Norman TR, Burrows GD. Pharmacological treatment of panic disorder. Int Clin Psychopharmacol 1986 Jan;1(1):3–16.

Judd FK, Norman TR, Burrows GD. Pharmacotherapy of panic disorder. Int Rev Psychiatry 1990;2(3–4):399–409.

Klein DF. Psychopharmacologic treatment of panic disorder. Psychosomatics 1984;25(10 Suppl):32–6.

Liebowitz MR. Tricyclic antidepressants and monoamine oxidase inhibitors in the treatment of panic disorder: brief review. Psychopharmacol Bull 1989;25(1):17–20.

Liebowitz MR, Fyer AJ, Gorman J, Klein DF. Recent developments in the understanding and pharmacotherapy of panic attacks. Psychopharmacol Bull 1986;22(3):792–6.

Lydiard RB. Pharmacological treatment. Psychiatr Ann 1988 Aug;18(8):468–72.

Lydiard RB, Roy-Byrne PP, Ballenger JC. Recent advances in the psychopharmacological treatment of anxiety disorders. Hosp Community Psychiatry 1988 Nov;39(11):1157–65.

Philipp M, Maier W, Buller R. Pharmacotherapy of panic attacks. Pharmacopsychiatry 1988 Nov;21(6):281–2.

Sheehan DV. Monoamine oxidase inhibitors and alprazolam in the treatment of panic disorder and agoraphobia. Psychiatr Clin North Am 1985 Mar;8(1):49–62.

Sheehan DV, Sheehan KH. Pharmacological treatment of panic and anxiety disorders. ISI Atlas Sci Pharmacol 1987;1(3):254–6.

Stewart RS. Pharmacologic treatment of panic disorder and agoraphobia. Hosp Formul 1990;25(4):416–22.

Tiller JW. The new and newer antianxiety agents. Med J Aust 1989 Dec 4–18;151(11–12):697–701.

Treatment of syndromes or of symptoms in psychiatry? Lancet 1988;2(8607):373–4.

Psychosocial

Cognitive-Behavior Therapies

Barlow DH. Behavioral conception and treatment of panic. Psychopharmacol Bull 1986;22(3):802–6.

Barlow DH. In defense of panic disorder with agoraphobia and the behavioral treatment of panic: A comment on Kleiner. Behavior Ther 1986 May;9(5):99–100.

Barlow DH. Long-term outcome for patients with panic disorder treated with cognitive-behavioral therapy. J Clin Psychiatry 1990 Dec;51 Suppl A: 17–23.

Barlow DH, Craske MG, Cerny JA, Klosko JS. Behavioral treatment of panic disorder. Behav Ther 1989;20(2):261–82.

Borden JW, Clum GA, Broyles SE, Watkins PL. Coping strategies and panic. J Anxiety Disord 1988;2(4):339–52.

Clark DM. A cognitive approach to panic. Behav Res Ther 1986;24(4):461–70.

Clark DM, Salkovskis PM, Chalkley AJ. Respiratory control as a treatment for panic attacks. J Behav Ther Exp Psychiatry 1985 Mar;16(1):23–30.

Clum GA, Borden JW. Etiology and treatment of panic disorders. Prog Behav Modif 1989;24:192–222.

Craske MG, Street L, Barlow DH. Instructions to focus upon or distract from internal cues during exposure treatment of agoraphobic avoidance. Behav Res Ther 1989;27(6):663–72.

Dattilio FM. Symptom induction and de-escalation in the treatment of panic attacks. J Ment Health Couns 1990 Oct;12(4):515–9.

Dattilio FM. The use of paradoxical intention in the treatment of panic attacks. J Couns Dev 1987 Oct;66(2):102–3.

de Ruiter C, Ryken H, Garssen B, Kraaimaat F. Breathing retraining, exposure and a combination of both, in the treatment of panic disorder with agoraphobia. Behav Res Ther 1989;27(6):637–55.

Frances A, Shear MK, Fyer MR. "Relaxation-induced panic (RIP): When resting isn't peaceful": Commentary. Integr Psychiatry 1987 Dec;5(4):295–6.

Gelder MG. Psychological treatment of panic anxiety. Psychiatr Ann 1990 Sep;20(9):529–32.

Gilbert C. Skin conductance feedback and panic attacks. Biofeedback Self Regul 1986 Sep;11(3):251–4.

Gitlin B, Martin J, Shear MK, Frances A, Ball G, Josephson S. Behavior therapy for panic disorder. J Nerv Ment Dis 1985 Dec;173(12):742–3.

Hegel MT, Abel GG, Etscheidt M, Cohen-Cole S, Wilmer CI. Behavioral treatment of angina-like chest pain in patients with hyperventilation syndrome. J Behav Ther Exp Psychiatry 1989 Mar;20(1):31–9.

Hibbert GA, Chan M. Respiratory control: its contribution to the treatment of panic attacks. A controlled study. Br J Psychiatry 1989 Feb;154:232–6.

Klosko JS, Barlow DH. Cognitive-behavioral treatment of panic attacks. J Integr Eclectic Psychother 1987 Winter;6(4):462–9.

Laraia MT, Stuart GW, Best CL. Behavioral treatment of panic-related disorders: a review. Arch Psychiatr Nurs 1989 Jun;3(3):125–33.

Levis DJ. Treating anxiety and panic attacks: The conflict model of Implosive Therapy. J Integr Eclectic Psychother 1987 Winter;6(4):450–61.

Lindemann C. "Relaxation-induced panic (RIP): When resting isn't peaceful": Commentary. A. Integr Psychiatry 1987 Jun;5(2):109–10.

Marchione KE, Michelson L, Greenwald M, Dancu C. Cognitive behavioral treatment of agoraphobia. Behav Res Ther 1987;25(5):319–28.

Marks IM. Behavioral aspects of panic disorder. Am J Psychiatry 1987 Sep;144(9):1160–5.

Marriott P. Panic and phobic disorders. Current cognitive behavioral strategies. Aust Fam Physician 1990 Sep;19(9):1357, 1360–2, 1365–70.

McNamee G, O'Sullivan G, Lelliott P, Marks I. Telephone-guided treatment for housebound agoraphobics with panic disorder: Exposure vs. relaxation. Behav Ther 1989;20(4):491–7.

Michelson L, Marchione K, Greenwald M, Glanz L, Testa S, Marchione N. Panic disorder: cognitive-behavioral treatment. Behav Res Ther 1990;28(2):141–51.

Öst LG. A maintenance program for behavioral treatment of anxiety disorders. Behav Res Ther 1989;27(2):123–30.

Öst LG. Applied relaxation in the treatment of panic disorder. Special Issue: Applied relaxation: Method and applications. Scand J Behav Ther 1988;17(2):111–24.

Öst LG. Applied relaxation vs progressive relaxation in the treatment of panic disorder. Behav Res Ther 1988;26(1):13–22.

Öst LG. Coping techniques in the treatment of anxiety disorders: Two controlled case studies. Behav Psychother 1985;13(2):154–61.

Putkonen AR. Behavior therapy of panic disorders. Proceedings of the World Psychiatric Association on the Psychopathology of Panic Disorders: Many faces of panic disorder (1988, Espoo, Finland). Psychiatr Fenn 1989;Suppl:127–32.

Rapee RM. A case of panic disorder treated with breathing retraining. J Behav Ther Exp Psychiatry 1985 Mar;16(1):63–5.

Rapee RM, Barlow DH. Cognitive-behavioral treatment. Psychiatr Ann 1988 Aug;18(8):473–7.

Salkovskis PM, Clark DM, Hackmann A. Treatment of panic attacks using cognitive therapy without exposure or breathing retraining. Behav Res Ther 1991;29(2):161–6.

Salkovskis PM, Jones DR, Clark DM. Respiratory control in the treatment of panic attacks: replication and extension with concurrent measurement of behavior and pCO2. Br J Psychiatry 1986 May;148:526–32.

Schwartz RM, Michelson L. States-of-mind model: Cognitive balance in the treatment of agoraphobia. J Consult Clin Psychol 1987 Aug;55(4):557–65.

Shear MK, Ball G, Josephson S. An empirically developed cognitive-behavioral treatment of panic. J Integr Eclectic Psychother 1987 Winter;6(4):421–33.

Sokol L, Beck AT, Greenberg RL, Wright FD, Berchick RJ. Cognitive therapy of panic disorder. A nonpharmacological alternative. J Nerv Ment Dis 1989 Dec;177(12):711–6.

Swinson RP, Kuch K. Behavioral psychotherapy of agoraphobia/panic disorder. Special Issue: Behavioral psychotherapy into the 1990's. Int Rev Psychiatry 1989;1(3):195–205.

Tarrier N, Main CJ. Applied relaxation training for generalized anxiety and panic attacks: the efficacy of a learnt coping strategy on subjective reports. Br J Psychiatry 1986 Sep;149:330–6.

Watkins PL, Sturgis ET, Clum GA. Guided imaginal coping: an integrative treatment for panic disorder. J Behav Ther Exp Psychiatry 1988 Jun;19(2):147–55.

Wells A. Panic disorder in association with relaxation induced anxiety: An attentional training approach to treatment. Behav Ther 1990;21(3):273–80.

Other Psychotherapies

Borkovec TD, Mathews AM. Treatment of nonphobic anxiety disorders: A comparison of nondirective, cognitive, and coping desensitization therapy. J Consult Clin Psychol 1988 Dec;56(6):877–84.

Bourne S. Panic attacks: New approaches to an old problem. Br J Psychiatry 1987 Feb;150:265–6.

Craske MG, Burton T, Barlow DH. Relationships among measures of communication, marital satisfaction and exposure during couples treatment of agoraphobia. Behav Res Ther 1989;27(2):31–140.

Der DF, Lewington P. Rational self-directed hypnotherapy: a treatment for panic attacks. Am J Clin Hypn 1990 Jan;32(3):160–7.

Feist E. An innovative program for the treatment of panic attacks: A case study. Aust J Clin Hypnother Hypnosis 1986 Sep;7(2):122–6.

Katschnig H. Strategies for treating primary and secondary symptoms of panic disorder: A conceptual framework. Proceedings of the World Psychiatric Association on the Psychopathology of Panic Disorders: Many faces of panic disorder (1988, Espoo, Finland). Psychiatr Fenn 1989;Suppl:112–9.

Leistikow D. Panic disorder: An in utero problem. Med Hypnoanal J 1987 Mar;2(1):25–31.

Martinsen EW, Hoffart A, Solberg OY. Aerobic and non-aerobic forms of exercise in the treatment of anxiety disorders. Stress Med 1989;5(2):115–20.

Matez A. The rapid treatment of fear, panic and phobia disorders using hypnoanalysis . . . with illustrative case history summaries. J Am Acad Med Hypnoanal 1986 Dec;1(2):68–87.

Milrod B, Shear MK. Psychodynamic treatment of panic: three case histories. Hosp Community Psychiatry 1991 Mar;42(3):311–2.

Sartory G, Olajide D. Vagal innervation techniques in the treatment of panic disorder. Behav Res Ther 1988;26(5):431–4.

Silber A. Panic attacks facilitating recall and mastery: implications for psychoanalytic technique. J Am Psychoanal Assoc 1989;37(2):337–64.

Stoeri JH. Psychoanalytic psychotherapy with panic states: A case presentation. Psychoanal Psychol 1987;4(2):101–13.

Straub JH. An eclectic counseling approach to the treatment of panics. J Integr Eclectic Psychother 1987 Winter;6(4):434–49.

Wolfe BE. Phobias, panic and psychotherapy integration. J Integr Eclectic Psychother 1989 Fall;8(3):264–76.

Reviews

McNally RJ. Psychological approaches to panic disorder: a review. Psychol Bull 1990 Nov;108(3):403–19.

Combined Treatments

Beitman BD, Basha IM, Trombka LH. Panic attacks and their treatment: An introduction. J Integr Eclect Psychother 1987 Winter;6(4):412–20.

Burrows GD. Managing long-term therapy for panic disorder. J Clin Psychiatry 1990 Nov;51 Suppl: 9–12.

Clum GA. Psychological interventions vs. drugs in the treatment of panic. Behav Ther 1989;20(3):429–57.

Harnett DS. Panic disorder: integrating psychotherapy and psychopharmacology. Psychiatr Med 1990;8(3):211–22.

Judd FK, Burrows GD. Panic and phobic disorders—are psychological or pharmacological treatments effective? Aust N Z J Psychiatry 1986 Sep;20(3):342–8.

Klosko JS, Barlow DH, Tassinari R, Cerny JA. A comparison of alprazolam and behavior therapy in treatment of panic disorder. J Consult Clin Psychol 1990 Feb;58(1):77–84.

Kupfer DJ. Lessons to be learned from long-term treatment of affective disorders: potential utility in panic disorder. J Clin Psychiatry 1991 Feb;52 Suppl:12–6; discussion 17.

Marks I. Behavioral and drug treatments of phobic and obsessive-compulsive disorders. Psychother Psychosom 1986;46(1–2):35–44.

Mattick RP, Andrews G, Hadzi-Pavlovic D, Christensen H. Treatment of panic and agoraphobia. An integrative review. J Nerv Ment Dis 1990 Sep;178(9):567–76.

Mavissakalian M. Differential effects of imipramine and behavior therapy on panic disorder with agoraphobia. Psychopharmacol Bull 1989;25(1):27–9.

Mavissakalian M. Sequential combination of imipramine and self-directed exposure in the treatment of panic disorder with agoraphobia. J Clin Psychiatry 1990 May;51(5):184–8.

Mavissakalian MR, Jones BA. Antidepressant drugs plus exposure treatment of agoraphobia/panic and obsessive-compulsive disorders. Special Issue: Behavioral psychotherapy into the 1990's. Int Rev Psychiatry 1989;1(3):275–81.

Michelson LK, Marchione K. Behavioral, cognitive, and pharmacological treatments of panic disorder with agoraphobia: critique and synthesis. J Consult Clin Psychol 1991 Feb;59(1):100–14.

Nagy LM, Krystal JH, Woods SW, Charney DS. Clinical and medication outcome after short-term alprazolam and behavioral group treatment in panic disorder. 2.5 year naturalistic follow-up study. Arch Gen Psychiatry 1989 Nov;46(11):993–9.

Pecknold JC. Behavioral and combined therapy in panic states. Prog Neuropsychopharmacol Biol Psychiatry 1987;11(2–3):97–104.

Sheehan DV, Soto S. Recent developments in the treatment of panic disorder. Acta Psychiatr Scand Suppl 1987;335:75–85.

Smith GR, O'Rourke DF, Parker PE, Ford CV, et al. Panic and nausea instead of grief in an adolescent. J Am Acad Child Adolesc Psychiatry 1988 Jul;27(4):509–13.

Taylor CB, King R, Margraf J, Ehlers A, Telch M, Roth WT, Agras WS. Use of medication and in vivo exposure in volunteers for panic disorder research. Am J Psychiatry 1989 Nov;146(11):1423–6.

Tobena A, Sanchez R, Pose R, Masana J, et al. Brief treatment with alprazolam and behavioral guidance in panic disorder. Anxiety Res 1990 Nov;3(3):163–74.

Treatment outlines for the management of anxiety states. Aust N Z J Psychiatry 1985;19(2):138–51.

Tyrer P, Seivewright N, Murphy S, Ferguson B, Kingdon D, Barczak P, Brothwell J, Darling C, Gregory S, Johnson AL. The Nottingham study of neurotic disorder: comparison of drug and psychological treatments. Lancet 1988 Jul 30;2(8605):235–40.

Mechanism of Action of Treatments

Adler CM, Craske MG, Kirshenbaum S, Barlow DH. 'Fear of panic': an investigation of its role in panic occurrence, phobic avoidance, and treatment outcome. Behav Res Ther 1989;27(4):391–6.

Argyle N. The nature of cognitions in panic disorder. Behav Res Ther 1988;26(3):261–4.

Breslow MF, Fankhauser MP, Potter RL, Meredith KE, Misiaszek J, Hope DG Jr. Role of gamma-aminobutyric acid in antipanic drug efficacy. Am J Psychiatry 1989 Mar; 146(3):353–6.

Carr DB, Sheehan DV, Surman OS, Coleman JH, Greenblatt DJ, Heninger GR, Jones KJ, Levine PH, Watkins WD. Neuroendocrine correlates of lactate-induced anxiety and their response to chronic alprazolam therapy. Am J Psychiatry 1986 Apr;143(4):483–94.

Charney DS, Heninger GR. Noradrenergic function and the mechanism of action of anti-anxiety treatment. I. The effect of long-term alprazolam treatment. Arch Gen Psychiatry 1985 May;42(5):458–67.

Charney DS, Heninger GR. Noradrenergic function and the mechanism of action of anti-anxiety treatment. II. The effect of long-term imipramine treatment. Arch Gen Psychiatry 1985 May;42(5):473–81.

Charney DS, Heninger GR. Serotonin function in panic disorders. The effect of intravenous tryptophan in healthy subjects and patients with panic disorder before and during alprazolam treatment. Arch Gen Psychiatry 1986 Nov;43(11):1059–65.

Clum GA, Pendrey D. Depression symptomatology as a non-requisite for successful treatment of panic with antidepressant medications. J Anxiety Disord 1987;1(4):337–44.

Coryell W, Noyes R Jr, Schlechte J. The significance of HPA axis disturbance in panic disorder. Biol Psychiatry 1989 Apr 15;25(8):989–1002.

Den Boer JA, Westenberg HG. Serotonin function in panic disorder: a double blind placebo controlled study with fluvoxamine and ritanserin. Psychopharmacology (Berl) 1990;102(1):85–94.

Edlund MJ, Swann AC. Low MHPG and continuing treatment in panic disorder. Prog Neuropsychopharmacol Biol Psychiatry 1989;13(5):701–7.

Eriksson E. Brain neurotransmission in panic disorder. Acta Psychiatr Scand Suppl 1987;335:31–7.

Eriksson E, Carlsson M, Nilsson C, Soderpalm B. Does alprazolam, in contrast to diazepam, activate alpha 2-adrenoceptors involved in the regulation of rat growth hormone secretion? Life Sci 1986 Apr 21;38(16):1491–8.

Eriksson E, Westberg P, Thuresson K, Modigh K, Ekman R, Widerlov E. Increased cerebrospinal fluid levels of endorphin immunoreactivity in panic disorder. Neuropsychopharmacology 1989 Sep;2(3):225–8.

Friedman S. Assessing the marital environment of agoraphobics. J Anxiety Disord 1990;4(4):335–40.

Fyer AJ, Gorman JM, Liebowitz MR, et al. Sodium lactate infusion, panic attacks, and ionized calcium. Biol Psychiatry 1984;19(10):1437–47.

George DT, Ladenheim JA, Nutt DJ. Effect of pregnancy on panic attacks. Am J Psychiatry 1987 Aug;144(8):1078–9.

Goodman WK, Charney DS. Therapeutic applications and mechanisms of action of monoamine oxidase inhibitor and heterocyclic antidepressant drugs. J Clin Psychiatry 1985 Oct;46(10 Pt 2):6–24.

Gorman JM, Fyer AJ, Ross DC, Cohen BS, Martinez JM, Liebowitz MR, Klein DF. Normalization of venous pH, pCO_2, and bicarbonate levels after blockade of panic attacks. Psychiatry Res 1985 Jan;14(1):57–65.

Klein DF. The pathophysiology of panic anxiety. J Clin Psychiatry 1991;52(2 Suppl):10–1.

Lepola U, Jolkkonen J, Rim:on R, Riekkinen P. Long-term effects of alprazolam and imipramine on cerebrospinal fluid monoamine metabolites and neuropeptides in panic disorder. Neuropsychobiology 1989;21(4):182–6.

Ley R. Dyspneic-fear and catastrophic cognitions in hyperventilatory panic attacks. Behav Res Ther 1989;27(5):549–54.

Lingjaerde O. Lactate-induced panic attacks: possible involvement of serotonin reuptake stimulation. Acta Psychiatr Scand 1985 Aug;72(2):206–8.

Lopez AL, Kathol RG, Noyes R Jr. Reduction in urinary free cortisol during benzodiazepine treatment of panic disorder. Psychoneuroendocrinology 1990;15(1):23–8.

Louie AK, Lannon RA, Ketter TA. Treatment of cocaine-induced panic disorder. Am J Psychiatry 1989 Jan;146(1):40–4.

Marazziti D. Imipramine binding in panic disorder. Pharmacopsychiatry 1989 May; 22(3):128–9.

Marazziti D, Rotondo A, Placidi GF, Perugi G, Cassano GB, Pacifici GM. Binding of imipramine to platelet membranes is reduced in panic attacks. Fundam Clin Pharmacol 1988;2(2):69–75.

Marazziti D, Rotondo A, Placidi GF, Perugi G, Cassano GB, Pacifici GM. Imipramine binding in platelets of patients with panic disorder. Pharmacopsychiatry 1988 Jan;21(1):47–9.

Redmond DE Jr. The possible role of locus coeruleus noradrenergic activity in anxiety-panic. Clin Neuropharmacol 1986;9 Suppl 4:40–2.

Shear MK, Fyer AJ, Ball G, Josephson S, Fitzpatrick M, Gitlin B, Frances A, Gorman J, Liebowitz M, Klein DF. Vulnerability to sodium lactate in panic disorder patients given cognitive-behavioral therapy. Am J Psychiatry 1991 Jun;148(6):795–7.

Yeragani VK, Balon R, Pohl R, Berchou R, Merlos B, Weinberg P. Lactate induced panic and beta–2 adrenergic activation. Pharmacopsychiatry 1990 Jul;23(4):198.

Agoraphobia

Agoraphobia. Lancet 1988 Oct 15;2(8616):881–2.

Alfin PL. Agoraphobia: A study of family of origin characteristics and relationship patterns. Smith Coll Stud Soc Work 1987 Mar;57(2):134–54.

Ambrosini P. Imipramine binding in agoraphobia. Psychiatry Res 1986 Jun;18(2):189–90.

Anton RF, Ballenger JC, Lydiard RB, Laraia MT, Howell EF, Gold PW. CSF prostaglandin-E in agoraphobia with panic attacks. Biol Psychiatry 1989 Jul;26(3):257–64.

Arnow BA, Taylor CB, Agras WS, Telch MJ. Enhancing agoraphobic treatment outcome by changing couple communication patterns. Behav Ther 1985;16(5):452–67.

Arntz A, Van den Hout MA, Lousberg R, Schouten E. Is the match/mismatch model based on a statistical artefact? Behav Res Ther 1990;28(3):249–53.

Arrindell WA, Emmelkamp PM, Sanderman R. Marital quality and general life adjustment in relation to treatment outcome in agoraphobia. Adv Behav Res Ther 1986;8(3):139–85.

Arrindell WA, Sanderman R, Van der Molen H, Van der Ende J, et al. The structure of assertiveness: A confirmatory approach. Behav Res Ther 1988;26(4):337–9.

Ascher LM, Schotte DE, Grayson JB. Enhancing effectiveness of paradoxical intention in treating travel restriction in agoraphobia. Behav Ther 1986 Mar;17(2):124–30.

Badalamenti AF. Psychopharmacology of agoraphobia and a hypothesis of Sigmund Freud. Dyn Psychother 1985 Fall-Winter;3(2):159–68.

Barlow DH, Hallam RS. Anxiety: Psychological perspectives on panic and agoraphobia. Behav Res Ther 1986;24(6):693–6.

Baum M. An animal model for agoraphobia using a safety-signal analysis. Behav Res Ther 1986;24(1):87–9.

Beckfield DF. Importance of altering global response style in the treatment of agoraphobia. Psychother Theory Res Pract Train 1987;24(4):752–8.

Bennun I. A composite formulation of agoraphobia. Am J Psychother 1986 Apr;40(2):177–88.

Biran M. Cognitive and exposure treatment for agoraphobia: Reexamination of the outcome research. J Cogn Psychother 1988 Fall;2(3):165–78.

Biran MW. Two-stage therapy for agoraphobia. Am J Psychother 1987 Jan;41(1):127–36.

Blanco IM. Comments on "From Symmetry to Asymmetry" by Klaus Fink. Int J Psychoanal 1989;70 (Pt 3):491–8.

Bowen RC, D'Arcy C, South MN, Hawkes JE. The effects of a nurse therapist conducted behavioral agoraphobia treatment program on medical utilization. J Anxiety Disord 1990;4(4):341–9.

Brown R, Munjack D, McDowell D. Agoraphobia with and without current panic attacks. Psychol Rep 1989 Apr;64(2):503–6.

Burgess PM. Toward resolution of conceptual issues in the assessment of belief systems in rational-emotive therapy. J Cogn Psychother 1990 Summer;4(2 Spec Iss):171–84.

Burns LE, Thorpe GL, Cavallaro LA. Agoraphobia 8 years after behavioral treatment: A follow-up study with interview, self-report, and behavioral data. Behav Ther 1986 Nov;17(5):580–91.

Butler G, Gelder M. Problem-solving: Not a treatment for agoraphobia: A reply to D'Zurilla (1985). Behav Ther 1985 Nov;16(5):548–50.

Cerny JA, Barlow DH, Craske MG, Himadi WG. Couples treatment of agoraphobia: A two-year follow-up. Behav Ther 1987 Fall;18(4):401–15.

Chambless DL. Measurement effects on outcome of treatment for agoraphobia. Behav Ther 1989 Summer;20(3):465–6.

Chambless DL. Spacing of exposure sessions in treatment of agoraphobia and simple phobia. Behav Therapy 1990 Spring;21(2):217–29.

Chambless DL, Caputo GC, Jasin SE, Gracely EJ, Williams C. The Mobility Inventory for Agoraphobia. Behav Res Ther 1985;23(1):35–44.

Chambless DL, Goldstein AJ, Gallagher R, Bright P. Integrating behavior therapy and psychotherapy in the treatment of agoraphobia. Psychotherapy 1986;23(1):150–9.

Chambless DL, Mason J. Sex, sex-role stereotyping and agoraphobia. Behav Res Ther 1986;24(2):231–5.

Chambless DL, Woody SR. Is agoraphobia harder to treat? A comparison of agoraphobics' and simple phobics' response to treatment. Behav Res Ther 1990;28(4):305–12.

Comings DE, Comings BG. Hereditary agoraphobia and obsessive-compulsive behavior in relatives of patients with Gilles de la Tourette's syndrome. Br J Psychiatry 1987 Aug;151:195–9.

Cottraux J, Mollard E, Duinat-Pascal A. Agoraphobia with panic attacks and social phobia: A comparative clinical and psychometric study. Psychiatr Psychobiol 1988;3(1):49–56.

Covelli V, Maffione AB, Jirillo E. Effects of in vivo administration of timostimolina (TP-1) on the immune system from patients with phobic disorders. New Trends Exp Clin Psychiatry 1988 Oct-Dec;4(4):213–21.

Cox DJ, Ballenger JC, Laraia M, Hobbs WR, Peterson GA, Hucek A. Different rates of improvement of different symptoms in combined pharmacological and behavioral treatment of agoraphobia. J Behav Ther Exp Psychiatry 1988 Jun;19(2):119–26.

Craske MG, Sanderson WC, Barlow DH. How do desynchronous response systems relate to the treatment of agoraphobia? A follow-up evaluation. Behav Res Ther 1987;25(2):117–22.

D'Zurilla TJ. Problem-solving: Still a promising treatment strategy for agoraphobia. Behav Ther 1985 Nov;16(5):545–8.

de Moor W. The topography of agoraphobia. Am J Psychotherapy 1985 Jul;39(3):371–88.

Dewey D, Hunsley J. The effects of marital adjustment and spouse involvement on the behavioral treatment of agoraphobia: A meta-analytic review. Anxiety Res 1990;2(2):69–83.

Diamond DB. Panic attacks, hypochondriasis, and agoraphobia: a self-psychology formulation. Am J Psychother 1985 Jan;39(1):114–25.

Diamond DB. Psychotherapeutic approaches to the treatment of panic attacks, hypochondriasis and agoraphobia. Br J Med Psychol 1987 Mar;60(Pt 1):79–84.

Eaton WW, Keyl PM. Risk factors for the onset of Diagnostic Interview Schedule/DSM-III agoraphobia in a prospective, population-based study. Arch Gen Psychiatry 1990 Sep;47(9):819–24.

Elsenga S, Emmelkamp PM. Behavioral treatment of an incest-related trauma in an agoraphobic client. J Anxiety Disord 1990;4(2):151–62.

Emanuele MA, Brooks MH, Gordon DL, Braithwaite SS. Agoraphobia and hyperthyroidism. Am J Med 1989 Apr;86(4):484–6.

Emmelkamp PM, Brilman E, Kuiper H, Mersch PP. The treatment of agoraphobia: A comparison of self-instructional training, rational emotive therapy, and exposure in vivo. Behav Modif 1986 Jan;10(1):37–53.

Emmelkamp PM, Mersch PP, Vissia E. The external validity of analogue outcome research: evaluation of cognitive and behavioral interventions. Behav Res Ther 1985;23(1):83–6.

Evans L, et al. Plasma serotonin levels in agoraphobia. Am J Psychiatry 1985 Feb;142(2):267.

Evans L, Kenardy J, Schneider P, Hoey H. Effect of a selective serotonin uptake inhibitor in agoraphobia with panic attacks. A double-blind comparison of zimeldine, imipramine and placebo. Acta Psychiatr Scand 1986 Jan;73(1):49–53.

Evans LE, Oei TP, Hoey H. Prescribing patterns in agoraphobia with panic attacks. Med J Aust 1988 Jan 18;148(2):74–7.

Faravelli C, Webb T, Ambonetti A, Fonnesu F, Sessarego A. Prevalence of traumatic early life events in 31 agoraphobic patients with panic attacks. Am J Psychiatry 1985 Dec;142(12):1493–4.

Fava GA, Kellner R, Zielezny M, Grandi S. Hypochondriacal fears and beliefs in agoraphobia. J Affective Disord 1988 May-Jun;14(3):239–44.

Fava GA, Zielezny M, Luria E, Canestrari R. Obsessive-compulsive symptoms in agoraphobia: changes with treatment. Psychiatry Res 1988 Jan;23(1):57–63.

Filewich RJ. Treatment of the agoraphobic dental patient. Dent Clin North Am 1988 Oct;32(4):723–33.

Fink K. From symmetry to asymmetry. Int J Psychoanal 1989;70(Pt 3):481–9.

Finkel JA. Diazepam in a patient with chronic schizophrenia complicated by agoraphobia. J Clin Psychiatry 1987 Jan;48(1):33–4.

Fodor IG. Cognitive/behavior therapy for agoraphobic women: Toward utilizing psychodynamic understanding to address family belief systems and enhance behavior change. Special Issue: Women, power, and therapy: Issues for women. Women Ther 1987 Spring-Summer;6(1-2):103–23.

Franklin JA. A 6-year follow-up of the effectiveness of respiratory retraining, in-situ isometric relaxation, and cognitive modification in the treatment of agoraphobia. Behav Modif 1989 Apr;13(2):139–67.

Franklin JA. The changing nature of agoraphobic fears. Br J Clin Psychol 1987 May;26(Pt 2):127–33.

Friedman S. Implications of object-relations theory for the behavioral treatment of agoraphobia. Am J Psychother 1985 Oct;39(4):525–40.

Friedman S. Technical considerations in the behavioral-marital treatment of agoraphobia. Am J Fam Ther 1987 Summer;15(2):111–22.

Frustaci J. A survey of agoraphobics in self-help groups. Smith Coll Stud Social Work 1988 Jun;58(3):193–211.

Gerew AB, Romney DM, Leboeuf A. Synchrony and desynchrony in high and low arousal subjects undergoing therapeutic exposure. J Behav Ther Exp Psychiatry 1989 Mar;20(1):41–8.

Ghosh A, Marks IM. Self-treatment of agoraphobia by exposure. Behav Ther 1987 Winter;18(1):3–16.

Gloger S, Grunhaus L, Gladic D, O'Ryan F, Cohen L, Codner S. Panic attacks and agoraphobia: low dose clomipramine treatment. J Clin Psychopharmacol 1989 Feb;9(1):28–32.

Goldberg C. Agoraphobia: Contributing factors, phobic situations, and exposure in vivo. Psychol Rep 1986 Aug;59(1):143–60.

Goldberg C. Biological model of agoraphobia: a comment. Psychol Rep 1988 Oct;63(2):571–8.

Gournay KJ. The base for exposure treatment in agoraphobia: some indicators for nurse therapists and community psychiatric nurses. J Adv Nurs 1991 Jan;16(1):82–91.

Greenberg D, Belmaker RH. DDAVP as a possible method to enhance positive benefit of behavior therapy. Br J Psychiatry 1985 Dec;147:713–5.

Gustavson B, Jansson L, Jerremalm A, Öst LG. Therapist behavior during exposure treatment of agoraphobia. Behav Modif 1985 Oct;9(4):491–504.

Haimo S, Blitman F. The effects of assertive training on sex role concept in female agoraphobics. Women Ther 1985 Summer;4(2):53–61.

Hamann MS, Mavissakalian M. Discrete dimensions in agoraphobia: a factor analytic study. Br J Clin Psychol 1988 May;27(Pt 2):137–44.

Hazell J, Wilkins AJ. A contribution of fluorescent lighting to agoraphobia. Psychol Med 1990 Aug;20(3):591–6.

Herod EL. An agoraphobic patient with dental anxiety: report of case. J Am Dent Assoc 1988 Jun;116(7):860–1.

Himadi WG. Safety signals and agoraphobia. J Anxiety Disord 1987;1(4):345–60.

Himadi WG, Boice R, Barlow DH. Assessment of agoraphobia: II. Measurement of clinical change. Behav Res Ther 1986;24(3):321–32.

Himadi WG, Boice R, Barlow DH. Assessment of agoraphobia: Triple response measurement. Behav Res Ther 1985;23(3):311–23.

Himadi WG, et al. The relationship of marital adjustment to agoraphobia treatment outcome. Behav Res Ther 1986;24(2):107–15.

Hoffart A, Matinsen EW. Exposure-based integrated vs. pure psychodynamic treatment of agoraphobic inpatients. Psychotherapy 1990 Summer;27(2):210–8.

Holden AE, Barlow DH. Heart rate and heart rate variability recorded in vivo in agoraphobics and nonphobics. Behav Ther 1986 Jan;17(1):26–42.

Horn TL. Agoraphobia. Am Fam Physician 1985 Jul;32(1):165–73.

Jackson HJ, Elton V. A multimodal approach to the treatment of agoraphobia: four case studies. Can J Psychiatry 1985 Nov;30(7):539–43.

Jacobson NS, Holtzworth-Munroe A, Schmaling KB. Marital therapy and spouse involvement in the treatment of depression, agoraphobia, and alcoholism. J Consult Clin Psychol 1989 Feb;57(1):5–10.

Jacobson NS, Wilson L, Tupper C. The clinical significance of treatment gains resulting from exposure-based interventions for agoraphobia: A reanalysis of outcome data. Behav Ther 1988 Fall;19(4):539–54.

James JE. Desensitization treatment of agoraphobia. Br J Clin Psychol 1985 May;24(Pt 2):133–4.

Jansson L, Jerremalm A, Öst LG. Applied relaxation in the treatment of agoraphobia: Two experimental case studies. Scand J Behav Ther 1985;14(4):169–76.

Jansson L, Jerremalm A, Öst LG. Follow-up of agoraphobic patients treated with exposure in vivo or applied relaxation. Br J Psychiatry 1986 Oct;149:486–90.

Jansson L, Öst LG, Jerremalm A. Prognostic factors in the behavioral treatment of agoraphobia. Behav Psychother 1987 Jan;15(1):31–44.

Johnston DG, Troyer IE, Whitsett SF. Clomipramine treatment of agoraphobic women. An eight-week controlled trial. Arch Gen Psychiatry 1988 May;45(5):453–9.

Kaplan SP. Agoraphobia in a rehabilitation medicine setting: A case report. J Couns Psychology 1987 Apr;34(2):132–5.

Katerndahl DA. Factors in the panic-agoraphobia transition. J Am Board Fam Pract 1989 Jan-Mar;2(1):10–6.

Kay G. Mental health. Joyful strategies. Nurs Times 1990 Mar 14–20;86(11):69–71.

Kenardy J, Evans L, Oei TPS. The importance of cognitions in panic attacks. Behav Ther 1988;19(3):471–83.

Kenardy J, Oei TP, Evans L. Neuroticism and age of onset for agoraphobia with panic attacks. J Behav Ther Exp Psychiatry 1990 Sep;21(3):193–7.

Klein DF, Klein HM. The substantive effect of variations in panic measurement and agoraphobia definition. J Anxiety Disord 1989;3(1):45–56.

Klein DF, Ross DC, Cohen P. Panic and avoidance in agoraphobia. Application of path analysis to treatment studies. Arch Gen Psychiatry 1987 Apr;44(4):377–85.

Kleiner L, Marshall WL. Relationship difficulties and agoraphobia. Clin Psychol Rev 1985;5(6):581–95.

Kleiner L, Marshall WL, Spevack M. Training in problem-solving and exposure treatment for agoraphobics with panic attacks. J Anxiety Disord 1987;1(3):219–38.

Klerman GL. Current trends in clinical research on panic attacks, agoraphobia, and related anxiety disorders. J Clin Psychiatry 1986 Jun;47 Suppl: 37–9.

Koehler K, Vartzopoulos D, Ebel H. Agoraphobia and depression: relationships and severity in hospitalized women. Compr Psychiatry 1986 Nov-Dec;27(6):533–9.

Koksal F, Power KG. Four Systems Anxiety Questionnaire (FSAQ): A self-report measure of somatic, cognitive, behavioral, and feeling components. J Pers Assess 1990 Summer;54(3–4):534–45.

Kopp M, Gruzelier J. Electrodermally differentiated subgroups of anxiety patients and controls. II: Relationships with auditory, somatosensory and pain thresholds, agoraphobic fear, depression and cerebral laterality. Int J Psychophysiol 1989 Mar;7(1):65–75.

Kopp MS. Psychophysiological characteristics of anxiety patients and controls. Psychother Psychosom 1989;52(1–3):74–9.

Kopp MS, Mihaly K, Linka E, Bitter I. Electrodermally differentiated subgroups of anxiety patients. I. Automatic and vigilance characteristics. Int J Psychophysiol 1987 May; 5(1):43–51.

Last CG, Barlow DH, O'Brien GT. Assessing cognitive aspects of anxiety. Stability over time and agreement between several methods. Behav Modif 1985 Jan;9(1):72–93.

Laybourne PC Jr, Redding JG. Agoraphobia. Is fear the basis of symptoms? Postgrad Med 1985 Oct;78(5):109–12, 114, 117–8.

Lazarus AA. Treating agoraphobia: Behavioral/multimodal perspectives. Psychother Priv Pract 1986 Fall;4(3):11–23.

Lazarus AA, Messer SB. Clinical choice points: Behavioral versus psychoanalytic interventions. Psychotherapy 1988 Spring;25(1):59–70.

LeBoeuf A. Relaxation-induced anxiety in an agoraphobic population. Perceptual Motor Skills 1986 Jun;62(3):910.

Lelliott PT, Marks IM, Monteiro WO, et al. Agoraphobics 5 years after imipramine and exposure. Outcome and predictors. J Nerv Ment Dis 1987;175(10):599–605.

Lewis DA. "Imipramine binding in agoraphobia": Reply. Psychiatry Res 1986 Jun; 18(2):191–2.

Lewis DA, Noyes R Jr, Coryell W, Clancy J. Tritiated imipramine binding to platelets is decreased in patients with agoraphobia. Psychiatry Res 1985 Sep;16(1):1–9.

Ley R. Agoraphobia, the panic attack and the hyperventilation syndrome. Behav Res Ther 1985;23(1):79–81.

Ley R. Blood, breath, and fears: A hyperventilation theory of panic attacks and agoraphobia. Clin Psychol Rev 1985;5(4):271–85.

Liddell A, Acton B. Agoraphobics' understanding of the development and maintenance of their symptoms. J Behav Ther Exp Psychiatry 1988 Dec;19(4):261–6.

Liddell A, Bilsbury CD, Rattenbury C. Concordance and discordance of cognitive, behavioral and somatic self-ratings as a function of exposure: A Discan analysis. Behav Res Ther 1987;25(5):425–8.

Liddell A, et al. Compliance as a factor in outcome with agoraphobic clients. Behav Res Ther 1986;24(2):217–20.

Lydiard RB. Desipramine in agoraphobia with panic attacks: an open, fixed-dose study. J Clin Psychopharmacol 1987 Aug;7(4):258–60.

Mackay W, Liddell A. An investigation into the matching of specific agoraphobic anxiety response characteristics with specific types of treatment. Behav Res Ther 1986; 24(3):361–4.

Mali D, Hudson KJ. A note on waiting list attrition. Behav Change 1988;5(4):171–4.

Marcus HP, Runge CM. Community-based services for agoraphobics. Families Society 1990 Dec;71(10):602–6.

Margraf J, Ehlers A, Taylor CB, Arnow B, Roth WT. Guttman scaling in agoraphobia: cross-cultural replication and prediction of treatment response patterns. Br J Clin Psychol 1990 Feb;29(Pt 1):37–41.

Marks I, O'Sullivan G. Drugs and psychological treatments for agoraphobia/panic and obsessive-compulsive disorders: a review. Br J Psychiatry 1988 Nov;153:650–8.

Matte Blanco I. Comments on "From symmetry to asymmetry" by Klaus Fink. Int J Psychoanal 1989;70(3):491–8.

Mattimore-Knudson RS. Reality Therapy via proxy for paranoia and agoraphobia. Clin Gerontol 1986 Feb;4(3):58–61.

Mavissakalian M. Clinically significant improvement in agoraphobia research. Behav Res Ther 1986;24(3):369–70.

Mavissakalian M. Imipramine in agoraphobia. Compr Psychiatry 1986 Jul-Aug;27(4):401–6.

Mavissakalian M. Initial depression and response to imipramine in agoraphobia. J Nerv Ment Dis 1987 Jun;175(6):358–61.

Mavissakalian M. Male and female agoraphobia: are they different? Behav Res Ther 1985;23(4):469–71.

Mavissakalian M. The placebo effect in agoraphobia—II. J Nerv Ment Dis 1988 Jul; 176(7):446–8.

Mavissakalian M. The placebo effect in agoraphobia. J Nerv Ment Dis 1987 Feb;175(2):95–9.

Mavissakalian M. The relationship between panic, phobic and anticipatory anxiety in agoraphobia. Behav Res Ther 1988;26(3):235–40.

Mavissakalian M. Trimodal assessment in agoraphobia research: Further observations on heart rate and synchrony/desynchrony. J Psychopathol Behav Asses 1987 Mar;9(1):89–98.

Mavissakalian M, Hamann MS. Assessment and significance of behavioral avoidance in agoraphobia. J Psychopathol Behav Assess 1986 Dec;8(4):317–27.

Mavissakalian M, Hamann MS. DSM-III personality disorder in agoraphobia. Compr Psychiatry 1986 Sep-Oct;27(5):471–9.

Mavissakalian M, Michelson L. Agoraphobia: relative and combined effectiveness of therapist-assisted in vivo exposure and imipramine. J Clin Psychiatry 1986 Mar;47(3):117–22.

Mavissakalian M, Michelson L. Two-year follow-up of exposure and imipramine treatment of agoraphobia. Am J Psychiatry 1986 Sep;143(9):1106–12.

Mavissakalian M, Perel J. Imipramine in the treatment of agoraphobia: dose-response relationships. Am J Psychiatry 1985 Sep;142(9):1032–6.

Mayerhoff D, Vital-Herne J, Lesser M, Brenner R. Alprazolam-induced manic reaction. N Y State J Med 1986 Jun;86(6):320.

McConaghy N, Silove D, Hall W. Behavior completion mechanisms, anxiety and agoraphobia. Aust N Z J Psychiatry 1989 Sep;23(3):373–8.

McNally RJ, Foa EB. Cognition and agoraphobia: Bias in the interpretation of threat. Special Issue: Anxiety: Cognitive factors and the anxiety disorders. Cogn Ther Res 1987 Oct;11(5):567–81.

McNally RJ, Lorenz M. Anxiety sensitivity in agoraphobics. J Behav Ther Exp Psychiatry 1987 Mar;18(1):3–11.

Michelson L. Treatment consonance and response profiles in agoraphobia: The role of individual differences in cognitive, behavioral and physiological treatments. Behav Res Ther 1986;24(3):263–75.

Michelson L, et al. The role of self-directed in vivo exposure in cognitive, behavioral, and psychophysiological treatments of agoraphobia. Behav Ther 1986 Mar;17(2):91–108.

Michelson L, Marchione K, Marchione N, Testa S, Mavissakalian M. Cognitive correlates and outcome of cognitive, behavioral and physiological treatments of agoraphobia. Psychol Rep 1988 Dec;63(3):999–1004.

Michelson L, Mavissakalian M. Psychophysiological outcome of behavioral and pharmaco-logical treatments of agoraphobia. J Consult Clin Psychol 1985 Apr;53(2):229–36.

Michelson L, Mavissakalian M, Marchione K. Cognitive, behavioral, and psychophysiological treatments of agoraphobia: A comparative outcome investigation. Behav Ther 1988;19(2):97–120.

Michelson L, Mavissakalian M, Marchione K. Cognitive and behavioral treatments of agoraphobia: Clinical, behavioral, and psychophysiological outcomes. J Consult Clin Psychol 1985;53(6):913–25.

Michelson L, Mavissakalian M, Marchione K, Ulrich RF, Marchione N, Testa S. Psycho-physiological outcome of cognitive, behavioral and psychophysiologically-based treat-ments of agoraphobia. Behav Res Ther 1990;28(2):127–39.

Milne G. Hypnosis in the treatment of single phobia and complex agoraphobia: A series of case studies. Aust J Clin Exp Hypnosis 1988 May;16(1):53–65.

Miranda D, Doctor RM. Agoraphobia: A review of research and treatment. Phobia Pract Res J 1989 Spring-Summer;2(1):37–55.

Monteiro W, Marks IM, Ramm E. Marital adjustment and treatment outcome in agorapho-bia. Br J Psychiatry 1985 Apr;146:383–90.

Moran C. Depersonalization and agoraphobia associated with marijuana use. Br J Med Psychol 1986 Jun;59(Pt 2):187–96.

Moran C, Andrews G. A familial occurrence of agoraphobia. Br J Psychiatry 1985;146:262–7.

Nicholson RC. How the significant other can help an agoraphobic patient. Emphasis Nurs 1985;1(2):57–65.

Norton GR, Allen GE, Walker JR. Predicting treatment preferences for agoraphobia. Behav Res Ther 1985;23(6):699–701.

Noyes R, Chaudry DR, Domingo DV. Pharmacologic treatment of phobic disorders. J Clin Psychiatry 1986 Sep;47(9):445–52.

Oatley K, Hodgson D. Influence of husbands on the outcome of their agoraphobic wives' therapy. Br J Psychiatry 1987 Mar;150:380–6.

Ogles BM, Lambert MJ, Weight DG, Payne IR. Agoraphobia outcome measurement: A review and meta-analysis. Psychol Assess 1990 Sep;2(3):317–25.

Öst LG. Psychophysiological assessment of agoraphobia. J Psychophysiol 1990;4(4):315–9.

Öst LG. The Agoraphobia Scale: An evaluation of its reliability and validity. Behav Res Ther 1990;28(4):323–9.

Öst LG. Ways of acquiring phobias and outcome of behavioral treatments. Behav Res Ther 1985;23(6):683–9.

Perlmutter RA. Psychopharmacology of attachment: Effects of successful agoraphobia treatment on marital relationships. Fam Syst Med 1990 Fall;8(3):279–84.

Persson G, Nordlund CL. Agoraphobics and social phobics: differences in background factors, syndrome profiles and therapeutic response. Acta Psychiatr Scand 1985 Feb;71(2):148–59.

Peterson GA, Ballenger JC, Cox DP, Hucek A, Lydiard RB, Laraia MT, Trockman C. The dexamethasone suppression test in agoraphobia. J Clin Psychopharmacol 1985 Apr;5(2):100–2.

Phillipson H. The use of O.R.T. as a facilitator of maturational processes: Some implications for a range of applications with special reference to subliminal activation of preconscious processing. Special Issue: Object Relations Technique. Br J Proj Psychol 1988 Jun; 33(1):84–105.

Pollack MH, Sachs GS, Tesar GE, Shushtari J, Herman JB, Otto MW, Rosenbaum JF. Pilot outreach services to homebound agoraphobic patients. Hosp Community Psychiatry 1991 Mar;42(3):315–7.

Pollard CA. Respiratory distress during panic attacks associated with agoraphobia. Psychol Rep 1986 Feb;58(1):61–2.

Pollard CA, Henderson JG, Frank M, Margolis RB. Help-seeking patterns of anxiety-disordered individuals in the general population. J Anxiety Disord 1989;3(3):131–8.

Pollard CA, Pollard HJ, Corn KJ. Panic onset and major events in the lives of agoraphobics: a test of contiguity. J Abnorm Psychol 1989 Aug;98(3):318–21.

Pyke JM, Longdon M. Agoraphobia. Can Nurse 1985 Jun;81(6):18–21.

Pyke RE, Greenberg HS. Norepinephrine challenges in panic patients. J Clin Psychopharmacol 1986 Oct;6(5):279–85.

Rachman S, Craske M, Tallman K, Solyom C. Does escape behavior strengthen agoraphobic avoidance? A replication. Behav Ther 1986;17(4):366–84.

Rifkin A, Pecknold JC, Swinson RP, Ballenger JC, Burrows GD, Noyes R, DuPont RL, Lesser I. Sequence of improvement in agoraphobia with panic attacks. J Psychiatr Res 1990;24(1):1–8.

Rohrbaugh M, Shean GD. Anxiety disorders: An interactional view of agoraphobia. J Psychother Fam 1987 Fall;3(3):65–85.

Rose SD. Group exposure: A method of treating agoraphobia. Special Issue: Group work with the emotionally disabled. Soc Work Groups 1990;13(1):37–51.

Roth WT, Telch MJ, Taylor CB, Agras WS. Autonomic changes after treatment of agoraphobia with panic attacks. Psychiatry Res 1988 Apr;24(1):95–107.

Roth WT, Telch MJ, Taylor CB, Sachitano JA, Gallen CC, Kopell ML, McClenahan KL, Agras WS, Pfefferbaum A. Autonomic characteristics of agoraphobia with panic attacks. Biol Psychiatry 1986 Oct;21(12):1133–54.

Sakol MS, Power KG. The effects of long-term benzodiazepine treatment and graded withdrawal on psychometric performance. Psychopharmacology 1988 May;95(1):135–8.

Sartory G, Master D, Rachman S. Safety-signal therapy in agoraphobics: a preliminary test. Behav Res Ther 1989;27(2):205–9.

Schneider P, Evans L, Ross-Lee L, Wiltshire B, Eadie M, Kenardy J, Hoey H. Plasma biogenic amine levels in agoraphobia with panic attacks. Pharmacopsychiatry 1987 May;20(3):102–4.

Shean G, Uchenwa U. Interpersonal style and anxiety. J Psychol 1990 Jul;124(4):403–8.

Southworth S, Kirsch I. The role of expectancy in exposure-generated fear reduction in agoraphobia. Behav Res Ther 1988;26(2):113–20.

Stanton HE. Treating phobias rapidly with Bandler's theater technique. Aust J Clin Exp Hypnosis 1988 Nov;16(2):153–60.

Surman OS, Williams J, Sheehan DV, Strom TB, Jones KJ, Coleman J. Immunological response to stress in agoraphobia and panic attacks. Biol Psychiatry 1986 Jul;21(8-9):768–74.

Taylor IL. The reactive effect of self-monitoring of target activities in agoraphobics: A pilot study. Scand J Behav Ther 1985;14(1):17–22.

Telch MJ, et al. Combined pharmacological and behavioral treatment for agoraphobia. Behav Res Therapy 1985;23(3):325–35.

Thomson G. Agoraphobia: The etiology and treatment of an attachment/separation disorder. Trans Anal J 1986 Jan;16(1):11–7.

Thorpe GL, Freedman EG, Lazar JD. Assertiveness training and exposure in vivo for agoraphobics. Behav Psychother 1985 Apr;13(2):132–41.

Thorpe GL, Hecker JE, Cavallaro LA, Kulberg GE. Insight versus rehearsal in cognitive-behavior therapy: A crossover study with sixteen phobics. Behav Psychother 1987 Oct;15(4):319–36.

Thyer BA. Agoraphobia: a superstitious conditioning perspective. Psychol Rep 1986 Feb;58(1):95–100.

Thyer BA. Community-based self-help groups for the treatment of agoraphobia. J Soc Welf 1987 Sep;14(3):135–41.

Thyer BA, Himle J. Temporal relationship between panic attack onset and phobic avoidance in agoraphobia. Behav Res Ther 1985;23(5):607–8.

Trull TJ, Nietzel MT, Main A. The use of meta-analysis to assess the clinical significance of behavior therapy for agoraphobia. Behav Ther 1988 Fall;19(4):527–38.

Turner SM, Stanley MA, Beidel DC, Bond L. The Social Phobia and Anxiety Inventory: Construct validity. J Psychopathol Behav Assess 1989 Sep;11(3):221–34.

Viswanathan R, Kachur EK. Development of agoraphobia after surviving cancer. Gen Hosp Psychiatry 1986 Mar;8(2):127–32.

Vital-Herne J, Brenner R, Lesser M. Another case of alprazolam withdrawal syndrome. Am J Psychiatry 1985 Dec;142(12):1515.

Wardle J. Behavior therapy and benzodiazepines: Allies or antagonists? World Congress of Behavior Therapy (1988, Edinburgh, Scotland). Br J Psychiatry 1990 Feb;156:163–8.

Wardle J, Ahmad T, Hayward P. Anxiety sensitivity in agoraphobia. J Anxiety Disord 1990;4(4):325–33.

Watts FN. Attentional strategies and agoraphobic anxiety. Behav Psychother 1989 Jan;17(1):15–26.

What precipitates agoraphobia? Lancet 1990 Jun 2;335(8701):1314–5.

Williams KE, Chambless DL. The relationship between therapist characteristics and outcome of in vivo exposure treatment for agoraphobia. Behav Therapy 1990 Winter;21(1):111–6.

Williams SL. Guided mastery treatment of agoraphobia: beyond stimulus exposure. Prog Behav Modif 1990;26:89–121.

Williams SL, Kinney PJ, Falbo J. Generalization of therapeutic changes in agoraphobia: the role of perceived self-efficacy. J Consult Clin Psychol 1989 Jun;57(3):436–42.

Williams SL, Kleifield E. Transfer of behavioral change across phobias in multiply phobic clients. Behav Modif 1985 Jan;9(1):22–31.

Williams SL, Zane G. Guided mastery and stimulus exposure treatments for severe performance anxiety in agoraphobics. Behav Res Ther 1989;27(3):237–45.

Winter D, Gournay K. Construction and constriction in agoraphobia. Br J Med Psychol 1987 Sep;60(Pt 3):233–44.

Wood AV. Hypnosis and audio tapes as a treatment for agoraphobia. Aust J Clin Hypnother Hypnosis 1986 Sep;7(2):100–4.

Woods SW, Charney DS, Loke J, Goodman WK, Redmond DE Jr, Heninger GR. Carbon dioxide sensitivity in panic anxiety. Ventilatory and anxiogenic response to carbon dioxide in healthy subjects and patients with panic anxiety before and after alprazolam treatment. Arch Gen Psychiatry 1986 Sep;43(9):900–9.

Woods SW, Charney DS, McPherson CA, Gradman AH, Heninger GR. Situational panic attacks. Behavioral, physiologic, and biochemical characterization. Arch Gen Psychiatry 1987 Apr;44(4):365–75.

Yager EK. Treating agoraphobia with hypnosis, subliminal therapy and paradoxical intention. Med Hypnoanal J 1988 Dec;3(4):156–60.

Zarate R, Craske MG, Barlow DH. Situational exposure treatment versus panic control treatment for agoraphobia. A case study. J Behav Ther Exp Psychiatry 1990 Sep; 21(3):211–24.

Zgourides GD, Warren R, Englert ME. Further evidence of construct validity for the Agoraphobic Cognitions Questionnaire and the Body Sensations Questionnaire. Psychol Rep 1989 Apr;64(2):590.

Zoldak W. Agoraphobia, fear of the marketplace. Emot First Aid J Crisis Interv 1986 Summer;3(2):15–8.

Reviews

Abstracts from Panic and Anxiety: a Decade of Progress. An international conference. June 19-22, 1990, Geneva, Switzerland. J Psychiatr Res 1990;24 Suppl 1:1–103.

Bittikofer F, Kane CA. Panic disorder. West J Med 1987;146(3):353–4.

Chambless DL. Update on panic disorder and agoraphobia. Curr Opin Psychiatry 1990;3(6):790–4.

Crowe RR, Noyes R Jr. Panic disorder and agoraphobia. Dis Mon 1986 Jul;32(7):389–444.

Dilsaver SC. Panic disorder. Am Fam Physician 1989 Jun;39(6):167–72.

Fyer AJ. Agoraphobia. Mod Probl Pharmacopsychiatry 1987;22:91–126.

Hasan MK, Mooney RP. Panic disorder: a review. Compr Ther 1986 Aug;12(8):3–7.

Heninger GR. Recent research on the neurobiology of panic. Curr Opin Psychiatry 1989;2(1):112–6.

Katon W. Panic disorder: epidemiology, diagnosis, and treatment in primary care. J Clin Psychiatry 1986 Oct;47 Suppl:21–30.

Klerman GL. Conclusions. Panic disorder: Strategies for long-term treatment. J Clin Psychiatry 1991;52(2 Suppl):33.

Lum LC. Hyperventilation syndromes in medicine and psychiatry: a review. J R Soc Med 1987 Apr;80(4):229–31.

Maser JD, Woods SW. The biological basis of panic: psychological interactions. Psychiatr Med 1990;8(3):121–147.

Mathis JL. Panic disorder with agoraphobia. N C Med J 1988 Oct;49(10):521–2.

O'Boyle M. Panic disorder: diagnosis and treatment. Tex Med 1989 Aug;85(8):46–9.

Panic disorder. Proceedings of a symposium. Gothenburg, Sweden, September 18-19, 1986. Acta Psychiatr Scand Suppl 1987;335:1–98.

Panic disorder: diathesis and treatment issues. 143rd annual meeting of the American Psychiatric Association, New York, N.Y., May 12–17, 1990. Proceedings. J Clin Psychiatry 1990 Dec;51 Suppl A:3–47.

Parker G, Curtis J. Panic disorder. Psychiatr Dev 1987 Autumn;5(3):265–77.

Raj A, Sheehan DV. Panic anxiety: diagnosis, etiology, and treatment. Compr Ther 1986 Oct;12(10):7–15.

Rosenbaum JF. Panic disorder: Diathesis and treatment issues. J Clin Psychiatry 1990;51(12 Suppl A):3–4.

Roth M, Argyle N. Anxiety, panic and phobic disorders: an overview. J Psychiatr Res 1988;22 Suppl 1:33–54.

Sargent M. Panic disorder. Hosp Community Psychiatry 1990 Jun;41(6):621–3.

Uhde TW, Maser JD. NIMH report. Current perspectives on panic disorder and agoraphobia. Hosp Community Psychiatry 1985 Nov;36(11):1153–4.

Books and Book Chapters

Achte K, Tamminen T, Laaksonen R, editors. Many faces of panic disorder. Proceedings of the WPA Symposium on the Psychopathology of Panic Disorder; 1988 Aug 26–27; Espoo, Finland. Helsinki: Foundation of Psychiatric Research in Finland; 1989. 158 p. (Psychiatria Fennica supplementum; 1989).

Albu M, Zellner A, Ackenheil M, Braune S, Engel RR. Do anxiety patients differ in autonomic base levels and stress response from normal controls? In: Hand I, Wittchen HU, editors. Panic and phobias 2: treatments and variables affecting course and outcome. Berlin: Springer-Verlag; 1988. p. 171–9.

American Psychiatric Association. Diagnostic and statistical manual of mental disorders. 3rd ed. rev. Washington, DC: The Association; 1987. 300.21 Panic disorder with agoraphobia, 300.01 Panic disorder without agoraphobia; p. 235–9.

American Academy of Clinical Psychiatrists. Update on anxiety and panic disorders. Annual meeting of the American Academy of Clinical Psychiatrists; 1985 Oct 9; San Francisco. [Memphis (TN): Physicians Postgraduate Press; c1986]. 39 p. (Journal of clinical psychiatry; vol. 47, no. 6, suppl.).

Andrews G, Moran C. Exposure treatment of agoraphobia with panic attacks: are drugs essential? In: Hand I, Wittchen HU, editors. Panic and phobias 2: treatments and variables affecting course and outcome. Berlin: Springer-Verlag; 1988. p. 89–99.

Anton RF. Prostaglandins—relationship to the central-nervous-system and the platelet in panic disorder. In: Ballenger JC, editor. Neurobiology of panic disorder. New York: Wiley-Liss; 1990. p. 349–64.

Baker R. Introduction: where does "panic disorder" come from? In: Baker R, editor. Panic disorder: theory, research, and therapy. New York: Wiley; c1989. p. 1–12.

Baker R. Personal accounts of panic. In: Baker R, editor. Panic disorder: theory, research and therapy. New York: Wiley; 1989. p. 67–88.

Baker R. Synthesis. In: Baker R, editor. Panic disorder: theory, research and therapy. New York: Wiley; 1989. p. 325–44.

Baker R, editor. Panic disorder: theory, research, and therapy. New York: Wiley; c1989. 350 p.

Ballenger JC. Treatment of panic disorder and agoraphobia. In: Coryell W, Winokur G, editors. The clinical management of anxiety disorders. New York: Oxford University Press; 1991. p. 41–62.

Ballenger JC, Burrows G, DuPont R, Lesser IM, Noyes R, Pecknold J, Rifkin A, Swinson R. Aprazolam in panic disorder and agoraphobia. Results from a multicenter trial. 1. Efficacy of short-term treatment. In: Ballenger JC, editor. Clinical aspects of panic disorder. New York: Wiley-Liss; 1990. p. 219–38.

Ballenger JC, editor. Clinical aspects of panic disorder. New York: Wiley-Liss; c1990. 328 p. (Frontiers of clinical neuroscience; vol. 9).

Ballenger JC, editor. Neurobiology of panic disorder. New York: Wiley-Liss; c1990. 391 p. (Frontiers of clinical neuroscience; vol. 8).

Barlow DH. A psychological model of panic. In: Shaw BF, Segal ZV, Vallis TM, Cashman FE, editors. Anxiety disorders: psychological and biological perspectives. New York: Plenum; 1986. p. 93–114.

Barlow DH. Anxiety and its disorders: the nature and treatment of anxiety and panic. New York: Guilford Press; c1988. 698 p.

Barlow DH. Current models of panic disorder and a view from emotion theory. In: Frances AJ, Hales RE, editors. American Psychiatric Press review of psychiatry. Vol. 7. Washington: American Psychiatric Press; 1988. p. 10–28.

Barlow DH. Panic disorder – foreword. In: Frances AJ, Hales RE, editors. American Psychiatric Press review of psychiatry. Vol. 7. Washington: American Psychiatric Press; 1988. p. 5–9.

Barlow DH, Cerny JA. Psychological treatment of panic. New York: Guilford Press; c1988. 227 p.

Barlow DH, Craske MG. The phenomenology of panic. In: Rachman S, Maser JD, editors. Panic: psychological perspectives. Hillsdale (NJ): Lawrence Erlbaum Associates; 1988. p. 11–36.

Barreto E, Amado H. Identifying panic disorders. In: Munoz RA, editor. Treating anxiety disorders. San Francisco: Jossey-Bass, Inc.; 1986. p. 31–44. (New directions for mental health services; no. 32).

Beck AT. Cognitive approaches to panic disorder: theory and therapy. In: Rachman S, Maser JD, editors. Panic: psychological perspectives. Hillsdale (NJ): Lawrence Erlbaum Associates; 1988. p. 91–109.

Beck AT, Emery G. Anxiety disorders and phobias: a cognitive perspective. New York: Basic Books; c1985. 343 p.

Beitman BD, Mukerji V, Flaker G, Trombka LH, Basha IM. Panic disorder in cardiology patients with atypical chest pain. In: Ballenger JC, editor. Clinical aspects of panic disorder. New York: Wiley-Liss; 1990. p. 111–40.

Bradley SJ. Panic disorder in children and adolescents—a review with examples. In: Feinstein SC, Esman AH, Looney JG, et al., editors. Adolescent psychiatry. Vol. 17, Developmental and clinical studies. Chicago: University of Chicago Press; 1990. p. 433–50.

Brown JT. Panic attacks. In: Walker JI, Brown JT, Gallis HA, editors. The complicated medical patient: new approaches to psychomedical syndromes. New York: Human Sciences Press; 1987. p. 174–86.

Buller R, Maier W, Benkert O. Factors relevant to lactate response in panic disorder. In: Hand I, Wittchen HU, editors. Panic and phobias 2: treatments and variables affecting course and outcome. Berlin: Springer-Verlag; 1988. p. 167–70.

Cassano GB, Deltito JA. Standard therapies for panic disorder. In: Lader MH, Davies HC, editors. Drug treatment of neurotic disorders: focus on alprazolam. Proceedings of an international symposium; 1984 Nov 14–15; Vienna, Austria. New York: Churchill Livingstone; 1986. p. 166–72.

Cassano GB, Petracca A, Perugi G, Nisita C, Musetti L, Mengali F, McNair DM. Comparative evaluation of clomipramine and imipramine in panic disorder: preliminary report of a naturalistic treatment trial. In: Racagni G, Smeraldi E, editors. Anxious depression: assessment and treatment. New York: Raven Press; 1987. p. 181–8.

Chambless DL. Cognitive mechanisms in panic disorder. In: Rachman S, Maser JD, editors. Panic: psychological perspectives. Hillsdale (NJ): Lawrence Erlbaum Associates; 1988. p. 205–17.

Chambless DL, Gracely EJ. Prediction of outcome following in vivo exposure treatment of agoraphobia. In: Hand I, Wittchen HU, editors. Panic and phobias 2: treatments and variables affecting course and outcome. Berlin: Springer-Verlag; 1988. p. 209–20.

Charney DS, Woods SW, Krystal JH, Nagy LM, Heninger GR. Hypotheses relating serotonergic dysfunction to the etiology and treatment of panic and generalized anxiety disorders. In: Coccaro EF, Murphy DL, editors. Serotonin in major psychiatric disorders. Washington: American Psychiatric Press; 1990. p. 127–52.

Charney DS, Woods SW, Price LH, Goodman WK, Glazer WM, Heninger GR. Noradrenergic dysregulation in panic disorder. In: Ballenger JC, editor. Neurobiology of panic disorder. New York: Wiley-Liss; 1990. p. 91–106.

Clark DM. A cognitive model of panic attacks. In: Rachman S, Maser JD, editors. Panic: psychological perspectives. Hillsdale (NJ): Lawrence Erlbaum Associates; 1988. p. 71–89.

Clark DB, Taylor CB, Hayward C. Naturalistic assessment of the physiology of panic. In: Ballenger JC, editor. Clinical aspects of panic disorder. New York: Wiley-Liss; 1990. p. 83–98.

Cowley DS, Roy-Byrne PP. Panic disorder and hyperventilation syndrome: implications of recent research. In: Roy-Byrne PP, editor. Anxiety: new findings for the clinician. Washington: American Psychiatric Press; 1989. p. 19–42.

Craske MC. Cognitive-behavioral treatment of panic. In: Frances AJ, Hales RE, editors. American Psychiatric Press review of psychiatry. Vol. 7. Washington: American Psychiatric Press; 1988. p. 121–37.

Crowe RR. Molecular genetics and panic disorder. New approaches to an old problem. In: Ballenger JC, editor. Neurobiology of panic disorder. New York: Wiley-Liss; 1990. p. 59–70.

Crowe RR, Noyes R Jr, Persico T, Wilson AF, Elston RC. Genetic studies of panic disorder and related conditions. In: Dunner DL, Gershon ES, Barrett JE, editors. Relatives at risk for mental disorder. New York: Raven Press; 1988. p. 73–85.

Crowe RR, Noyes R. Panic disorder and agoraphobia. Chicago: Year Book Medical Publishers; c1986. (Disease-a-month; vol. 32, no. 7).

Dager SR, Roth WT. Panic disorder and cardiac fears: is there reason to worry? In: Roy-Byrne PP, editor. Anxiety: new findings for the clinician. Washington: American Psychiatric Press; 1989. p. 99–120.

Dencker SJ, Holmberg G, editors. Panic disorder: proceedings of a symposium; 1986 Sep 18–19; Gothenburg, Sweden. Copenhagen: Munksgaard; 1987. 98 p. (Acta Psychiatrica Scandinavica; vol. 76, Suppl. no. 335).

Durham RC. Cognitive therapy of panic disorder. In: Baker R, editor. Panic disorder: theory, research and therapy. New York: Wiley; 1989. p. 261–80.

Eaton WW, Dryman A, Weissman MM. Panic and phobia: the diagnosis of panic disorder and phobic disorder. In: Robins LN, Regier DA, editors. Psychiatric disorders in America: the Epidemiologic Catchment Area study. New York: The Free Press; 1991. p. 155–79.

Ehlers A, Margraf J. The psychophysiological model of panic attacks. In: Emmelkamp PMG, Everaerd WTAM, Kraaimaat FW, van Son MJM, editors. Fresh perspectives on anxiety disorders. Berwyn (PA): Swets North America; 1989. p. 1–29.

Emmellkamp PMG. Marital quality and treatment outcome in anxiety disorders. In: Hand I, Wittchen HU, editors. Panic and phobias 2: treatments and variables affecting course and outcome. Berlin: Springer-Verlag; 1988. p. 233–9.

Fiegenbaum W. Long-term efficacy of ungraded versus graded massed exposure in agoraphobia. In: Hand I, Klerman HU, editors. Panic and phobias 2: treatments and variables affecting course and outcome. Berlin: Spinger-Verlag; 1988. p. 83–8.

Fischer M, Hand I, Angenendt J, Buttner-Westphal H. Failures in exposure treatment of agoraphobia: evaluation and prediction. In: Hand I, Wittchen HU, editors. Panic and phobias 2: treatments and variables affecting course and outcome. Berlin: Springer-Verlag; 1988. p. 195–208.

Foa EB. What cognitions differentiate panic disorder from other anxiety disorders? In: Hand I, Wittchen HU, editors. Panic and phobias 2: treatments and variables affecting course and outcome. Berlin: Springer-Verlag; 1988. p. 159–66.

Fontaine R. The role of the primary care physician in the treatment of panic disorder. In: Walker JR, Norton GR, Ross CA, editors. Panic disorder and agoraphobia: a comprehensive guide for the practitioner. Pacific Grove (CA): Brooks/Cole Pub. Co.; c1991. p. 352–67.

Freedman RR. Ambulatory monitoring findings on panic. In: Baker R, editor. Panic disorder: theory, research and therapy. New York: Wiley; 1989. p. 51–66.

Fyer AJ. Effects of discontinuation of antipanic medication. In: Hand I, Wittchen HU, editors. Panic and phobias 2: treatments and variables affecting course and outcome. Berlin: Springer-Verlag; 1988. p. 47–53.

Fyer AJ, Sandberg D. Pharmacologic treatment of panic disorder. In: Frances AJ, Hales RE, editors. American Psychiatric Press review of psychiatry. Vol. 7. Washington: American Psychiatric Press; 1988. p. 88–120.

Fyer AJ, Sandberg D, Klein DF. The pharmacologic treatment of panic disorder and agoraphobia. In: Walker JR, Norton GR, Ross CA, editors. Panic disorder and agoraphobia: a comprehensive guide for the practitioner. Pacific Grove (CA): Brooks/Cole Pub. Co.; c1991. p. 211–51.

Gentil V. The aversive system, 5-HT and panic attacks—commentary. In: Simon P, Soubrie P, Wildlocher D, editors. Selected models of anxiety, depression and psychosis. Vol. 1, Animal models of psychiatric disorders. Basel: Karger; 1988. p. 142–5.

Gold PW, Pigott TA, Kling MA, Brandt HA, Kalogeras K, Demitrack MA, Geracioti TD. Hypothalamic pituitary-adrenal axis in panic disorder. In: Ballenger JC, editor. Neurobiology of panic disorder. New York: Wiley-Liss; 1990. p. 313–20.

Goodwin DW. Anxiety. New York: Oxford Univ. Press; 1986. Chapter 12, Panic disorder; p. 112–22.

Gorman JM. Panic disorders. In: Klein DF, editor. Anxiety. New York: Karger; 1987. p. 36–90. (Modern problems of pharmacopsychiatry; vol. 22).

Gorman JM, Papp L, Klein DF. Biological models of panic disorder. In: Burrows GD, Roth M, Noyes R, editors. Neurobiology of anxiety. Amsterdam: Elsevier; 1990. p. 59–78.

Gorman JM, Papp LA. Respiratory physiology of panic. In: Ballenger JC, editor. Neurobiology of panic. New York: Wiley-Liss; 1990. p. 187–204.

Gournay K, editor. Agoraphobia: current perspectives on theory and treatment. New York: Routledge; 1989. 243 p.

Hallam RS. Anxiety: psychological perspectives on panic and agoraphobia. Orlando: Academic Press; 1985. 210 p.

Hallam R. Classification and research into panic. In: Baker R, editor. Panic disorder: theory, research and therapy. New York: Wiley; 1989. p. 93–105.

Hand I, Angenendt J, Fischer M, Wilke C. Exposure in-vivo with panic management for agoraphobia: treatment rationale and longterm outcome. In: Hand I, Wittchen HU, editors. Panic and phobias: empirical evidence of theoretical models and long-term effects of behavioral treatments. Berlin: Springer-Verlag; 1986. p. 104–27.

Hand I, Wittchen HU, editors. Panic and phobias: empirical evidence of theoretical models and longterm effects of behavioral treatments. 15th congress of the European Association of Behavior Therapy; 1985; Munich, Germany. Berlin: Springer-Verlag; c1986. 130 p.

Hand I, Wittchen HU, editors. Panic and phobias 2: treatments and variables affecting course and outcome. Berlin: Springer-Verlag; 1988. 275 p.

Hayward C, Clark DB, Taylor CB. Panic disorder, anxiety, and cardiovascular risk. In: Ballenger JC, editor. Clinical aspects of panic disorder. New York: Wiley-Liss; 1990. p. 99–110.

Hecker JE, Thorpe GL. Agoraphobia and panic: a guide to psychological treatment. Boston: Allyn and Bacon; 1991.

Heninger GR. A biologic perspective on comorbidity of major depressive disorder and panic disorder. In: Maser JD, Cloninger CR, editors. Comorbidity of mood and anxiety disorders. Washington: American Psychiatric Press; 1990. p. 381–401.

Hoehn-Saric R, McLeod RD. Panic and generalized anxiety disorders. In: Last CG, Hersen M, editors. Handbook of anxiety disorders. New York: Pergamon Press; 1988. p. 109–26.

Hoffmann-La Roche Limited. Panic disorder: relative merits of pharmacotherapy and psychotherapy; summary proceedings of the satellite symposium, 141st American Psychiatric Association Annual Meeting; 1988 May 8; Montreal. Mississauga (ONT): MES Medical Education Services; c1988. 20 p.

Hollander E, Levin AP, Liebowitz MR. Biological tests in the differential diagnosis of anxiety disorders. In: Ballenger JC, editor. Clinical aspects of panic disorder. New York: Wiley-Liss; 1990. p. 31–46.

Hsiao JK, Potter WZ. Mechanisms of action of antipanic drugs. In: Ballenger JC, editor. Clinical aspects of panic disorder. New York: Wiley-Liss; 1990. p. 297.

Jacob RG, Lilienfeld SO. Panic disorder: diagnosis, medical assessment, and psychological assessment. In: Walker JR, Norton GR, Ross CA, editors. Panic disorder and agoraphobia: a comprehensive guide for the practitioner. Pacific Grove (CA): Brooks/Cole Pub. Co.; c1991. p. 61–102.

Jacob RG, Turner SM. Panic disorder—diagnosis and assessment. In: Frances AJ, Hales RE, editors. American Psychiatric Press review of psychiatry. Vol. 7. Washington: American Psychiatric Press; 1988. p. 67–87.

Kagan J, Reznick JS, Snidman N, Johnson MO, Gibbons J, Gersten M, Biederman J, Rosenbaum JF. Origins of panic disorder. In: Ballenger JC, editor. Neurobiology of panic disorder. New York: Wiley-Liss; 1990. p. 71–90.

Kaplan HS. Sexual aversion, sexual phobias, and panic disorder. New York: Brunner/Mazel; c1987. 158 p.

Katon W. Panic disorder in the medical setting. Washington: American Psychiatric Press; c1990. 147 p.

Katon W. Patients with unexplained cardiac symptoms: relationship to panic disorder. In: Roy-Byrne PP, editor. Anxiety: new findings for the clinician. Washington: American Psychiatric Press; 1989. p. 1–18.

Katschnig H, Amering M. Panic attacks and panic disorders in cross-cultural-perspective. In: Ballenger JC, editor. Clinical aspects of panic disorder. New York: Wiley-Liss; 1990. p. 67–82.

Kellner C, Roybyrne PP. Computed-tomography and magnetic-resonance-imaging in panic disorder. In: Ballenger JC, editor. Neurobiology of panic disorder. New York: Wiley-Liss; 1990. p. 271–80.

King R, Margraf J, Ehlers A, Maddock R. Panic disorder: overlap with symptoms of somatization disorder. In: Hand I, Wittchen HU, editors. Panic and phobias: empirical evidence of theoretical models and long-term effects of behavioral treatments. Berlin: Springer-Verlag; 1986. p. 72–7.

Klein DF, Klein HM. The definition and psychopharmacology of spontaneous panic and phobia. In: Tyrer P, editor. Psychopharmacology of anxiety. New York: Oxford Univ. Press; 1989. p. 135–62.

Klein DF, Klein HM. The nosology, genetics, and theory of spontaneous panic and phobia. In: Tyrer P, editor. Psychopharmacology of anxiety. New York: Oxford Univ. Press; 1989. p. 163–95.

Klerman GL. Diagnosis of panic states: a North American view. In: Lader MH, Davies HC, editors. Drug treatment of neurotic disorders: focus on alprazolam. Proceedings of an international symposium; 1984 Nov 14–15; Vienna, Austria. New York: Churchill Livingstone; 1986. p. 151–9.

Klerman GL. History and development of modern concepts of anxiety and panic. In: Ballenger JC, editor. Clinical aspects of panic disorder. New York: Wiley-Liss; 1990. p. 3–12.

Klosko JS, Barlow DH, Tassinari RB, Cerny JA. Comparison of alprazolam and cognitive behavior therapy in the treatment of panic disorder: a preliminary report. In: Hand I, Wittchen HU, editors. Panic and phobias 2: treatments and variables affecting course and outcome. Berlin: Springer-Verlag; 1988. p. 54–65.

Knapp S, VandeCreek L. Diagnosis and treatment selection for anxiety disorders. Sarasota (FL): Professional Resource Exchange, Inc.; 1989. Panic attacks and agoraphobia; p. 24–35.

Lader M. The biology of panic disorder: a long-term view and critique. In: Walker JR, Norton GR, Ross CA, editors. Panic disorder and agoraphobia: a comprehensive guide for the practitioner. Pacific Grove (CA): Brooks/Cole Pub. Co; c1991. p. 150–74.

Lader MH, Davies HC, editors. Drug treatment of neurotic disorders: focus on alprazolam: proceedings of an international symposium; 1984 Nov 14–15; Vienna, Austria. Edinburgh: Churchill Livingstone; 1986. 186 p.

Lang PJ. Fear, anxiety, and panic: context, cognition, and visceral arousal. In: Rachman S, Maser JD, editors. Panic: psychological perspectives. Hillsdale (NJ): Lawrence Erlbaum Associates; 1988. p. 219–36.

Leckman JF, Clubb MM, Pauls DL. Comorbidity of panic disorder and major depression— a review of epidemiologic and genetic data. In: Ballenger JC, editor. Clinical aspects of panic disorder. New York: Wiley-Liss; 1990. p. 141–50.

Lepola U. Panic disorder: a clinical, neurochemical, neurophysiological, and neu-
roradiological study. Kuopio: University of Kuopio, Dept. of Neurology; 1990. 163 p.
(Neurologian klinikan julkaisusarja; no. 19).

Lesser IM. Panic disorder and depression—co-occurrence and treatment. In: Ballenger JC,
editor. Clinical aspects of panic disorder. New York: Wiley-Liss; 1990. p. 181–94.

Ley R. Panic disorder: a hyperventilation interpretation. In: Michelson L, Ascher LM,
editors. Anxiety and stress disorders: cognitive-behavioral assessment and treatment.
New York: Guilford Press; 1987. p. 191–212.

Liebowitz MR, Fyer AJ, Gorman JM, Campeas R, Levin A, Davies SR, Klein DF. Alprazolam
in the treatment of panic disorders. In: Lader MH, Davies HC, editors. Drug treatment
of neurotic disorders: focus on alprazolam. Proceedings of an international symposium;
1984 Nov 14–15; Vienna, Austria. New York: Churchill Livingstone; 1986. p. 173–7.

Lydiard RB, Ballenger JC, Laraia MT, Fossey M, Howell EF, Peterson G, Hucek A, Lack CR.
Effects of chronic alprazolam and imipramine treatment of catecholamine function in
patients with agoraphobia with panic attacks or panic disorder. In: Ballenger JC, editor.
Clinical aspects of panic disorder. New York: Wiley-Liss; 1990. p. 239–50.

Maier W, Buller R, Hallmayer J. Comorbidity of panic disorder and major depression:
results from a family study. In: Hand I, Wittchen HU, editors. Panic and phobias 2:
treatments and variables affecting course and outcome. Berlin: Springer-Verlag; 1988. p.
181–5.

Malcolm R, Ballenger JC, Brady K, Hodges R. Benzodiazepine abuse. In: Ballenger JC,
editor. Clinical aspects of panic disorder. New York: Wiley-Liss; 1990. p. 273–80.

Margraf J, Ehlers A. Biological models of panic disorder and agoraphobia—theory and
evidence. In: Burrows GD, Roth M, Noyes R, editors. Neurobiology of anxiety. Amsterdam: Elsevier; 1990. p. 79–140.

Margraf J, Ehlers A. Etiological models of panic—medical and biological aspects. In: Baker
R, editor. Panic disorder: theory, research and therapy. New York: Wiley; 1989. p.
145–203.

Margraf J, Ehlers A. Etiological models of panic—psychophysiological and cognitive aspects. In: Baker R, editor. Panic disorder: theory, research and therapy. New York:
Wiley; 1989. p. 205–31.

Margraf J, Ehlers A, Roth WT. Panic attacks: theoretical models and empirical evidence. In:
Hand I, Wittchen HU, editors. Panic and phobias: empirical evidence of theoretical
models and long-term effects of behavioral treatments. Berlin: Springer-Verlag; 1986. p.
31–43.

Marks I. Agoraphobia and panic disorder. In: Baker R, editor. Panic disorder: theory,
research and therapy. New York: Wiley; 1989. p. 107–15.

Marks IM. Diagnosis of panic states: a European view. In: Lader MH, Davies HC, editors.
Drug treatment of neurotic disorders: focus on alprazolam. Proceedings of an international symposium; 1984 Nov 14–15; Vienna, Austria. New York: Churchill Livingstone;
1986. p. 160–5.

Marks IM. Fears, phobias, and rituals: panic, anxiety, and their disorders. New York:
Oxford University Press; 1987. 682 p.

Marks I, O'Sullivan G. Anti-anxiety drug and psychological treatment effects in agoraphobia/panic and obsessive-compulsive disorders. In: Tyrer P, editor. Psychopharmacology of anxiety. New York: Oxford Univ. Press; 1989. p. 196–242.

Maser JD, Cloninger CR, editors. Comorbidity of mood and anxiety disorders. Washington (DC): American Psychiatric Press; 1990. 869 p.

Marshall WL. An appraisal of expectancies, safety signals, and the treatment of panic disorder patients. In: Rachman S, Maser JD, editors. Panic: psychological perspectives. Hillsdale (NJ): Lawrence Erlbaum Associates; 1988. p. 305–20.

Mathew RJ, Wilson WH. Cerebral blood-flow in anxiety and panic. In: Ballenger JC, editor. Neurobiology of panic disorder. New York: Wiley-Liss; 1990. p. 281–312.

Mathews A. Cognitive factors in the treatment of anxiety states. In: Hand I, Wittchen HU, editors. Panic and phobias 2: treatments and variables affecting course and outcome. Berlin: Springer-Verlag; 1988. p. 75–82.

Mavissakalian M. Agoraphobia. In: Beitman BD, Klerman GL, editors. Integrating pharmacotherapy and psychotherapy. Washington: American Psychiatric Press, Inc.; 1991. p. 165–81.

Mavissakalian M. Differential efficacy between tricyclic antidepressants and behavior therapy of panic disorder. In: Ballenger JC, editor. Clinical aspects of panic disorder. New York: Wiley-Liss; 1990. p. 195–210.

Mavissakalian M. Relationship of dose plasma-concentrations of imipramine to the treatment of panic disorder with agoraphobia. In: Ballenger JC, editor. Clinical aspects of panic disorder. New York: Wiley-Liss; 1990. p. 211–8.

Mavissakalian M. The mutually potentiating effects of imipramine and exposure in agoraphobia. In: Hand I, Wittchen HU, editors. Panic and phobias 2: treatments and variables affecting course and outcome. Berlin: Springer-Verlga; 1988. p. 36–43.

McFadyen M. The cognitive invalidation approach to panic. In: Baker R, editor. Panic disorder: theory, research and therapy. New York: Wiley; 1989. p. 281–99.

McGlynn TJ, Metcalf HL, editors. Diagnosis and treatment of anxiety disorders: a physician's handbook. [Washington]: American Psychiatric Press; 1989. Panic disorder with or without agoraphobia; p. 67–76.

McLean JN, Knights SA. Phobics and other panic victims: a practical guide for those who help them. New York: Continuum; 1989. 179 p.

Mellman TA, Uhde TW. Sleep in panic and generalized anxiety disorders. In: Ballenger JC, editor. Neurobiology of panic disorder. New York: Wiley-Liss; 1990. p. 365.

Michelson L. Cognitive, behavioral, and psychophysiological treatments and correlates of panic. In: Rachman S, Maser JD, editors. Panic: psychological perspectives. Hillsdale (NJ): Lawrence Erlbaum Associates; 1988. p. 137–65.

Michelson L. Cognitive-behavioral assessment and treatment of agoraphobia. In: Michelson L, Ascher LM, editors. Anxiety and stress disorders: cognitive-behavioral assessment and treatment. New York: The Guilford Press; 1987. p. 213–79.

Nesse RM, Cameron OG, Green MA, Kuttesch DA. Panic disorder and agoraphobia. In: Howells JG, editor. Modern perspectives in the psychiatry of neuroses. New York: Mazel; 1989. p. 130–52. (Modern perspectives in psychiatry; vol. 12).

Norman TR, Burrows GD, Judd FK. Towards a biochemistry of panic disorders—a critique of platelet studies. In: Burrows GD, Roth M, Noyes R, editors. Neurobiology of anxiety. Amsterdam: Elsevier; 1990. p. 245–68.

Norton GR, Walker JR, Ross CA. Panic disorder and agoraphobia: an introduction. In: Walker JR, Norton GR, Ross CA, editors. Panic disorder and agoraphobia: a comprehensive guide for the practitioner. Pacific Grove (CA): Brooks/Cole Pub. Co.; c1991. p. 3–15.

Noyes R, Garvey MJ, Cook BL. Benzodiazepines other than alprazolam in the treatment of panic disorder. In: Ballenger JC, editor. Clinical aspects of panic disorder. New York: Wiley-Liss; 1990. p. 251–8.

Nutt DJ. Basic mechanisms of benzodiazepine tolerance, dependence, and withdrawal. In: Ballenger JC, editor. Clinical aspects of panic disorder. New York: Wiley-Liss; 1990. p. 281–96.

Öst LG. Panic disorder, agoraphobia, and social phobia. In: Turpin G, editor. Handbook of clinical psychophysiology. Chichester (Sussex, United Kingdom): Wiley; 1989. p. 309–28.

Pauls DL, DiBenedetto AM. The familial relationship between panic disorder and major depressive disorder. In: Racagni G, Smeraldi E, editors. Anxious depression: assessment and treatment. New York: Raven Press; 1987. p. 73–80.

Pecknold JC. Serotonin abnormalities in panic disorder. In: Ballenger JC, editor. Neurobiology of panic disorder. New York: Wiley-Liss; 1990. p. 121–42.

Peter H, Hand I. Patterns of patient-spouse interaction in agoraphobics: assessment by Camberwell Family Interview (CFI) and impact on outcome of self-exposure treatment. In: Hand I, Wittchen HU, editors. Panic and phobias 2: treatments and variables affecting course and outcome. Berlin: Springer-Verlag; 1988. p. 240–51.

Pohl R, Yeragani V, Balon R, Ortiz A, Aleem A. Isoproterenol-induced panic—a beta-adrenergic model of panic anxiety. In: Ballenger JC, editor. Neurobiology of panic disorder. New York: Wiley-Liss; 1990. p. 107–20.

Rachman S. Panics and their consequences: a review and prospect. In: Rachman S, Maser JD, editors. Panic: psychological perspectives. Hillsdale (NJ): Lawrence Erlbaum Associates; 1988. p. 259–303.

Rachman S, Maser JD, editors. Panic: psychological perspectives. Hillsdale (NJ): Lawrence Erlbaum Associates; 1988. 373 p.

Rachman S, Maser JD. Panic: psychological contributions. In: Rachman S, Maser JD, editors. Panic: psychological perspectives. Hillsdale (NJ): Lawrence Erlbaum Associates; 1988. p. 1–10.

Rainey JM, Manov G, Aleem A, Toth A. Relationships between posttraumatic-stress-disorder and panic disorder—concurrent psychiatric-illness, effects of lactate infusions, and erythrocyte lactate production. In: Ballenger JC, editor. Clinical aspects of panic disorder. New York: Wiley-Liss; 1990. p. 47–56.

Rapee RM, Barlow DH. Psychological treatment of unexpected panic attacks: cognitive/behavioral components. In: Baker R, editor. Panic disorder: theory, research and therapy. New York: Wiley; 1989. p. 239–59.

Rapee RM, Barlow DH. The cognitive-behavioral treatment of panic attacks and agoraphobic avoidance. In: Walker JR, Norton GR, Ross CA, editors. Panic disorder and agoraphobia: a comprehensive guide for the practitioner. Pacific Grove (CA): Brooks/Cole Pub. Co.; c1991. p. 252–305.

Raskin A. Role of depression in the antipanic effects of antidepressant drugs. In: Ballenger JC, editor. Clinical aspects of panic disorder. New York: Wiley-Liss; 1990. p. 169–80.

Reiamn EM. PET, panic disorder, and normal anticipatory anxiety. In: Ballenger JC, editor. Neurobiology of panic disorder. New York: Wiley-Liss; 1990. p. 245–70.

Reichler RJ, Sylvester CE, Hyde TS. Biological studies on offspring of panic disorder probands. In: Dunner DL, Gershon ES, Barrett JE, editors. Relatives at risk for mental disorder. New York: Raven Press; 1988. p. 103–25.

Reiman EM. Contributions to the development and treatment of panic disorder: toward a piece of mind and brain. In: Beitman BD, Klerman GL, editors. Integrating pharmacotherapy and psychotherapy. Washington: American Psychiatric Press, Inc.; 1991. p. 423–34.

Reiman EM. Positron emission tomography in the study of panic disorder and anticipatory anxiety. In: Burrows GD, Roth M, Noyes R, editors. Neurobiology of anxiety. Amsterdam: Elsevier; 1990. p. 289–306.

Rosenbaum JF, Tesar GE. Clonazepam and other anticonvulsants. In: Ballenger JC, editor. Clinical aspects of panic disorder. New York: Wiley-Liss; 1990. p. 259–72.

Roy-Byrne P, editor. Anxiety: new findings for the clinician. Washington: American Psychiatric Press; c1989. 204 p. (Clinical practice; no. 5).

Salkovskis PM. Phenomenology, assessment, and the cognitive model of panic. In: Rachman S, Maser JD, editors. Panic: psychological perspectives. Hillsdale (NJ): Lawrence Erlbaum Associates; 1988. p. 111–36.

Sandberg DP, Liebowitx MR. Potential mechanisms for sodium lactates induction of panic. In: Ballenger JC, editor. Neurobiology of panic disorder. New York: Wiley-Liss; 1990. p. 155–72.

Schatzberg AF, Herrygers EJ, Rege GC, editors. Anxiety disorders, panic attacks, and phobias: proceedings of the Key Biscayne Research Conference on Anxiety Disorders, Panic Attacks, and Phobias; 1982 Dec 9–11; Key Biscayne, FL. New York: Pergamon Press; 1988. 114 p. (Journal of psychiatric research; vol. 22, suppl. 1).

Scrignar CB. From panic to peace of mind: overcoming panic and agoraphobia. New Orleans (LA): Bruno Press; 1991.

Seligman MEP. Competing theories of panic. In: Rachman S, Maser JD, editors. Panic: psychological perspectives. Hillsdale (NJ): Lawrence Erlbaum Associates; 1988. p. 321–9.

Shear MK. Cognitive and biological models of panic: toward an integration. In: Rachman S, Maser JD, editors. Panic: psychological perspectives. Hillsdale (NJ): Lawrence Erlbaum Associates; 1988. p. 51–70.

Shear MK. Panic disorder. In: Beitman BD, Klerman GL, editors. Integrating pharmacotherapy and psychotherapy. Washington: American Psychiatric Press, Inc.; 1991. p. 143–64.

Shear MK. The psychodynamic approach in the treatment of panic disorder. In: Walker JR, Norton GE, Ross CA, editors. Panic disorder and agoraphobia: a comprehensive guide for the practitioner. Pacific Grove (CA): Brooks/Cole Pub. Co.; c1991. p. 335–51.

Shear MK, Ball GG, Josephson S, Gitlin. Cognitive-behavioral treatment of panic. In: Hand I, Wittchen HU, editors. Panic and phobias 2: treatments and variables affecting course and outcome. Berlin: Springer-Verlag; 1988. p. 66–74.

Shear MK, Barlow D. Panic disorder—afterword. In: Frances AJ, Hales RE, editors. American Psychiatric Press review of psychiatry. Vol. 7. Washington: American Psychiatric Press; 1988. p. 138–46.

Shear MK, Fyer MR. Biological and psychopathologic findings in panic disorder. In: Frances AJ, Hales RE, editors. American Psychiatric Press review of psychiatry. Washington: American Psychiatric Press; 1988. p. 29–53.

Sheehan DV, Raj BA. Panic disorder. In: Thase ME, Edelstein BA, Hersen M, editors. Handbook of outpatient treatment of adults: nonpsychotic mental disorders. New York: Plenum; 1990. p. 177–208.

Sheehan DV, Raj BA. Treatment of the difficult case with panic disorder. In: Walker JR, Norton GR, Ross CA, editors. Panic disorder and agoraphobia: a comprehensive guide for the practitioner. Pacific Grove (CA): Brooks/Cole Pub. Co.; c1991. p. 368–97.

Stein MB, Uhde TW. Panic disorder and major depression—lifetime relationship and biological markers. In: Ballenger JC, editor. Clinical aspects of panic disorder. New York: Wiley-Liss; 1990. p. 151–68.

Stern EM, editor. Psychotherapy and the terrorized patient. New York: Haworth Press; c1985. 116 p. (The psychotherapy patient; vol. 1, no. 4).

Swinson RP, Kuch K. Clinical-features of panic and related disorders. In: Ballenger JC, editor. Clinical aspects of panic disorder. New York: Wiley-Liss; 1990. p. 13–30.

Swinson RP, Kuch K, Antony MM. Combining pharmacotherapy and behavioral therapy for panic disorder and agoraphobia. In: Walker JR, Norton GR, Ross CA, editors. Panic disorder and agoraphobia: a comprehensive guide for the practitioner. Pacific Grove (CA): Brooks/Cole Pub. Co.; c1991. p. 306–34.

Sylvester CE, Hyde TS, Reichler RJ. Clinical psychopathology among children of adults with panic disorder. In: Dunner DL, Gershon ES, Barrett JE, editors. Relatives at risk for mental disorder. New York: Raven Press; 1988. p. 87–102.

Taylor CB, Arnow B. The nature and treatment of anxiety disorders. New York: The Free Press; 1988. Chapter 7, Panic disorder (uncomplicated); p. 137–82.

Taylor CB, Arnow B. The nature and treatment of anxiety disorders. New York: The Free Press; 1988. Chapter 8, Agoraphobia (Panic disorder with agoraphobia); p. 183–229.

Teasdale J. Cognitive models and treatments for panic: a critical evaluation. In: Rachman S, Maser JD, editors. Panic: psychological perspectives. Hillsdale (NJ): Lawrence Erlbaum Associates; 1988. p. 189–203.

Telch MJ. Combined pharmacological and psychological treatments for panic sufferers. In: Rachman S, Maser JD, editors. Panic: psychological perspectives. Hillsdale (NJ): Lawrence Erlbaum Associates; 1988. p. 167–87.

Thorpe GL, Hecker JE. Psychosocial aspects of panic disorder. In: Walker JR, Norton GR, Ross CA, editors. Panic disorder and agoraphobia: a comprehensive guide for the practitioner. Pacific Grove (CA): Brooks/Cole Pub. Co.; c1991. p. 175–207.

Thyer BA. Treating anxiety disorders: a guide for human service professionals. Newbury Park (CA): Sage Publications; 1987. Chapter 4, Agoraphobia and panic disorder: diagnosis, etiology, and assessment; p. 61–75.

Thyer BA. Treating anxiety disorders: a guide for human service professionals. Newbury Park (CA): Sage Publications; 1987. Chapter 5, Agoraphobia and panic disorder: treatment strategies; p. 76–91.

Torgerson S. Twin studies in panic disorder. In: Ballenger JC, editor. Neurobiology of panic disorder. New York: Wiley-Liss; 1990. p. 51–8.

Tuma AH, Maser JD, editors. Anxiety and the anxiety disorders. Hillsdale (NJ): Lawrence Erlbaum Associates. 1020 p.

Turner SM, Beidel DC, Jacob RG. Assessment of panic. In: Rachman S, Maser JD, editors. Panic: psychological perspectives. Hillsdale (NJ): Lawrence Erlbaum Associates; 1988. p. 37–50.

Tyrer P. Classification of neurosis. Chichester (Sussex, United Kingdom): Wiley; 1989. Panic and generalized anxiety disorder, p. 17–41.

Uhde TW. Caffeine provocation of panic—a focus on biological mechanisms. In: Ballenger JC, editor. Neurobiology of panic disorder. New York: Wiley-Liss; 1990. p. 219–44.

Uhde TW, Roy-Byrne PP, Vittone BJ, Boulenger JP, Post RM. Phenomenology and neurobiology of panic disorder. In: Tuma AH, Maser J, editors. Anxiety and the anxiety disorders. Hillsdale (NJ): Lawrence Erlbaum Associates; 1985. p. 557–76.

Uhde TW, Stein MB. Biology and pharmacological treatment of panic disorder. In: Hand I, Wittchen HU, editors. Panic and phobias 2: treatments and variables affecting course and outcome. Berlin: Springer-Verlag; 1988. p. 18–35.

Uhde TW, Tancer ME. Chemical models of panic: a review and critique. In: Tyrer P, editor. Psychopharmacology of anxiety. New York: Oxford University Press; 1989. p. 109–31.

van den Hout MA. Panic, perception, and pCO2. In: Hand I, Wittchen HU, editors. Panic and phobias 2: treatments and variables affecting course and outcome. Berlin: Springer-Verlag; 1988. p. 117–28.

van den Hout MA. The explanation of experimental panic. In: Rachman S, Maser JD, editors. Panic: psychological perspectives. Hillsdale (NJ): Lawrence Erlbaum Associates; 1988. p. 237–57.

van der Molen GM, Merckelbach H, Jansen A, van den Hout MA. Panic, phobia and hypocapnia: an interwoven triad. In: Emmelkamp PMG, Everaerd WTAM, Kraaimaat FW, van Son MJM, editors. Fresh perspectives on anxiety disorders. Berwyn (PA): Swets North America; 1989. p. 45–58.

Vanggaard T. Panic: the course of a psychoanalysis. Vanggaard J, translator. New York: W.W. Norton; c1989. 144 p. Translation of: Angst.

Von Korff M, Eaton WW. Epidemiologic findings on panic. In: Baker R, editor. Panic disorder: theory, research and therapy. New York: Wiley; 1989. p. 35–50.

Walker L, Ashcroft G. Pharmacological approaches to the treatment of panic. In: Baker R, editor. Panic disorder: theory, research and therapy. New York: Wiley; 1989. p. 301–14.

Walker JR, Norton GR, Ross CA, editors. Panic disorder and agoraphobia: a comprehensive guide for the practitioner. Pacific Grove (CA): Brooks/Cole Pub. Co.; c1991. 575 p.

Waring H. The nature of panic attack symptoms. In: Baker R, editor. Panic disorder: theory, research and therapy. New York: Wiley; 1989. p. 17–34.

Weeks C. The key to resisting relapse in panic. In: Baker R, editor. Panic disorder: theory, research and therapy. New York: Wiley; 1989. p. 315–23.

Weissman MM. Epidemiology of panic disorder and agoraphobia. In: Ballenger JC, editor. Clinical aspects of panic disorder. New York: Wiley-Liss; 1990. p. 57–66.

Weissman MM. The epidemiology of panic disorder and agoraphobia. In: Frances AJ, Hales RE, editors. American Psychiatric Press review of psychiatry. Vol. 7. Washington: American Psychiatric Press; 1988. p. 54–66.

Westphal CFO. Agoraphobie with commentary: the beginnings of agoraphobia. Schumacher MT, translator. Lanham (MD): University Press of America; c1988. 99 p.

Wittchen HU. Epidemiology of panic attacks and panic disorders. In: Hand I, Wittchen HU, editors. Panic and phobias: empirical evidence of theoretical models and long-term effects of behavioral treatments. Berlin: Springer-Verlag; 1986. p. 18–28.

Wittchen HU, Essau CA. The epidemiology of panic attacks, panic disorder, and agoraphobia. In: Walker JR, Norton GR, Ross CA, editors. Panic disorder and agoraphobia: a comprehensive guide for the practitioner. Pacific Grove (CA): Brooks/Cole Pub. Co.; c1991. p. 103–49.

Woods SW, Charney DS. Biologic responses to panic anxiety elicited by nonpharmacologic means. In: Ballenger JC, editor. Neurobiology of panic disorder. New York: Wiley-Liss; 1990. p. 205–18.

Zal HM. Panic disorder: the great pretender. New York: Plenum Press; c1990. 232 p.

Zane MD. A contextual approach to panic. In: Baker R, editor. Panic disorder: theory, research and therapy. New York: Wiley; 1989. p. 117–40.

Zitrin CM. New perspectives on the treatment of panic and phobic disorders. In: Shaw BF, Segal ZV, Vallis TM, Cashman FE, editors. Anxiety disorders: psychological and biological perspectives. New York: Plenum; 1986. p. 179–202.

Audiovisuals

Anxiety disorders: generalized anxiety, agoraphobia, and obsessive compulsive anxiety [videorecording]. [Chapel Hill (NC)]: University of North Carolina at Chapel Hill, School of Medicine, Medical Sciences Teaching Laboratories; c1988. 2 videocassettes (77 min.): sound, color; 3/4 in. + 1 guide. (Simulated psychiatric profiles; 3).

Panic [videorecording]. Dartmouth Hitchcock Medical Center, producer. [Princeton (NJ)]: Films for the Humanities and Sciences; c1990. 1 videocassette (26 min.): sound, color; 1/2 in.

Panic disorder, the nameless fear [videorecording]. Fogelson DL. Secaucus (NJ): Network for Continuing Medical Education; 1986. 1 videocassette (18 min.): sound, color; 3/4 in. + 1 booklet. (NCME telecourse; no. 492).

Panic/Panic disorders [slide]. Jones BA, Mavissakalian M. [Columbus (OH): Ohio Medical Education Network; 1989]. 18 slides: color + 1 sound cassette (60 min.: 1 7/8 ips) + 1 guide. (OMEN; no. 14).

Phobias and panic disorders [videorecording]. Uhde T, National Institutes of Health, Office of Clinical Reports and Inquiries. [Los Angeles]: Hospital Satellite Network; c1985. [1 videocassette (58 min.): sound, color; 3/4 in].

Index

*Page numbers printed in **boldface** type refer to tables or figures.*